Cardiac Transplantation

Books Available in Cardiovascular Clinics Series

Cardiac Transplantation

Mark E. Thompson, M.D. / Editor

Associate Professor of Medicine
Division of Cardiology
University of Pittsburgh School of Medicine
Pittsburgh, Pennsylvania

CARDIOVASCULAR CLINICS
Albert N. Brest, M.D. / Editor-in-Chief

James C. Wilson Professor of Medicine
Director, Division of Cardiology
Jefferson Medical College
Philadelphia, Pennsylvania

 F. A. DAVIS COMPANY ● Philadelphia

Printed in the United States of America

Last digit indicates print number: 10 9 8 7 6 5 4 3 2 1

Printed on acid-free paper effective with Volume 17, Number 1.

NOTE: As new scientific information becomes available through basic and clinical research, recommended treatments and drug therapies undergo changes. The author(s) and publisher have done everything possible to make this book accurate, up-to-date, and in accord with accepted standards at the time of publication. However, the reader is advised always to check product information (package inserts) for changes and new information regarding dose and contraindications before administering any drug. Caution is especially urged when using new or infrequently ordered drugs.

Library of Congress Cataloging in Publication Data

Cardiovascular clinics. 20/2
    Philadelphia, F. A. Davis, 1969–
      v. ill. 27 cm.
      Editor: v. 1-   A. N. Brest
      Key title: Cardiovascular clinics, ISSN 0069-0384.
      1. Cardiovascular system—Diseases—Collected works.   I.
Brest, Albert N., ed.
      [DNLM: W1 CA77N]
    RC681.A1C27   616.1   70-6558
    ISBN 0-8036-8477-0   MARC-S

Preface

Cardiac transplantation has recently entered the third decade of clinical applicability. During this period of time, the procedure has progressed from one of limited experimental availability—during which the current basis for clinical practice was established—to one that is generally accepted as a suitable alternative for the management of refractory congestive heart failure, now limited by a suitable number of donors. The first chapter of this book, by Lansman and associates, summarizes the developmental history of cardiac and cardiopulmonary transplantation, both of which have revolutionized the approach to management of patients with end-stage failure of these organs.

The second chapter reviews the experimental and pathophysiologic basis for transplantation. Dr. Uretsky provides clinical and physiologic correlates of the transplanted heart, and insight into the importance of these factors in the postoperative assessment of these patients. Similarly, Dr. Theodore reviews the extensive Stanford experience with the preoperative and postoperative evaluation of pulmonary physiology in patients undergoing cardiopulmonary transplantation. This chapter also describes the clinical features of obliterative bronchiolitis, a devastating postoperative complication occurring in approximately one third of recipients. The long-term consequences of rejection and immunosuppression are superbly described by Dr. Billingham in her summary of the pathology observed in patients undergoing cardiac and cardiopulmonary transplantation. Finally, Drs. Duquesnoy and Cramer outline the immunologic mechanisms that are intimately involved whenever transplantation is undertaken. Fundamental research must be directed toward selective inhibition of the immunologic responses of the transplanted organ. Elucidation of such an approach, in contrast to the present-day practice of nonspecific inhibition of the immune system, is required in order to decrease postoperative complications that now invariably occur.

The next section of the book is directed toward a discussion of the clinical aspects of cardiac transplantation. The criteria for recipient selection are summarized by Drs. Hastillo and Hess. These guidelines have changed little since their establishment based on the early Stanford experience. The major change to recipient selection has been that of extending the upper age limit to 60 to 65 years. The chapter prepared by Dr. Fragomeni and colleagues provides current information regarding the national effort to increase the donor supply and establish an equitable system for distributing available organs. The role of the United Network for Organ Sharing in this process is described. The inevitable consequence of a lack of sufficient donors is reflected in the high death rate—estimated to be in excess of 50 percent—experienced by potential recipients awaiting cardiac transplantation.

The operative technique is described by Dr. Bolman. In his chapter, he emphasizes the importance of proper preoperative preparation of the recipient, as well as the technical aspects of the procedure. For those patients with a higher pulmonary vascular resistance, the alternative of heterotopic cardiac transplantation is also discussed. Drs. O'Connell and Renlund describe the clinical assessment of rejection and review current immunosuppressive protocols designed to control this immunologic phenomenon. These authors have had extensive experience with the use of monoclonal antibodies in prevention and treatment of rejection. Likewise, the trend toward the use of triple immunosuppressive therapy using a lower dose of cyclosporine in an effort to reduce the side effects of this agent is discussed.

Infectious complications have been an inevitable concomitant of the transplantation procedure. Dr. Dummer describes his intimate personal knowledge of infection in transplant recipients and provides invaluable guidance for the diagnosis and treatment of such infections in these patients.

In spite of the enthusiasm with which cyclosporine was heralded as a major advance in immunosuppression, experience has revealed major long-term complications associated with its administration. The inevitable development of hypertension and renal failure is described by Dr. Shapiro and associates and by Dr. Greenberg. Both chapters deal with the longitudinal clinical correlates of cyclosporine administration and strategies to treat the hypertension and ameliorate the nephrotoxicity of this drug. The development of accelerated coronary atherosclerosis represents an additional major cause of late morbidity and mortality in patients undergoing transplantation. The clinical manifestations of this complication and therapeutic implications are presented in the chapter prepared by Dr. Eich and colleagues.

Dr. Thompson and coworkers outline an approach to management and long-term followup of patients undergoing cardiac transplantation. The ultimate benefit derived by recipients depends in large part on successful management of the numerous postoperative complications that arise.

The final section of this book is devoted to a discussion of patients who require special consideration for a transplant procedure. Dr. Fricker and associates describe experience with cardiac transplantation in the pediatric population. Special attention is given to the quality of life in these young patients, as well as to the role of transplantation in neonates. Drs. Bahnson and Gordon provide a thoughtful discussion of the issues relating to the transplantation of the heart and another major organ, such as the liver or kidney. This chapter provides sage counsel as to when consideration should be given to transplantation of multiple organs, and a realistic assessment of the results that may be expected.

A personal perspective on combined cardiopulmonary transplantation and single and double lung transplantation is provided by Dr. Griffith. During this first decade of development, these operations may be viewed as being at the same state of evolution as was cardiac transplantation in the early 1970s. The major problems to be overcome are a lack of suitable donors, organ preservation, the development of techniques to diagnose pulmonary rejection, and the long-term consequences of infection and rejection.

The editors are pleased to present this contemporary summary of cardiac and cardiopulmonary transplantation. To the extent that there is overlap in the subject matter, the reader has the opportunity to appreciate the areas of agreement and controversy as they presently exist in this complex and rapidly evolving field. The distinguished contributors to this book have provided a comprehensive review of the subject. Each author has made major contributions to the field of transplantation and is currently actively engaged in the clinical practice of transplantation.

Our thanks are extended to each of these busy individuals who devoted a precious portion of their free time to the preparation of the manuscripts that comprise this text. We hope that this book will provide the stimulus for continued research in the field of transplantation, an up-to-date reference for the reader, and encouragement for patients and families who must make the courageous decision to undergo transplantation.

Finally, our gratitude is extended to those families who have unselfishly granted permission for organ donation—the gift of life.

Mark E. Thompson

Editor's Commentary

During the past 20 years, CARDIOVASCULAR CLINICS has covered virtually every aspect of cardiology and has aimed to put into clinical perspective each of the various advances in this field as they have developed. Although affecting fewer patients than some of the other achievements of the past two decades, no development has been more monumental or more dramatic than heart transplantation, in which life is literally restored to an otherwise end-stage cardiac patient. Thus, it is especially gratifying to present this particular volume, which covers the entire spectrum of issues affecting cardiac transplantation, from physiology and pathology to immunologic and clinical aspects. I am very grateful to Mark Thompson for his insightful guidance in the development of this material, and both of us are deeply indebted to the contributing authors for their superb contributions.

Albert N. Brest, M.D.
Editor-in-Chief

Contributors

Henry T. Bahnson, M.D.
Professor of Surgery
University of Pittsburgh School of Medicine
Pittsburgh, Pennsylvania

Glenn R. Barnhart, M.D.
Surgical Specialists, Inc.
Norfolk General Hospital
Norfolk, Virginia

Margaret E. Billingham, M.B., B.S., F.R.C.Path.
Professor of Pathology
Stanford University Medical School
Stanford, California

R. Morton Bolman III, M.D.
Professor and Chief
Division of Cardiovascular and Thoracic Surgery
Department of Surgery
University of Minnesota Medical School
Director
Minnesota Heart and Lung Institute
Minneapolis, Minnesota

Donald V. Cramer, D.V.M., Ph.D.
Associate Professor of Pathology
University of Pittsburgh School of Medicine
Pittsburgh, Pennsylvania

J. Stephen Dummer, M.D.
Associate Professor of Medicine and Surgery
University of Pittsburgh School of Medicine
Pittsburgh, Pennsylvania

René J. Duquesnoy, Ph.D.
Professor of Pathology
University of Pittsburgh School of Medicine
Pittsburgh, Pennsylvania

David M. Eich, M.D.
Department of Medicine
Division of Cardiology
Medical College of Virginia
Virginia Commonwealth University
Richmond, Virginia

M. Arisan Ergin, M.D., Ph.D.
Associate Professor
Division of Cardiothoracic Surgery
Department of Surgery
The Mount Sinai Medical Center
New York, New York

Luis Sergio Fragomeni, M.D.
Visiting Professor
University of Minnesota Medical School
Minneapolis, Minnesota

F. Jay Fricker, M.D.
Associate Professor of Pediatrics
University of Pittsburgh School of Medicine
Children's Hospital of Pittsburgh
Pittsburgh, Pennsylvania

Robert D. Gordon, M.D.
Associate Professor of Surgery
University of Pittsburgh School of Medicine
Pittsburgh, Pennsylvania

Arthur Greenberg, M.D.
Associate Professor of Medicine
Renal-Electrolyte Division
Department of Medicine
University of Pittsburgh School of Medicine
Pittsburgh, Pennsylvania

Randall Griepp, M.D.
Professor of Surgery
Chief, Division of Cardiothoracic Surgery
The Mount Sinai Medical Center
New York, New York

Bartley P. Griffith, M.D.
Professor of Surgery
University of Pittsburgh School of Medicine
Pittsburgh, Pennsylvania

Andrea Hastillo, M.D.
Associate Professor of Medicine
Division of Cardiology
Medical College of Virginia
Virginia Commonwealth University
Richmond, Virginia

Alain Heroux, M.D.
Department of Medicine
Division of Cardiology
Medical College of Virginia
Virginia Commonwealth University
Richmond, Virginia

Michael L. Hess, M.D.
Professor of Medicine
Division of Cardiology
Medical College of Virginia
Virginia Commonwealth University
Richmond, Virginia

Danna E. Johnson, M.D.
Assistant Professor of Pathology
Department of Pathology
Medical College of Virginia
Virginia Commonwealth University
Richmond, Virginia

Michael P. Kaye, M.D.
Professor of Surgery
University of Minnesota Medical School
Minneapolis, Minnesota

Daijin Ko, Ph.D
Assistant Professor of Statistics
Medical College of Virginia
Virginia Commonwealth University
Richmond, Virginia

Steven L. Lansman, M.D., Ph.D.
Assistant Professor of Surgery
Division of Cardiothoracic Surgery
The Mount Sinai Medical Center
New York, New York

Richard R. Lower, M.D.
  Professor and Chairman
  Division of Cardiothoracic Surgery
  Medical College of Virginia
  Virginia Commonwealth University
  Richmond, Virginia

R.L. Nigalye, M.B., B.S.
  Division of Clinical Pharmacology/Hypertension
  University of Pittsburgh School of Medicine
  Pittsburgh, Pennsylvania

John B. O'Connell, M.D.
  Associate Professor of Medicine
  Division of Cardiology
  University of Utah School of Medicine
  Medical Director
  Utah Cardiac Transplant Program
  Salt Lake City, Utah

Dale G. Renlund, M.D.
  Assistant Professor of Medicine
  Division of Cardiology
  University of Utah School of Medicine
  Medical Co-Director
  Utah Cardiac Transplant Program
  Salt Lake City, Utah

Sheelah Rider-Katz, R.N.
  Clinical Transplant Coordinator
  Division of Cardiothoracic Surgery
  Medical College of Virginia
  Virginia Commonwealth University
  Richmond, Virginia

Gayl Rogers, R.N., B.A.N., M.B.A.
  Organ and Tissue Procurement Director
  St. Paul American Red Cross
  St. Paul, Minnesota

Gale H. Rutan, M.D., M.P.H.
  Assistant Professor of Medicine
  Division of Clinical Pharmacology/Hypertension
  University of Pittsburgh School of Medicine
  Pittsburgh, Pennsylvania

Alvin P. Shapiro, M.D.
Professor of Medicine
Division of Clinical Pharmacology/Hypertension
University of Pittsburgh School of Medicine
Director, Internal Medicine Residency Program
Shadyside Hospital
Pittsburgh, Pennsylvania

James Theodore, M.D.
Associate Professor of Medicine
Division of Respiratory Medicine
Stanford University School of Medicine
Stanford, California

James A. Thompson, M.D.
Associate Professor of Medicine
Division of Cardiology
Medical College of Virginia
Virginia Commonwealth University
Richmond, Virginia

Mark E. Thompson, M.D.
Associate Professor of Medicine
Division of Cardiology
University of Pittsburgh School of Medicine
Pittsburgh, Pennsylvania

Alfredo Trento, M.D.
Director, Heart Transplant Program
Cedars-Sinai Medical Center
Los Angeles, California

Barry F. Uretsky, M.D.
Associate Professor of Medicine
University of Pittsburgh School of Medicine
Pittsburgh, Pennsylvania

Contents

PART 1

History

CHAPTER 1

The History of Heart and Heart-Lung Transplantation

Steven L. Lansman, M.D., Ph.D.
M. Arisan Ergin, M.D., Ph.D.
Randall B. Griepp, M.D.

Clinical heart and heart-lung transplantation, once thought "a fantastic speculation for the future,"[1] is grounded in a 60-year history of experimental efforts. Clinical application awaited solutions to certain "key" problems, characterized by Shumway as "some problems which require solution before the golden moment in tissue transplantation is upon us."[2] These include (1) technique, (2) recipient and graft protection during transfer, (3) physiology of the transplanted heart, (4) immunology, and (5) legal/logistic problems. This chapter reviews some of the major experimental and clinical contributions toward solving these problems.

Experimental efforts have been categorized into three historically overlapping types—those involving heterotopic, nonauxiliary models; heterotopic, auxiliary models; and orthotopic models (Fig. 1–1).

EXPERIMENTAL TRANSPLANTATION

HETEROTOPIC, NONAUXILIARY TRANSPLANTATION

The first cardiac transplant was performed by Alexis Carrel and C. C. Guthrie at the University of Chicago in 1905.[3] Seeking to establish techniques of vascular anastomoses, "the replantation of a limb, the transplantation of the heart and kidney, and the replantation of the thyroid gland were performed." The full description of their heart transplant experiment is as follows:

> The heart of a small dog was extirpated and transplanted into the neck of a larger one by anastomosing the cut ends of the jugular vein and the carotid artery to the aorta, the pulmonary artery, one of the vena cava and a pulmonary vein. The circulation was reestablished

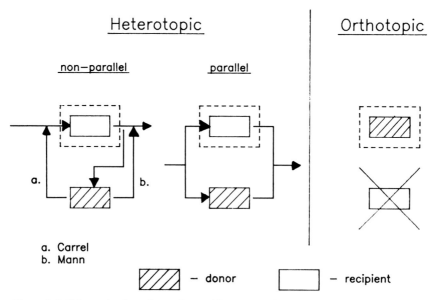

Figure 1–1. Schematization of experimental heart transplant models. The Carrel model (a) and the Mann model (b) of graft outflow are shown.

through the heart, about an hour and 15 minutes after the cessation of the beat; 20 minutes after the reestablishment of the circulation, the blood was actively circulating through the coronary system. A small opening being made through the wall of a small branch of the coronary vein, an abundant dark hemorrhage was produced. Then strong fibrillar contractions were seen. Afterward contractions of the auricles appeared, and, about an hour after the operation, effective contractions of the ventricles began. The transplanted heart beat at the rate of 88 per minute, while the rate of the normal heart was 100 per minute. A little later tracings were taken. Owing to the fact that the operation was made without aseptic technique, coagulation occurred in the cavities of the heart after about two hours, and the experiment was interrupted.[3]

Although the exact details of their experiment are not known, the most likely arrangement of anastomoses is depicted in Figure 1–2. In this model, atrial inflow under arterial pressure combined with aortic outflow under venous pressure provided a most unfavorable gradient for perfusion of the myocardium. However, this experiment addressed several "key" problems discussed earlier. A technically feasible model was demonstrated wherein all four chambers had pumping function and, perhaps most important, the heart survived an ischemic period—it was separated from its blood supply, sutured into the circulation of a second animal and recovered organized contractions; subsequent investigators would examine means of "myocardial preservation" during the ischemic transfer period. Last, rudimentary physiologic observations on the transplanted heart were made.

The next reference to mammalian cardiac transplantation in the medical literature was in 1933 by Mann.[4] Seeking a denervated heart model, technical aspects of transplanting the canine heart into the carotid-jugular circulation were

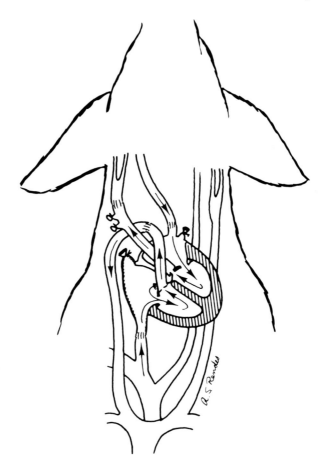

Figure 1–2. Possible anastomotic arrangement used by Carrel and Guthrie in 1905. (From Najarian, JS, and Simmons, RL (eds): Transplantation. Lea & Febiger, Philadelphia, 1972, p 532, with permission.)

studied. The most successful model (Fig. 1–3) was simple, with only the right ventricle functioning as a pump. However, the problem of coronary perfusion was solved, as arterial inflow was established via the donor coronary circulation and venous outflow via the donor coronary vein, pulmonary artery, and recipient jugular vein.

This model was reliably successful, the longest survival being 8 days, and the authors addressed several "key problems." Efforts at "myocardial preservation" included avoidance of air embolism and ventricular distension and well-documented observations on "the general behavior of the transplanted heart" were made; the heart rate was "surprisingly constant" at 100 to 130 beats/minute and the ECG was "surprisingly normal." Neural control mechanisms were postulated and the first observations of cardiac allograft rejection were made, as the authors noted, "histologically the heart was completely infiltrated with lymphocytes, large mononuclears and polymorphonuclears." They concluded:

> It is readily seen that the failure of the homotransplanted heart to survive is not due to the technique of transplantation but to some biologic factor which is probably identical to that which prevents survival of other homotransplanted tissues and organs.[4]

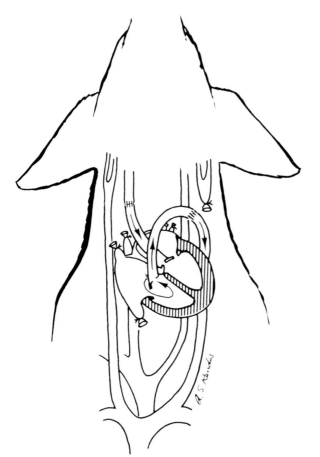

Figure 1-3. Anastomotic arrangement used by Mann and co-workers in 1933. (From Najarian, JS, Simmons, RL (eds): Transplantation. Philadelphia, Lea & Febiger, 1972, p 532, with permission.)

Interest in cardiac transplantation waned until Marcus, Wong, and Luisada,[1] working at the Chicago Medical School, reported their experience with a slightly modified Mann preparation (Marcus I technique). A subsequent modification (Marcus II technique) enabled pumping function in both right and left ventricles,[5] the donor left ventricle supplying blood to its own coronary arteries and to the recipient cerebral circulation. These investigators were interested in cardiac transplantation per se:

> The problem which we are attempting to explore can then be stated as follows: Can a combination of highly specialized tissues ... the heart be grafted in a mammalian animal? Can such a graft live in an homologous environment? Can such a graft actually function by receiving and delivering blood? Whether it might so function as to replace its counterpart in the host is a matter of fantastic speculation for the future.[1]

Marcus focused on donor graft preservation, attempting to improve survival. He cautioned that, "coronary artery air embolism spells quick and final defeat," and, concerned that autonomic stimulation might induce arrhythmias and ventricular distension, he performed bilateral donor cervical vagotomies and injected cocaine into the pericardium prior to harvesting. Most important, he felt, was the necessity to avoid any ischemic period, and an elaborate system was developed whereby the graft was cannulated and perfused by a third animal during transfer:

> The method we have called interim parabiotic perfusion; it is a homologous extracorporeal pump.[5]

Results were generally disappointing, demonstrating that more complicated procedures are not necessarily better ones, and maximum survival was only 48 hours. The authors noted that "perhaps the greatest deterrent to long term survival of the transplanted heart is the biologic problem of tissue specificity" and commented:

> . . . a transplanted heart or heart-lung preparation might be used for replacement of a diseased organ. The latter must be considered, at present, a fantastic dream, and does not fall within the scope of present considerations.[1]

The Mann preparation remained a valuable tool for evaluating the transplanted heart.[6,7] In 1953, Downie, working at the Ontario Veterinary College, reported excellent results with the original Mann technique, with 23 of 30 experiments successful, ischemic times ranging from 30 to 45 minutes, and maximum survival time 10 days.[8] Downie demonstrated that with simple techniques successful heterotopic transplantation was routinely possible and attributed his improved results to the use of penicillin and the availability of convenient, commercial suture material. Commenting upon possible clinical application, Downie stated:

> In the present state of knowledge it is not likely that homotransplantation of the usual tissues afflicted by disease will achieve great prominence clinically . . . homotransplantation of tissues has a melancholy record of failure in surgery. . . . The attempt to transplant tissues successfully from one subject to another is probably lacking in certain fundamental pieces of knowledge, much as is the case with our knowledge of carcinogenesis. In the one case we do not know why a cell continues to proliferate when it should not. In our case we do not know why a cell invites destruction when it ought to survive.[8]

The contribution of the Russian surgeon Demikhov to the evolution of thought in the field is obscure, inasmuch as most of his work was done in the Soviet Union when little scientific communication penetrated the Iron Curtain. In 1962, however, Demikhov published a volume documenting many interesting experiments, including "transplantation of the head," "transplantation of halves of the body," and "the surgical combination of two animals with the creation of a single circulation."[9] Among these projects were "experiments on the transplantation of a second, additional heart."[9] He states that he began his work in 1940 and by 1946 was performing canine heterotopic cardiac transplants to the inguinal region. Vascular anastomoses were made with collodian tube connectors and, later, with automatic staple devices. Twenty-four anatomic variants were tried and in 1956 an intrathoracic heterotopic graft continued to beat for 32 days.

Table 1–1. Maximum Survival in
Experimental, Heterotopic,
Nonauxiliary Transplantation

Authors	Date	Survival
Carrell, Guthrie[3]	1905	2 hours
Mann[4]	1933	8 days
Marcus, Wong, Luisada[1]	1951	2 days
Downie[8]	1953	10 days
Demikhov[9]	1956	32 days

Maximum survival of heterotopic, nonauxiliary cardiac transplants are reviewed in Table 1–1.

AUXILIARY, HETEROTOPIC TRANSPLANTATION

Heterotopic cardiac transplantation presented the possibility that an allograft might provide part or all of the recipient's circulatory requirement.

In 1953, Marcus reported a group of experiments[5] wherein "an attempt was made to transplant the heart with its own lesser circulation, the lungs" (Fig. 1–4). These heterotopic transplants are striking for two reasons: they represent the first successful heart-lung transplants reported in the Western medical literature and the first report of a transplanted heart supporting the recipient circulation. (As discussed below, Neptune reported similar accomplishments in 1953 with an orthotopic heart-lung transplant.) The heart-lung block was interposed in the abdominal circulation; donor lung ventilation was provided by a respirator; and, in such experiments, maximum survival was 9 hours. Recipient viability was maintained despite (1) ventilating the recipient lungs with nitrogen only, and oxygen supplied via the donor lungs; (2) temporary ligature of the recipient pulmonary artery; and (3) venous inflow occlusion of the recipient tricuspid valve. Despite the latter two manipulations, complete cardiopulmonary support was generated by the transplanted organs—in one case for as long as 75 minutes. In some of these experiments, the heart-lung block supported the recipient as the native mitral valve was explored via left atriotomy under inflow occlusion.

Demikhov's monograph[9] reported a long series of 250 experimental efforts at transplanting a "second, additional heart" to a heterotopic, intrathoracic position. In many experiments, the number of vascular anastomoses was reduced and the procedure expedited by transplanting the heart and lung as a unit; thus, "there would be no need to suture the numerous vessels connecting the heart to the lungs." The first success in this series was a heterotopic heart-lung transplant performed on June 30, 1946, which survived 9 hours and 26 minutes. On October 13, 1946, a dog survived a similar transplant, expiring on the fifth postoperative day due to "separation of the tracheobronchial suture line." Subsequently, tracheobronchial anastomoses were avoided by exteriorizing the donor trachea or by performing transplants whereby oxygenated blood perfused the donor lung, permitting ligation of the donor trachea altogether.

Between 1951 and 1955, Demikhov performed 22 experiments involving "replacement of the heart alone (without the lungs)."[9] Experiment 20 on January 11, 1955, was notable in that the recipient great vessels and mitral valve were

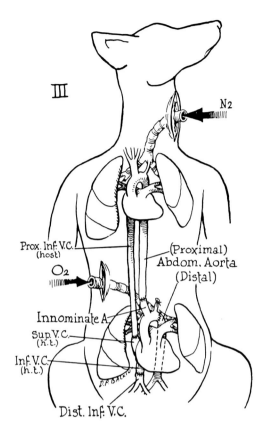

Figure 1–4. Anastomosis arrangement used by Marcus and co-workers in 1953 to perform the first functional heterotopic heart-lung transplant. (From Marcus et al.,[5] with permission.)

ligated, and circulation was maintained solely by the transplanted heart. The dog awoke from anesthesia, stood up, and drank, but died suddenly after 15.5 hours of auxiliary function, with death attributed to thrombosis of the superior vena caval anastomosis.

Reemtsma employed intrathoracic auxiliary heart transplants to document improved graft survival with immunosuppression,[10] and, in one of his series,[11] the recipient heart was fibrillated, transferring total circulatory function to the donor heart; maximum circulatory support was 4 hours.

In 1967 Johansson, Soderlund, and William-Olsson, at the Karlinska Institute in Stockholm, reported intrathoracic heterotopic transplants in which the graft functioned as an auxiliary left heart bypass pump,[12] and total left heart bypass was demonstrated by clamping the recipient aorta. Notably, during induced recipient heart fibrillation, adequate cardiac output was maintained for periods of up to 1 hour by donor left heart bypass, with pulmonary circulation maintained only passively by elevated central venous pressure.

Maximum support by auxiliary, heterotopic transplants are listed in Table 1–2.

ORTHOTOPIC TRANSPLANTATION

Between 1946 and 1951, Demikhov devised a technique of serially anastomosing vessels whereby donor and recipient perfusion might be maintained during orthotopic heart-lung transplantation.[9] In two such experiments performed in

Table 1–2. Maximum Support by Experimental, Auxiliary,
Heterotopic Transplantation

Authors	Date	Type	Survival (hr)
Marcus, Wong, Luisada[5]	1953	Heart/lung	1.25
Demikhov[9]	1955	Heart	15.5
McGough, Brewer, Reemtsma[11]	1966	Heart	4
Johansson, Soderlund, William-Olsson[12]	1967	Heart	1

1946, the recipients never left the operating table; however, the grafts did support the circulation, respectively, for 2 and 7 hours; on June 12, 1951, the procedure was performed on a "bitch called Damka" who recovered fully and survived 6 days postoperatively.

By the early 1950s, some "key problems," primarily technical and physiologic, had been addressed. However, the "orthotopic phase" of experimental transplantation awaited solutions to problems involving the "transfer period"—the period between donor heart excision and implantation. There were requirements for means of preserving the graft and maintaining the recipient during transfer and a simplified surgical technique to expedite the process.

In 1953, Neptune and associates[13] addressed these problems in their publication, "Complete Homologous Heart Transplantation." Clearly interested in heart transplantation per se, the authors attempted to simplify the procedure by transplanting an entire heart-lung block, thus avoiding the multiple pulmonary venous anastomoses. The problem of donor myocardial protection and recipient preservation were simultaneously solved as both animals were "placed in an ordinary beverage cooler for the production of hypothermia."

> By the use of hypothermia we have been able to completely stop all circulation for periods up to 30 minutes without subsequent morbidity or mortality. It occurred to us that such a period of time would be more than ample to perform a complete transplantation of the heart—removal of the recipient animal's heart and the substitution by a donor heart.[13]

The authors reported successful heart-lung transplantation in three dogs with survival of up to 6 hours with these techniques. Although subsequent technical developments obviated the need to transplant the entire heart-lung block, hypothermia has remained indispensible during cardiopulmonary bypass for recipient protection and during the ischemic period for donor graft preservation.

In 1957, Webb and Howard[14] reported on "Restoration of Function of the Refrigerated Heart," demonstrating that canine hearts, heparinized and flushed with potassium citrate, can survive for prolonged periods at low temperatures (4°C) and yet return to adequate function when transplanted heterotopically (Marcus II technique). Perhaps anticipating current long-distance procurement procedures, the authors commented:

> Demonstration that the heart can be maintained viable and functional for periods of at least 8 hours by refrigeration in a nutrient

medium has been of great value to us in experimental work in cardiac and cardiopulmonary transplants. When the problems of immunology are solved and transplantation becomes a clinical possibility, it will presumably require several hours for obtaining the heart, preparation of the recipient and total reimplantation. The practices outlined above would seem to make cardiac transplantation completely feasible so far as this time element is concerned.[14]

In the same year, Webb and Howard[15] reported six successful canine orthotopic heart-lung transplants. The recipient was maintained with cardiopulmonary bypass as the donor organs were inserted by coupling the cavae and suture anastomosing the aorta. Maximum survival was 22 hours, but a "physiological impass" was noted, as the dogs were never able to resume spontaneous respiration. Consequently the authors summarized:

Our experience indicated that transplantation of the heart with both lungs will not be practical. We have been unable in any of our various experiments to obtain restoration of normal respiratory function in the presence of total denervation of the lungs.[15]

In 1958, Goldberg, Berman, and Akman,[16] at the University of Maryland, reported the first orthotopic cardiac transplants in a series of three experiments. In terms of technique, the authors comment, "The chief innovation was transsection of the left auricle to circumvent the anastomoses of the several pulmonary veins." In other words, the recipient heart was excised so as to leave a posterior "cuff" of left atrium containing the openings of the multiple pulmonary veins, thus necessitating one large, relatively simple left atrial anastomosis rather than multiple, small pulmonary venous anastomoses. The cavae were reconnected with methyl-methacrylate tubes and the aorta and pulmonary arteries were suture-anastomosed. Ischemic times ranged between 25 and 33 minutes, and the longest meaningful support of the circulation by the allograft was approximately 20 minutes.

Webb, Howard, and Neely,[17] in 1959, using their previously described method of "refrigeration"[14] to preserve the donor heart and the pump-oxygenator to maintain the recipient, accomplished 12 successful orthotopic cardiac transplants. The aortic and pulmonary anastomoses were sutured, while the individual pulmonary veins were joined using vascular couplers. Ischemic times ranged from 2 to 4 hours; two dogs succumbed within minutes of surgery, and the remaining 10 survived for periods ranging from 30 to 450 minutes.

In 1959, Cass and Brock,[18] working at Guy's Hospital in London, reported six methods of cardiac excision and replacement. The first five were autotransplants, but the sixth was an orthotopic transplant, which was significant because the authors described a method in which the native heart was "separated from the venae cavae and pulmonary veins by dividing through the walls of the atria," thus forming both right and left atrial "cuffs." This was the first description of the now standard practice of combining the multiple pulmonary venous and vena caval anastomoses into two atrial anastomoses. Suture line bleeding limited the experiment's success, although the graft did maintain the circulation for 1 hour.

In 1960, Lower and Shumway[19] published a milestone report in orthotopic

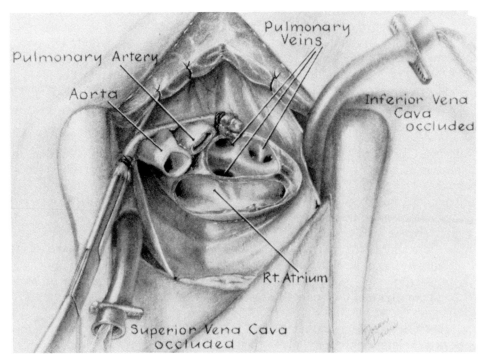

Figure 1–5. Essentials of the surgical technique used by Lower and Shumway in the first successful series of orthotopic canine cardiac transplants. Recipient pericardial cavity after removal of the recipient heart. Note the long stumps of the aorta and pulmonary artery and the combination of venous anastomoses into the atrial cuffs. (From Lower et al.,[20] with permission).

transplantation, integrating simplified techniques and strategies of recipient support and graft preservation into a single approach that permitted long-term success. Implantation was by suture anastomoses, and ischemic time, averaging 1 hour, was minimized by combining the pulmonary and caval anastomoses into two atrial "cuff" anastomoses (Fig. 1–5). Recipient protection was provided by cardiopulmonary bypass, with moderate hypothermia (30°C) induced by surface cooling, and graft preservation was provided by rapidly immersing the excised heart in iced saline (4°C).

Five of eight consecutive transplant recipients survived 6 to 21 days, eating and exercising normally in the postoperative period. This series represented the first description of a simple, routinely successful technique for mammalian orthotopic cardiac transplantation whereby recipients returned to normal activity, with their circulation supported by an orthotopic heart transplant.

No immunosuppression was given to these animals, and death was apparently due to rapid myocardial failure associated with massive infiltration of round cells and interstitial hemorrhage. The authors concluded:

> Observations on these animals suggest that, if the immunologic mechanisms of the host were prevented from destroying the graft, in all likelihood it would continue to function adequately for the normal life span of the animal.[19]

In 1961, Lower and colleagues[21] reported a series of canine heart-lung transplants wherein six recipients resumed spontaneous respiration, two of which were active and ambulatory until expiring on the fifth postoperative day of respiratory insufficiency attributed to rejection.

Kondo and coworkers,[22] in 1965, working at the Maimonides Hospital in Brooklyn, New York, used the technique of Lower and Shumway, but recipients, surface cooled to 16°C, underwent cardiac replacement during a 60-minute period of hypothermic circulatory arrest. In a series of 37 experiments, 18 animals survived more than one week, 12 more than 2 weeks, and one animal survived for 213 days. These experiments, performed on puppies, were conducted without immunosuppression, and the authors attributed long-term survival to relative immunologic incompetence of these very young animals.

Following the initial report by Lower and Shumway, a number of studies documenting successful orthotopic transplantation appeared during the early 1960s. Perhaps most significant was a report in 1965 by Lower, Dong, and Shumway[23] describing the use of the surface ECG as an indicator of rejection. During rejection episodes the ECG showed a definite drop in voltage, at which time the administration of azathioprine and methylprednisolone restored normal voltage. Using this test as a guide to intermittent administration of immunosuppressive therapy, survival time of 250 days in an adult dog was achieved.

Despite success in heart transplantation, long-term survival in experimental heart-lung transplantation was confounded by respiratory insufficiency, which followed pulmonary denervation in dogs. Eventually, it was observed that this problem did not occur in all mammals, and Castaneda and associates[24] demonstrated long-term survival with normal pulmonary function in primates following autotransplantation.

In 1980 Reitz and coworkers[25] published a landmark report documenting the operative technique and immunosuppressive regimen (cyclosporine and azathioprine) whereby long-term survival with normal pulmonary function was obtained with heart-lung allotransplantation in monkeys. Three of seven allotransplants survived long-term, with two alive at publication 9 to 10 months postoperatively.

A summary of experimental efforts in orthotopic transplantation is provided in Table 1–3.

Table 1–3. Maximum Survival in Experimental Orthotopic Transplantation

Authors	Date	Type	Survival
Demikhov[9]	1951	Heart/lung	6 days
Neptune, Cookson, Bailey[13]	1953	Heart/lung	6 hours
Webb, Howard[15]	1957	Heart/lung	22 hours
Goldberg, Berman, Akman[16]	1958	Heart	20 minutes
Webb, Howard, Neeley[17]	1959	Heart	7.5 hours
Cass, Brock[18]	1959	Heart	1 hour
Lower, Shumway[19]	1960	Heart	21 days
Lower, Shumway[21]	1961	Heart/lung	5 days
Kondo, Kantrowitz[22]	1965	Heart	213 days
Lower, Dong, Shumway[23]	1965	Heart	250 days
Reitz, Shumway[25]	1980	Heart/lung	311 days

CLINICAL TRANSPLANTATION

By the mid-1960s the stepwise progression of experimental contributions had provided solutions to many "key problems" facing cardiac transplantation. Shumway commented, "Enough has been achieved, in fact, to provoke expression of the concept that only the immunological barrier lies between this day and a radical new era in the treatment of cardiac diseases."[2]

Surgical techniques and methods of recipient support and myocardial protection had been described, observations regarding transplant cardiac allograft function had been reported, and fundamental means of diagnosing and treating rejection were available. Thus, the basis for clinical cardiac transplantation had been established in the experimental laboratory. Remaining problems to be addressed included legal and logistic issues involved in human cardiac transplantation.

In 1964, Hardy and his team,[26] working at the University Hospital in Jackson, Mississippi, indicated that progress in transplantation research "justified a planned approach directed toward eventual heart transplantation in man." Oddly, the "planned approach" dictated events so that the first human recipient of a cardiac transplant did not receive a human heart. It is interesting to review some of the early considerations surrounding this first human heart transplant:

> . . . considerable reflection was devoted to definition of the clinical circumstances under which heart transplantation might be ethically carried out . . . transplantation of the heart would involve basic emotional factors that could be exceeded only by those of the brain. . . . The donor heart presumably would be derived from a relatively young patient dying of brain damage and the recipient must be a patient dying of terminal myocardial failure. . . . But how soon after "death" of the donor could the heart be removed? If it were not done promptly, irreversible damage might have occurred. To minimize such damage it was planned to insert catheters into the femoral vessels and begin total body perfusion the instant death was announced . . . if the relatives were willing to permit use of the heart for transplantation, they probably would not object to heparinization and insertion of the peripheral catheters using local anesthesia at some point just prior to cardiorespiratory arrest.[26]

Conspicuous in this formulation is that "brain death" was not an accepted notion and that only cardiorespiratory arrest constituted death. Consequently, difficult logistic problems arose leading to usual solutions.

> By this stage of the program it has become abundantly clear that unless one were willing to halt mechanical support of respiration in a potential donor, it would be exceedingly unlikely that a potential recipient would die during the time a patient dying of myocardial insufficiency and shock could be kept on the pump oxygenator. Since we were not willing to stop the ventilator, we had concluded that a situation might rise in which the only heart available for transplantation would be that of a lower primate.[26]

The first patient considered for transplantation in January 1964 was a less than ideal recipient candidate by current standards. The patient, a 36-year old man presenting one year following surgical closure of a left ventricular knife wound, suffered recurrent embolization resulting in permanent right hemiplegia, severe mental impairment, urinary and fecal incontinence, amputation of the left leg for gangrene followed several months later by amputation of the right leg, and a recent "intra-abdominal catastrophe," thought to be improving. Anticipating that a transplant might be necessary and that a donor might not be available, the authors reasoned that the primate might prove an adequate donor:

> . . . we had purchased two large chimpanzees for possible use as kidney donors when no human donor kidney was available. . . . The cardiac output of the larger primate was 4.25 liters. . . . The patient, legless, weighed 73 lbs (33.1 kg) and the chimpanzee weighed 96 lb (43.5 kg).[26]

Fortunately, the patient did not require transplantation, but later in January 1964 a second "candidate" was referred. This patient, a 68-year old hypertensive man with lower leg gangrene, had recently been admitted pulseless and comatose. Management included vasopressors, tracheostomy, mechanical ventilation, femoral embolectomy and below-knee amputation. Elsewhere in the hospital a young patient was dying of irreversible brain damage, but the team faced the same dilemma:

> . . . experience with the previous case had underscored the fact that, for a homotransplant to succeed, the donor and the recipient must "die" at almost the same time; although this might occur, the chances that both prospective donor and prospective recipient would enter fatal collapse simultaneously were very slim . . . the prospective recipient went into terminal shock . . . and it was obvious that if heart transplantation were to be performed it must be done at once. Meanwhile, the condition of the prospective donor was not such that death appeared to be immediately imminent. At this time a tranquilizing drug was given to the larger of the two chimpanzees.[26]

Eventually, events forced a difficult decision, as "the patient was on cardiopulmonary bypass and the prospective human donor lingered on in the recovery ward. The larger chimpanzee had already been anesthetized in an adjacent operating room." It was decided to proceed using the primate heart. The suture technique of Lower and Shumway [19] was employed, but donor graft preservation was provided by retrograde coronary sinus perfusion with chilled, oxygenated blood. The transplant, which was technically satisfactory, was unable to maintain the circulatory load, and approximately 1 hour after cardiopulmonary bypass attempts at support were abandoned.

Interestingly, in 1966, the mirror image experiment was performed at the Medical College of Virginia by Lower.[27] Studies were performed on resuscitation of human cadaver hearts following kidney donor harvesting. In one such experiment, the resuscitated heart was successfully transplanted into a baboon. The large donor heart precluded closing the animal's chest, but satisfactory circulatory support was maintained for several hours until the experiment was electively terminated.

Although never reported in the medical literature, this experience was well known to several surgeons interested in cardiac transplantation and confirmed that the heart could be stopped, removed, resuscitated, and successfully transplanted.

On December 3, 1967, the first successful clinical cardiac transplant was performed by Christiaan N. Barnard at the Groote Schuur Hospital in Capte Town, South Africa.[28] In a paper entitled "The Operation," Barnard described the historic context in which the procedure took place:

> This achievement did not come as a surprise to the medical world. Steady progress towards this goal has been made by immunologists, biochemists, surgeons, and specialists in other branches of medical science all over the world during the past decades to ensure that this, the ultimate in cardiac surgery, would be a success.[28]

In the following paragraph, a somewhat broader perspective on transplantation was offered:

> The dream of the ancients from time immemorial has been the junction of portions of different individuals, not only to counteract disease, but also to combine the potentials of different species. This desire inspired the birth of many mythical creatures which were purported to have capabilities normally beyond the power of a single species. The modern world has inherited these dreams in the form of the sphinx, the mermaid and the chimerical forms of many heraldic beasts.[28]

A 54-year-old man dying of end-stage ischemic heart disease received the heart of a young man with severe brain injury, certified dead 5 minutes after the absence of ECG activity, spontaneous respirations, and reflexes. At that time the donor chest was opened and cardiopulmonary bypass was initiated to resuscitate the heart. The recipient recovered, but succumbed to pseudomonas pneumonia after 18 days.

Three days after this first cardiac transplant, Adrian Kantrowitz,[29] in Brooklyn, New York, transplanted the heart of an anencephalic infant into an 18-day-old child with Ebstein's anomaly using deep hypothermia and circulatory arrest. Although the procedure was technically satisfactory, the recipient developed unremitting acidosis and lived only 6½ hours postoperatively.

On September 15, 1968, the first clinical heart-lung transplant was performed by Denton Cooley.[30] The heart and lungs of a 2-month-old with an atrioventricular canal defect were replaced with those of an anencephalic infant donor, and the recipient survived 14 hours, succumbing to pulmonary insufficiency.

Failure to accept brain death as the standard for donation continued to hinder early clinical transplant efforts. Shumway commented in 1969:

> It should be underlined that no one can transplant a dead heart. The hearts which have been transplanted by surgeons all over the world could have been resuscitated in the donors, and the chests could have

been closed, leaving these hopelessly brain-injured persons to the fate of infection or peripheral vascular collapse. Death of the donor is a diagnosis which must be made by the neurological and neurosurgical team.[31]

No other cardiac transplants were done in 1967, but by the end of 1968, 102 had been performed in 17 countries. Early results were discouraging, with mean survival for the first 100 cardiac transplants being 29 days;[30] and by 1970 all but several institutions had abandoned the procedure. During the 1970s, clinical investigations, principally at Stanford University, steadily established key elements necessary for success in cardiac transplantation, and one-year survival increased from 22 percent in 1968 to 65 percent by 1978,[32] with rehabilitation to normal function in 90 percent.[33] Early clinical results,[34] infectious complications,[35] and hemodynamics of the transplanted heart were reported;[36,37] indications and contraindications for the procedure were defined[38] and donor management described.[39] The diagnosis of cardiac allograft rejection was greatly advanced by Dr. Philip Caves who developed a bioptome for obtaining repeated transvenous endomyocardial biopsies and Dr. Margaret Billingham, who described a histologic system for grading rejection in these specimens.[40] The treatment of rejection was greatly enhanced by the use of rabbit antithymocyte globulin;[41–43] and survival was prolonged by the control of graft arteriosclerosis[44] and the advent of cardiac retransplantation.[45] In addition, donor organ availability increased as the concept of "brain death" became accepted (Report Ad Hoc Committee Harvard),[46,47] and methods of long-distance procurement were developed.[48,49]

The 1980s has witnessed a worldwide wave of enthusiasm for cardiac transplantation, spurred by promising results with cyclosporine immunosuppression at Stanford University;[50] and computerized national procurement networks arose to help satisfy the growing demand for donors. In 1982, Reitz and coworkers[51] published the first successful clinical series of heart-lung transplants. Success was attributed to laboratory experience with primate cardiopulmonary transplants, and the use of cyclosporine.

SUMMARY

The current success of heart and heart-lung transplantation is grounded in a long progression of experimental and clinical advances. Beginning with an isolated heart transplant performed as a technical exercise in 1905, slowly accumulated experimental efforts yielded solutions to problems involving technique, recipient and graft protection, post-transplant function and immunology, and provided a foundation for subsequent clinical applications. Clinical studies augmented these observations and addressed legal and logistic issues involved in human transplantation.

REFERENCES

1. Marcus, E, Wong, SNT, and Luisada, AA: Homologous heart grafts: Transplantation of the heart in dogs. Surg Forum 2:212, 1951.
2. Shumway, NE and Lower, RR: Special problems in transplantation of the heart. Ann NY Acad Sci 120:773, 1964.

3. Carrel, A and Guthrie, CC: The transplantation of veins and organs. Am Med 10:1101, 1905.

4. Mann, FC, Priestley, JT, Markowitz, J, et al: Transplantation of the intact mammalian heart. Arch Surg 26:219, 1933.

5. Marcus, E, Wong, SNT, and Luisada, AA: Homologous heart grafts: Transplantation of the heart in dogs. Surg Forum 2:212, 1951.

6. Hairston, P: Heart transplantation: Past, present and future. J Thorac Cardiovasc Surg 50:1, 1965.

7. Cooper, DKC: Experimental development of cardiac transplantation. Br Med J 4:174, 1968.

8. Downie, HG: Homotransplantation of the dog heart. AMA Arch Surg 66:624, 1953.

9. Demikhov, VP: Experimental transplantation of vital organs. Haigh B. (trans), New York, Consultants' Bureau, 1962.

10. Reemtsma, K: The heart as a test organ in transplantation studies. Ann NY Acad Sci 120:778, 1964.

11. McGough, EC, Brewer, PL, and Reemtsma, K: The parallel heart: Studies

12. Johansson, L, Soderlund, S, and William-Olsson, G: Left heart bypass by means of a transplanted heart. Scand J Thor Cardiovasc Surg 1:23, 1967.

13. Neptune, WB, Cookson, BA, Bailey, CP, et al: Complete homologous heart transplantation. AMA Arch Surg 66:174, 1953.

14. Webb, WR and Howard, HS: Restoration of function of the refrigerated heart. Surg Forum 8:302, 1957.

15. Webb, WR and Howard HS: Cardio-pulmonary transplantation. Surg Forum 8:313, 1957.

16. Goldberg, M, Berman, EF, and Akman, LC: Homologous transplantation of the canine heart. J Internat Coll Surg 30:575, 1958.

17. Webb, WR, Howard, HS, and Neely, WA: Practical methods of homologous cardiac transplantation. J Thorac Surg 37:361, 1959.

18. Cass, MH and Brock, R: Heart excision and replacement. Guys Hosp Rep 108:285, 1959.

19. Lower, RR and Shumway, NE: Studies orthotopic homotransplantation of the canine heart. Surg Forum 11:18, 1960.

20. Lower, RR, Stofer, RC, and Shumway, NE: Homovital transplantation of the heart. J Thorac Cardiovasc Surg 41:196, 1961.

21. Lower, RR, Stofer, RC, Hurley, EJ, et al: Complete homograft replacement of the heart and both lungs. Surgery 50:842, 1961.

22. Kondo, Y, Grundel, FO, Chaptal, PA, et al: Immediate and delayed orthotopic homotransplantation of the heart. J Thorac Cardiovasc Surg 50:781, 1965a.

23. Lower, RR, Dong, E Jr, and Shumway, NE: Long-term survival of cardiac homografts. Surgery 58:110, 1965.

24. Castaneda, AE, Zamora, R, Schmidt-Habelmann, P, et al: Cardiopulmonary autotransplantation in primates (baboons): Late functional results. Surgery 72:1064, 1972.

25. Reitz, BA, Burton, NA, Jamieson, SW, et al: Heart and lung transplantation. J Thorac Cardiovasc Surg 80:360, 1980.

26. Hardy, JD, Chavez, CM, Kurrus, FD, et al: Heart transplantation in man. JAMA 188:114, 1964.

27. Griepp, RB and Ergin, MA: The history of experimental heart transplantation. Heart Transplant 3:145, 1984.

28. Barnard, CN: A human cardiac transplant: An interim report of a successful operation performed at Groote Schurr Hospital, Capetown. S Afr Med J 4:1271, 1967.

29. Kantrowitz, A, Huller, JD, Joos, H, et al: Transplantation of the heart in an infant and an adult. Am J Cardiol 22:782, 1968.

30. Cooley, DA, Bloodwell, RD, Hallman, GL, et al: Organ transplantation for advanced cardiopulmonary disease. Ann Thorac Surg 8:30, 1969.

31. Shumway, NE, Dong, E, and Stinson, B: Surgical aspects of cardiac transplantation in man. Bull NY Acad Med 45:387, 1969.

32. Griepp, RB: A decade of human heart transplantation. Transplant Proc 11:285, 1979.

33. Christopherson, LK, Griepp, RB, and Stinson, EB: Rehabilitation after cardiac transplantation. JAMA 236:2082, 1976.

34. Stinson, EB, Griepp, RB, Clark, DA, et al: Cardiac transplantation in man. VIII. Survival and function. J Thorac Cardiovasc Surg 60:303, 1970.

35. Stinson, EB, Bieber, CP, Griepp, RB, et al: Infectious complications after cardiac transplantation in man. Ann Intern Med 74:22, 1971.

36. Griepp, RB, Stinson, EB, Dong, E Jr, et al: Hemodynamic performance of the transplanted human heart. Surgery 70:88, 1971.

37. Stinson, EB, Griepp, RB, Schroeder, JS, et al: Hemodynamic observations one and two years after cardiac transplantation in man. Circulation 45:1183, 1972.
38. Griepp, RB, Stinson, EB, Dong, E Jr, et al: Determinants of operative risk in human heart transplantation. Am J Surg 122:192, 1971b.
39. Griepp, RB, Stinson, EB, Clark, DA, et al: Cardiac transplantation in man. IX. The cardiac donor. Surg Gynecol Obstet 133:792, 1971c.
40. Caves, PK, Billingham, ME, Stinson, EB, et al: Serial transvenous biopsy of the transplanted human heart: Improved management of acute rejection episodes. Lancet 1:821, 1974.
41. Griepp, RB, Stinson, EB, Dong, E Jr, et al: The use of antithymocyte globulin in human heart transplantation. Circulation 45–46 (Suppl I):147, 1972.
42. Bieber, CP, Griepp, RB, Oyer, PE, et al: Use of rabbit antithymocyte globulin in cardiac transplantation. Transplantation 22:478, 1976.
43. Baumgartner, WA, Reitz, BA, Bieber, CP, et al: Current expectations in cardiac transplantation. J Thorac Cardiovasc Surg 75:525, 1978.
44. Griepp, RB, Stinson, EB, Bieber, CP, et al: Control of graft arteriosclerosis in human heart transplant recipients. Surgery 81:262, 1977.
45. Copeland, JG, Griepp, RB, Bieber, CP, et al: Successful retransplantation of the human heart. J Thorac Cardiovasc Surg 73:242, 1977.
46. Report of the Ad Hoc Committee of the Harvard Medical School to Examine the Definition of Brain Death: A definition of irreversible coma. JAMA 205:85, 1968.
47. Black, PM: Brain death. N Engl J Med 299:338, 1978.
48. Watson, DC, Reitz, BA, Baumgartner, WA, et al: Distant heart procurement for transplantation. Surgery 86:56, 1979.
49. Thomas, FT, Szentpetery, SS, Mammana, RE, et al: Long-distance transportation of human hearts for transplantation. Ann Thorac Surg 26:344, 1978.
50. Oyer, PE, Stinson, EB, Jamieson, SA, et al: Cyclosporin A in cardiac allografting: A preliminary experience. Transplant Proc 15:1247, 1983.
51. Reitz, BA, Wallwork, MD, Hunt Ch B, et al: Heart-lung transplantation. N Engl J Med 306:557, 1982.

PART 2

Basic Mechanisms

CHAPTER 2

Physiology of the Transplanted Heart

Barry F. Uretsky, M.D.

The emergence of cardiac transplantation as an approach to terminal heart failure is due in large measure to the superb performance of the denervated, transplanted, immunologically suppressed heart. I have asked one of our transplant recipients at the University of Pittsburgh, Mr. William McGowan, Chief Executive Officer of MCI Corporation, to describe the differences between living with an ineffective pump (his own heart after myocardial infarction) and after the implantation of an effective one (the donor heart).

Eighteen years after starting MCI with three people, we finally achieved regulatory, legal, financial, organizational, and marketing success. We had developed worldwide long distance telephone service, 15,000 employees, and 3.5 billion dollars in revenues, and I had a heart attack. The initial prognosis was hopeful, but my physical condition deteriorated. I lost weight and appetite. I could not concentrate as in the past. My attempts to stay abreast of non-personal activities were intermittent at best. My physical stamina was eroding. Six further hospitalizations to stabilize drugs were unsuccessful. Days would all blur together and attention span was very short. I had to drop out of my exercise group when I could not keep up.

I was transferred to Pittsburgh 5 months after my heart attack. Ten days later I had my heart transplant. Within a week, I became aware that my world had changed. You feel that a miracle has truly happened. Every day is like a new and improved beginning. . . .

I returned to the office after 2 months, and was working full time in another 3 months. I felt more energy and enjoyment of my life, my family, and my business than before the heart attack. Now, 18 months later, except for taking medicines and having heart biopsies, there is no interference with life as I knew it and enjoyed it before the heart attack. . . .

Mr. McGowan's recovery is not unique. It is universally agreed that the general quality of life of the post-transplant patient is excellent, particularly in relation to preoperative status. Thus, description of cardiac physiology in the transplanted heart is more a description of the function of the denervated heart rather than clinical problems to be overcome because in the nonrejecting state the denervated transplanted heart has proven to be a durable and effective pump. There are, however, dangers to the continued effectiveness of the transplanted heart, which are discussed in the final part of this chapter.

Mann and coworkers[1] showed clearly as early as 1933 that a heart could be routinely transplanted from one animal to another and that cardiac function could be excellent following surgery. They observed ". . . it is readily seen that the failure of the homotransplanted heart to survive is not due to the technic of transplantation but to some biologic factor which is probably identical to that which prevents survival of other homotransplanted tissues and organs." That "biologic factor" is tissue rejection, discovered and extensively investigated over the last 30 years. Adequate (although still not ideal) immunosuppressive approaches have allowed cardiac transplantation to advance.

In the 1960s, autotransplantation—that is, removal and reimplantation of a heart into the same animal—was performed to determine the physiologic performance of the denervated organ.[2-6] Based on relatively normal function in this setting, orthotopic heart transplantation was performed between animals of the same species with and without immunosuppression.[7] This progressed to the human experiment[8] and has culminated at present in the routine surgical procedure of cardiac transplantation. The success of this approach is attested to by the major problem facing heart transplantation today—donor heart shortage.

EFFECTS OF AUTOTRANSPLANTATION

Stinson and associates[7] demonstrated an immediate depression of left ventricular function postoperatively, which was attributed to the period of ischemia during heart removal and reimplantation. Resting right and left heart pressures and cardiac output in the autotransplanted dog gradually return to levels similar to control animals. Approximation of normal cardiac function may require more than 1 month.[5,9] Resting heart rate is increased in the autotransplanted heart. Contractile indices in the denervated dog are similar to control subjects; the force interval relationship is preserved.[10] Exercise capacity appears comparable to that of normal animals.[11,12]

Daggett and colleagues[13] demonstrated that heart muscle from the autotransplanted denervated canine heart was similar to controls in regard to cardiac performance and oxygen consumption per gram of myocardial tissue. However, the hearts themselves were heavier than control hearts, and the mitochondria, viewed electron microscopically, were larger. The reason for these findings has not been clarified. Glycogen and hexokinase content have been reported to be higher in autotransplanted hearts than controls.[12,13] Differences have been attributed to lack of catecholamine stimulation of myocardial metabolic processes.

The ventricles and especially the atria have afferent neural fibers that are important in volume regulation. Thus, it might be expected that abnormalities of volume regulation may accompany cardiac denervation, a major component of experimental autotransplantation. Willman,[14] Dong,[15] and, more recently Parent[16] and their associates have demonstrated an increased blood volume in autotransplanted animals compared with controls. Evidence of fluid retention is frequently observed in the postoperative period in humans after cardiac transplantation. Cardiac deafferentation may be responsible at least in part. Gilmore and coworkers[17] have shown blunted diuretic and natriuretic responses to isooncotic volume expansion in animals with denervated hearts. The mechanism by which this occurs has not been clarified, but it may be related to a decrease in the opposition of sympathetic renal stimulation, which in essence may create a new volume steady state.[17,18] Further studies should help to clarify this subject.

Myocardial catecholamine levels are not measurable by 1 week after autotransplantation.[19]

RESTING HEMODYNAMICS IN THE TRANSPLANT HEART

Results of hemodynamics reported after transplantation may be divided into those from several days to several months after the procedure and those 6 months or more postoperatively.[20,21] Immediately postoperatively in experimental studies, cardiac index and diastolic compliance are reduced.[22] These abnormalities, which gradually improve over time, have been attributed to anoxic myocardial injury, similar to those found after autotransplantation. Tissue rejection causes a reduction in myocardial contractility, ventricular compliance, and cardiac performance, but these findings occur late (24 to 48 hours) in the course of the rejection process.

In the early period after transplantation in humans there are elevations in both right- and left-sided filling pressures, which gradually recede.[20] The reduction in right-sided pressures may relate to regression of pulmonary hypertension,[23] improvement in right ventricular ischemia that occurs during implantation, and decrease in tricuspid regurgitation.[23,24] Decreasing left-sided filling pressure may be secondary to recovery from left ventricular ischemia, which also occurs during implantation. Bhatia and coworkers found that systemic blood pressure, heart rate, and cardiac output remained constant from the early postoperative period to the end of the first year after transplantation.[23]

Resting hemodynamics reported at 6 months or longer in patients on immunosuppression with azathioprine and prednisone have shown relatively normal cardiac output and normal to slightly elevated pulmonary artery and pulmonary artery wedge pressures and left ventricular end-diastolic pressure.[24–28] Additionally, left ventricular volumes, ejection fraction and blood pressure have been reported to be normal.[29,30] Although these early studies showed relatively intact cardiac function, no study described a control group from the same hemodynamic laboratory for comparison.

Since the advent of cyclosporine immunosuppressive therapy, a major new hemodynamic abnormality has arisen—namely, systemic hypertension. One may propose that some elevation in left ventricular filling pressures and pulmonary artery wedge pressure with secondary elevations in pulmonary artery and right atrial pressures might occur on this basis. Our group, in fact, found mild to moderate elevations in these parameters, particularly when compared with a control group.[21] Furthermore, a decreased left ventricular ejection fraction[21,30] and reduced compliance [31] have been reported. A long-term hemodynamic comparison of groups treated with either azathioprine and prednisone or cyclosporine has been reported.[32] An elevated left ventricular end-diastolic pressure in the cyclosporine group was shown, which was higher than the azathioprine group, both at

1 and at 4 years.[32] We have previously attributed these findings in the cyclosporine group to the presence of increased afterload.[33] Although mean left ventricular ejection fraction falls within what has been considered the normal range, it is significantly lower than a control group studied by identical methods.[21,34] Left ventricular end-diastolic volume tends to be lower and end-systolic volume higher than in controls. The reason for these abnormalities is unclear. We have emphasized in the past the possibility that systemic hypertension may be an important factor in development of these abnormalities.[33] Another potential explanation includes the lack of sympathetic nervous system stimulation in the resting state, although in our original study, those on beta blockers showed similar ventricular function to those patients not on this therapy for hypertension.[21]

It has long been known that the native atria retain both electrical and mechanical activity at times far removed from the transplant procedure itself.[35] It has been demonstrated that the timing of the native atrial depolarization (and presumably contraction) affects parameters of diastolic function.[36] The data are consistent with the hypothesis that the atria continue to contract, and if contraction occurs in late systole (presumably raising left atrial pressure), isovolumic relaxation time and pressure half-time decrease and mitral valve inflow velocity increases.

Borow and associates[37] have shown that myocardial contractility, using the end-systolic dimension-pressure relationship, is similar to that in normal sub-

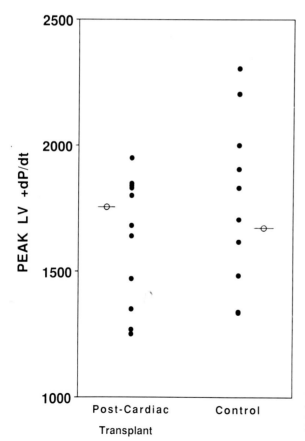

Figure 2–1. Peak rate of left ventricular pressure rise is shown in a group of transplant patients at least 1 year after operation and in a group of patients with atypical chest pain with normal coronary and ventricular angiography and hemodynamics at cardiac catheterization. Transplant patients show contractility similar to that of the control group.

jects. Additionally, we have shown that the peak rate of left ventricular pressure rise as a measure of contractility is similar in transplant patients and in control subjects (Fig. 2–1).[31]

The reversal of pulmonary hypertension is rapid, usually occurring within 2 weeks of transplantation.[23] The transpulmonary gradient (that is, mean pulmonary artery pressure minus mean pulmonary artery wedge pressure) tends to remain the same as before transplantation, suggesting that the fall in pulmonary artery pressure is directly related to the fall in left-sided filling pressure. Bhatia and coworkers[23] have also noted by echo/Doppler study that tricuspid regurgitation and right ventricular enlargement are frequently present after surgery. In Bhatia's series, approximately two thirds of patients immediately after transplantation had tricuspid regurgitation and right ventricular enlargement of some degree, decreasing to one third of patients by 1 year after transplantation. The etiology of these early problems is unknown but may be a combination of right ventricular ischemia during implantation, and the response to immediate pulmonary hypertension during implantation.

Diastolic relaxation characteristics of the transplanted heart also may be abnormal.[31] We have pointed out elsewhere the limitations of using the time constant of relaxation as a true measure of diastolic relaxation.[38] With these reservations in mind, it is reasonable to point out that the transplanted left ventricle appears to show a slower relaxation than a control group (Fig. 2–2).

Dagget's finding of a thickened ventricular myocardium[13] after autotransplantation emphasizes the possibility of a different pressure-volume relationship such that a fully preloaded ventricle might provoke higher filling pressure in the denervated left ventricle than in the normal heart. In favor of this hypothesis are

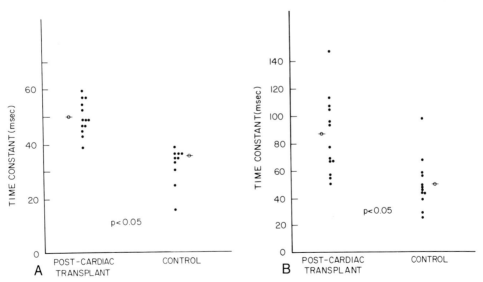

Figure 2–2. The time constant of relaxation is shown in a group of transplanted patients at least 1 year postoperatively and in the same group of controls as noted in Figure 2–1. A micromanometer-tipped catheter was utilized for measuring left ventricular pressure. Time constant was measured using a method that assumes left ventricular pressure falls to zero if filling does not occur (*A*) and a method that does not assume the lowest level of left ventricular pressure (*B*). Both methods show the transplanted heart relaxes more slowly than the control heart.

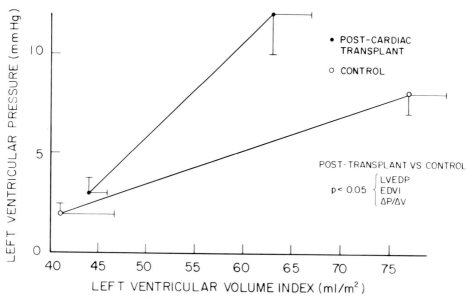

Figure 2–3. Left ventricular early and end-diastolic pressures and volumes are shown in a group of transplant patients and controls.[31] Although early left ventricular pressure and volume are similar in the two groups, left ventricular end-diastolic pressure is significantly higher than in controls, when left ventricular volume is slightly smaller in the transplant group. These data suggest increased stiffness in the transplanted ventricle.

data which show that left ventricular end-diastolic pressure is higher in transplants than controls, but left ventricular end-diastolic volume is actually smaller.[21] These data in effect demonstrate a shifting of the left ventricular pressure-volume relationship of the left ventricle up and to the left (Fig. 2–3).[31]

HEART RATE RESPONSE OF THE DENERVATED HEART

Resting Response

The resting heart rate in animals and humans is a complex interplay of the intrinsic sinus node function and the effects of the parasympathetic and sympathetic nervous systems. Jose[39] has discussed the concept of "intrinsic heart rate," demonstrating it by pharmacologic denervation of the sinus node with atropine and beta blockade. By this technique, sinus node firing is usually faster than that in the resting human, suggesting a predominance of parasympathetic over sympathetic tone. In the denervated transplanted heart, sinus rate is faster than in controls, approximating in most cases, the expected intrinsic rate described by Jose.

Small changes in sinus rate are typical of the innervated heart during the respiratory cycle.[10] It is not surprising, therefore, that the denervated heart typically shows a lack of sinus arrhythmia.[5,10,40] On the other hand, vigorous and chronic exercise training in cardiac transplant patients is associated with a decrease in the resting heart rate.[41] Furthermore, although over short periods there is little variation in heart rate, the heart rate may change by as much as 20 percent over a 24-hour period, as shown by Holter monitor.[42] These data imply that a circulating substance or substances, probably catecholamines, continue to influence sinus rate.

Exercise Response

Cannon[43] and Donald[5] and their colleagues first showed that heart rate after cardiac denervation rises in response to exercise. Unlike the innervated state, however, the rise in heart rate is delayed and requires a longer time to decrease following exercise (Fig. 2–4). This pattern of heart rate response has been shown by others in animal studies and in man.[2,29,44]

The mechanism of increasing heart rate has been extensively investigated. It is unlikely due to autonomic cardiac influences in that such increases in heart rate can be shown in animals as early as several weeks after autotransplantation at a time when there is no evidence of cardiac reinnervation.[45] Furthermore, there are no data to indicate that reinnervation in humans occurs, yet increased heart rate occurs both early and late after transplantation in response to exercise.

The Bainbridge reflex states that an increase in right atrial stretch causes cardioacceleration. The mechanism of this reflex has been investigated and appears to be mediated via the parasympathetic afferents and sympathetic efferents; it seems also that stretch of the sinus node or of the atrium independent of neural effects is unimportant in the promulgation of this response.[46] Thus, it is unlikely

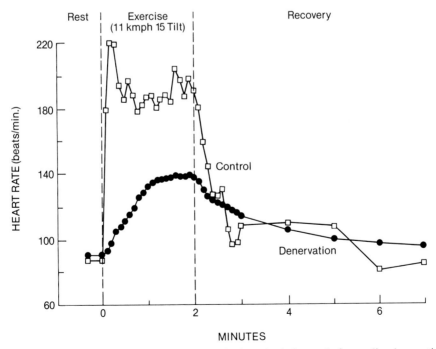

Figure 2–4. The heart rate increase with exercise in a dog before and after cardiac denervation is shown. Cardiac denervation produces a slower rise in heart rate with exercise and a slower decline in heart rate post-exercise. (From Donald and Shepherd[11] with permission.)

on theoretic grounds that volume loading via this reflex provokes the tachycardia observed during exercise. Furthermore, Donald and Shepherd[47] have shown that the increase in right atrial pressure occurs much earlier than the increase in heart rate during exercise, an atypical time course to be explained by the Bainbridge reflex. Donald and Shepherd[5] also have demonstrated that bilateral adrenalectomy does not prevent the rise in heart rate—strong evidence that release of adrenal catecholamines is not important in the heart rate response to exercise of the denervated heart.

Donald and coworkers[48] have demonstrated a marked deterioration in the maximal exercise performance of the exercising greyhound with beta blockade, which was associated with a marked attenuation in the heart rate response during exercise. These data provide strong evidence that circulating catecholamines are the stimulus by which the denervated sinus node increases its heart rate. The source of these catecholamines is likely to be from the peripheral nervous system in view of the maintenance of the tachycardia with adrenalectomy.[5] The plasma level of catecholamines probably represents more than simply a marker for the activity of the sympathetic nervous system.[49] Rather, such increased plasma levels probably are important for maximal exercise performance by increasing both inotropic and chronotropic cardiac responses.

Other data supporting the possibility of circulating catecholamines as the tachygenic substances have been provided by Cannom and associates.[50] An intravenous infusion of norepinephrine increases the sinus node firing rate and decreases atrioventricular nodal conduction time in the transplanted heart; these effects are blocked by propranolol. These data document the responsiveness of these sites in the denervated heart to circulating catecholamines.

CARDIAC OUTPUT RESPONSE TO EXERCISE

The mechanism of increased cardiac output after cardiac transplantation during supine bicycle exercise has been described. Using tantalum intramyocardial markers to define the left ventricular cavity, Pope and coworkers[29] demonstrated that mild to moderate exercise produces increases in left ventricular end-diastolic volume and stroke volume. Thus, the Frank-Starling mechanism is utilized early in exercise in the transplant patient while the heart rate accelerates only minimally. This response contrasts to normal subjects in whom in early moderate exercise left ventricular end-diastolic and stroke volumes change little and heart rate markedly accelerates.[51] At maximal exercise in transplant patients, however, the end-diastolic volume is similar to the resting end-diastolic volume. The heart rate increases and stroke volume and ejection fraction increase. Associated with these hemodynamic changes is a marked increase in circulated catecholamines, particularly norepinephrine.

Left ventricular filling pressure increases during mild to moderate supine exercise in transplant patients, which contrasts with the response in normal individuals.[26,27,52] This increase has been observed both in immunologically suppressed patients on azathioprine and prednisone as well as in cyclosporine-treated patients. The data of Pope and coworkers[29] and more recently Pflugfelder and associates,[44] suggest that the rise in end-diastolic volume is at least partially responsible for the increase in end-diastolic pressure noted in these studies. The differences in left ventricular pressure-volume relationships in normal subjects and transplant patients probably also account in part for these differences.

The response to isometric exercise in the transplanted patient is similar to that in the nontransplanted cardiac patient; that is, there is a rise in blood pressure and systemic vascular resistance with minimal change in cardiac output.[53] The major difference in these two groups is the minimal heart rate increase in the transplant patient, as would be expected because of cardiac denervation.

A relationship between systemic oxygen consumption and cardiac output has been described by Donald and Shepherd.[5] They demonstrated that a linear and comparable relationship of systemic oxygen consumption to cardiac output at submaximal work loads persists with cardiac denervation.

CAN MAXIMAL EXERCISE RESPONSE BE ACHIEVED IN THE DENERVATED HEART?

Donald and associates[54] demonstrated that maximal exercise performance is similar in innervated and autotransplanted denervated dogs. However, in denervated dogs (racing greyhounds) treated with beta blockade to total inhibition of isoproterenol-induced heart rate increase, maximal exercise response was affected adversely.[48] This worsening of maximal exercise performance was associated with a marked attenuation of the exercise-induced increase in heart rate.

Unlike Donald's comparable results in non–beta-blocked, autotransplanted and control animals, the maximal exercise response in transplanted humans is less clear. Savin and colleagues[55] showed a decreased maximal exercise capacity in comparison with age- and sex-matched controls. The authors pointed out that the differences may have been due to factors other than intrinsic cardiac performance. They suggested the possibility of proximal muscle weakness secondary to chronic steroids as a reason for the difference. The authors also suggested the possibility of a limited cardiac reserve as the reason for difference, which in turn they attributed to differences in maximal heart rate.

Bexton and associates[56] studied cardiac transplant patients' response to maximal exercise before and after beta blockade. Maximal exercise tolerance was significantly decreased after beta blockade, associated with an attenuation in exercise heart rate. The authors concluded that circulating catecholamines are necessary for maximal exercise response in the absence of cardiac innervation. They did not address, however, whether the decrease in maximal exercise tolerance was different from normal humans with an innervated heart.

McLaughlin and coworkers[57] demonstrated that left ventricular end-diastolic volume at maximal exercise capacity does not increase. This group noted that maximal exercise capacity was similar to a normal group. Maximal heart rate was increased less in transplants. Stroke volume and ejection fraction rose to a greater extent in the transplant group. To determine the importance of circulating catecholamines in this response, the authors atrially paced the same group of patients to identical heart rates as would occur during exercise. The mean cardiac output rose approximately 18 percent as opposed to 49 percent during exercise, suggesting a major role for catecholamine stimulation of the exercising heart. Pflugfelder and coworkers [44] using nuclear techniques confirmed the earlier exercise studies of McLaughlin[57] and Pope[29] and their colleagues. Unlike the earlier study of Savin and associates,[53] maximal exercise was similar to normal subjects in this study.

Yusuf and associates[58] showed similar exercise capacity in normal individuals and cardiac transplant patients. After beta blockade, maximal exercise capacity decreased but did so to a comparable degree as in normal subjects. Previous studies have suggested that beta blockade may decrease maximal exercise performance by as much as 10 to 40 percent.[59,60] Yusuf's data showed an approximately 10 to 15 percent decrease in exercise capacity, both in the transplant and normal group on beta blockers.

Kavanaugh and coworkers[41] have demonstrated a reduction in maximal exercise capacity in post-transplant patients versus an age- and sex-matched control group. It should be noted that this study came from the same institution as in Yusuf's study, in which no differences in exercise capacity had previously been noted. Kavanaugh's study showed that vigorous and chronic exercise training could increase maximal exercise tolerance, with the most compliant patients approaching normal values after exercise training. They attributed the lower peak performance to a relatively smaller muscle mass in the transplant group, which increased during exercise training. Nevertheless, peak systemic oxygen consumption still remained below control values overall, associated with a decreased peak heart rate and blood pressure compared with control subjects. Thus, a limitation in peak exercise capacity persisted. Whether it would be correctable by further exercise training or increase in lean muscle mass, or whether hemodynamic factors including attenuated heart rate or blood pressure response, myocardial stiffness, or an inappropriate lack of vasoconstriction in nonexercising vascular beds[61] may be responsible has still not been totally clarified. Thus, it cannot be stated with certainty at present whether a limitation of maximal exercise capacity is inherent with denervation per se in humans or if other correctable factors are responsible for this limitation that has been noted in some studies.

Schuler and colleagues[62] have demonstrated that at submaximal exercise levels, plasma catecholamines are higher in transplant patients than in normal control subjects, adding to the evidence that these circulating substances may be crucial in attempting to maintain normal exercise function.

RESPONSE OF THE DENERVATED HEART TO OTHER FORMS OF STRESS

Greenfield and associates[63,64] demonstrated that the increase in peak heart rate in dogs induced by breathing an hypoxic gas mixture or undergoing acute hemorrhage was reduced, suggesting the need for sympathetic efferents to maximize the stress heart rate response.

Tsakiris and coworkers[65] showed that acute hypertension is well tolerated in the denervated heart. The response is similar to that of normal dogs, with some decrease in cardiac output and a smaller increase in left ventricular end-diastolic pressure than in normal subjects. On the other hand, hypotension is less well tolerated, with a small increase in cardiac output due to less of an increase in heart rate than in normal subjects.

Mohanty and coworkers[61] have utilized heart transplantation as a model of ventricular deafferentation. The surgical technique of orthotopic heart transplantation permits a large portion of native atria with its accompanying sympathetic and parasympathetic fibers to remain. Using lower body negative pressure as a method of acute volume unloading, it was shown that a typical response to the maneuver—that is, a reduction in forearm blood flow and increase in forearm vascular resistance—was markedly impaired in this model, providing strong evidence for ventricular innervation, rather than atrial or pulmonary vascular innervation, as the afferent limb of the reflex. It is possible that the inability to vasoconstrict nonworking muscles may account in part for a limitation in maximal exercise capacity in humans, if, in fact, such does exist.

Deafferentation may be a mechanism for renal blood flow and resistance changes found in post-transplant patients. In patients on azathioprine and prednisone in whom renal function is apparently normal, blood flow is lower than normal and renal vascular resistance higher than normal.[18] These findings can be explained by increased sympathetic tone secondary to a decrease in central vagal inhibition of sympathetic stimulation of the kidneys.[18] It should be emphasized that definitive proof for this hypothesis is still required.

As Donald[66] has pointed out, the denervated heart appears to function adequately to stress with the possible exception of stress that requires an immediate tachycardic response.

ELECTRICAL ACTIVITY OF THE TRANSPLANTED HEART

Sinus Node Function

The native sinus node is still innervated and responds to sympathetic and parasympathetic input.[67] The native atrial electrical activity does not cross the suture line[67] and is of interest only insomuch as it demonstrates the effects of reflex stimuli at a time when the donor atria do not.

The denervated donor sinus node fires at a more rapid rate than its innervated counterpart.[5,21] This finding has been used as evidence that parasympathetic stimulation predominates in the maintenance of the resting heart rate in normal humans.

In two patients 1 to 2 years after transplantation, Cannom and associates[68] demonstrated sinus node recovery time comparable with normals. Bexton and colleagues[69] demonstrated by electrophysiologic techniques that a small incidence of sinus node dysfunction occurs (approximately 17 percent) after transplantation. Such patients may be identified by a lower heart rate than predicted by the method of Jose.[39] In clinical practice, this rate is generally under 70 beats per minute.

A few patients with sinus node dysfunction and disastrous consequences have been reported. Mackintosh and coworkers[70] reported a case of sinus node arrest and death of a patient while on ambulatory electrocardiographic monitoring. Autopsy revealed moderate tissue rejection. In the same series, Mackintosh reported a group with abnormal sinus node function shortly after transplantation who had a poor first year survival. It is not clear from this report, however, whether sinus node dysfunction was the cause of death or a marker of persistent rejection or other postoperative problem. Clark and colleagues[52] described three cases of sinus node dysfunction, one requiring a permanent pacemaker.

Atrioventricular Node

In three patients, Cannom and coworkers[68] showed atrioventricular nodal conduction time at rest and with atrial pacing to be similar to normal subjects. This finding suggested to the authors that parasympathetic stimulation of the atrioventricular node in the basal state is minimal. Bexton and associates[71] showed normal A-H and H-V intervals, again suggesting minimal parasympathetic effects at rest.

The atrioventricular node changes its conduction time relative to its rate of stimulation. Tuna and associates[72] recently demonstrated that such changes still occur in a denervated heart, produced either pharmacologically or surgically. These changes occur almost instantaneously in an innervated heart, but in a denervated heart require almost a minute or more to occur. Atropine has provoked this pattern,[73] which suggests the importance of parasympathetic innervation in this response. The electrical gatekeeper function of the atrioventricular node appears to be an intrinsic function, with autonomic innervation enhancing, but not critical, to this function.

IS DENERVATION PERMANENT IN THE TRANSPLANTED HEART?

Two groups have demonstrated reinnervation of both the sympathetic and parasympathetic cardiac nerves by 1 year after transplantation in some dogs who have undergone autotransplantation.[3,45,67] Several studies in humans, on the other hand, have been unable to show reinnervation at any point following transplantation up to at least 4 years.

IS THE DENERVATED HEART HYPERSENSITIVE TO CATECHOLAMINE STIMULATION?

Studies in this regard relate to the inotropic and chronotropic effects of catecholamines. There is, in fact, a leftward shift of the inotropic response curve with norepinephrine infusion in the denervated heart.[74] The mechanism is probably related to an inability of cardiac nerves to take up norepinephrine, inasmuch as the same response to a norepinephrine infusion can be elicited by adding cocaine (a norepinephrine neural uptake blocker) to an innervated heart.[74] On the other hand, a change in the myocardial contractile properties of the cell itself seems unlikely in view of a similar inotropic response to calcium in the innervated and in the denervated heart.[74] There also may be an up-regulation of beta receptors,[75,76] which may relate more to maintaining adequate inotropic reserve during stress.

Donald and Shepherd[77] demonstrated supersensitivity of the denervated heart to 1-norepinephrine in the heart rate response. Partial cardiac denervation (right cervical vagotomy, right stellate ganglionectomy) also produced hypersensitivity to norepinephrine. The authors proposed that denervation of the sinus node was responsible for this phenomenon. Borow and associates[37] tested the chronotropic response to dobutamine (5 μg/kg/min) in a group of transplant patients and normal controls pretreated with atropine. The increase in heart rate was greater in the transplant group. It has been proposed that the greater sensitivity might be related to up-regulation of beta receptors in the denervated sinus node.

ARRHYTHMIAS IN THE TRANSPLANTED HEART

Catecholamines may stimulate arrhythmias. Thus, cardiac denervation may be antiarrhythmogenic; experimental studies have tended to confirm this hypothesis.[78,79] Both Ebert[78] and Schaal and coworkers[79] reported that in the denervated dog, heart ventricular fibrillation occurred less frequently after acute coronary occlusion. On the other hand, early clinical reports have suggested that atrial and ventricular arrhythmias are a frequent manifestation in the transplanted heart.[80] Such reports preceded to a great extent the use of endomyocardial biopsy in the routine detection of preclinical rejection. It may be that such a high prevalence of arrhythmias was more a reflection of some degree of rejection, particularly in view of more recent reports that have found a relatively low prevalence of arrhythmias in the transplanted heart.[81]

Mason and coworkers[80] reported three sudden deaths following cardiac transplantation. All three patients had coronary artery disease, suggesting an ischemic origin to the presumed fatal arrhythmias.

In summary, existing data suggest that primary serious arrhythmic events in patients with cardiac transplantation are rare. Rather, malignant arrhythmias suggest the presence of tissue rejection, coronary artery disease, or ventricular dysfunction from other causes.

EFFECTS OF DRUGS ON THE TRANSPLANTED HEART

The transplanted heart should be considered denervated in terms of drug use. Thus, drugs that act primarily or totally through the autonomic nervous system will be ineffective. Drugs that have actions directly and via the autonomic nervous system will have only their direct actions expressed. Finally, with a drug that affects peripheral catecholamine release, it can be expected that such catecholamines will indirectly affect cardiac function.

Digoxin

Digoxin's effect on both the sinoatrial and atrioventricular nodes is mediated primarily via the parasympathetic nervous system. Thus, the electrical effects of digoxin on the transplanted heart are minimal.[82] On the other hand, the inotropic mechanism of digoxin is not mediated via the autonomic nervous system, and its inotropic effect probably remains intact in the transplanted heart.[83]

Atropine

Atropine, which exhibits tachygenic action based on its parasympatholytic mechanism, is ineffective in the transplanted donor sinus node.[25] It should be pointed out that atropine still increases the atrial rate of the native atrial remnant, but has no physiologic effect because the atrial impulse does not cross the suture line.

Quinidine and Disopyramide

Quinidine and disopyramide have vagolytic effects on the sinus and atrioventricular nodes, which would tend to increase the sinus rate and have minimal change on atrioventricular conduction. These effects should not be observed in the denervated heart. Rather, the direct effects of these two drugs—namely, slowing of the sinus rate and increasing atrioventricular conduction time—should be observed. Mason[84] and Bexton[85] and their colleagues confirmed these anticipated results.

Edrophonium

Edrophonium is a cholinesterase inhibitor that has no effect in the transplanted heart.[86]

Calcium Channel Blockers

The calcium channel blockers appear to slow the intrinsic firing rate and slow the A-H interval in vitro. In the innervated heart, nifedipine tends to speed up the sinus rate and decrease A-H conduction time, which has been attributed to activation of the sympathetic nervous system from systemic hypotension. Nifedipine in transplanted patients shows a minimal increase in heart rate coincident with the drop in systemic blood pressure with a minimal decrease in A-H interval.[87] Thus, doses in humans that produce a drop in blood pressure do not appear to evoke major changes in electrophysiologic properties of the denervated heart. The slight heart rate increase has been attributed to the effect of circulating catecholamines provoked by the drop in blood pressure. Verapamil produces a slight, insignificant increase in the A-H interval without changes in other intervals. Thus, two calcium channel blockers in current use appear not to induce any major electrophysiologic effects in the denervated heart in doses used in humans.

CORONARY ARTERY DYNAMICS

The coronary arteries are richly innervated and respond to both sympathetic and parasympathetic stimulation. Autoregulation, however, has been considered to be the dominant operative force in this regional bed. Thus, one might expect coronary blood flow to be commensurate with myocardial needs in the denervated heart. Maximal hyperemic response has been found to be comparable in denervated and control dogs.[88] In a small study in humans, Nitenberg and coworkers[89] demonstrated *increased* basal coronary blood flow compared with a normal group. Maximal coronary blood flow induced by dipyridamole was similar to normal subjects but the calculated coronary reserve was diminished owing entirely to increased resting blood flow. This increase was attributed to the increased myocardial oxygen requirement due to cyclosporine-induced elevated blood pressure compared with normals. Thus, this study suggests that coronary blood flow is appropriate for metabolic demands. Interestingly, in an animal study, coronary blood flow and myocardial oxygen utilization per gram of tissue were found to be lower in denervated dogs than in control subjects.[88] The authors suggested that this finding was secondary to the lack of sympathetic cardiac stimulation.

THE TRANSPLANTED HEART AS AN ENDOCRINE ORGAN

A 28 amino acid compound known as atrial natriuretic factor or peptide (ANF, ANP) is released from the mammalian heart, including the human heart, in response to localized atrial stretch.[90-93] Based on extensive animal experimentation, it is clear that the autonomic nervous system is not necessary for its release. Although unequivocal proof of the hormonal nature of this compound will probably require specific receptor antagonists, data have accumulated that this compound may play a role in sodium and water homeostasis via natriuresis and diuresis, and the inhibition of aldosterone and possible vasopressin secretion, and arterial vasodilation.[94-96]

One might postulate that ANP secretion after cardiac transplantation would be normal (considering local atrial stretch as unimpaired in the setting of transplant). Alternatively, one might speculate that cyclosporine might in some way inhibit ANP release, thus altering sodium excretion and vascular tone, promoting the hypertension and volume retention postoperatively encountered with the use of this agent. In fact, we and others[97-99] have shown that ANP plasma levels (which probably mirror ANP secretion) are elevated compared with normal control subjects.

There are several possible explanations for this increase. We have previously shown that both right and left atrial pressures are significantly elevated in cardiac transplant patients compared with a control group at a time distant from operation.[21] Thus, the elevation in ANP levels may simply reflect increased atrial stretch. Alternatively, even if one assumes that atrial stretch is similar to that in normal subjects, the actual surface area of the atria in the transplanted heart is greater than in normal subjects, inasmuch as some of the native atria and most of the donor atria are sutured together.[18] Thus, the total surface area of atrial cells secreting ANP may be greater than normal and may account for the higher levels (approximately 1.5 to 2 times normal levels). This latter explanation would be consistent with the findings of Magovern and associates,[98] who showed a higher ANP level at any level of right or left atrial pressure in transplant versus non-transplant surgical patients. A third explanation may be that at any level of atrial *pressure,* atrial *stretch* (the actual stimulus to ANP release) may be greater in transplant patients than nontransplant patients. In other words, atrial compliance may be increased in the transplant group. Finally, the possibility that prednisone may stimulate ANP production and release should be raised but very few data supportive of glucocorticoids as a major stimulus of ANP production or release have been forthcoming.[100]

The ability of a hormone system to respond to a specific stimulus is important in characterizing the intactness of the system. We have shown comparable increases in ANP secretion to volume loading in transplants as in normals (Fig.

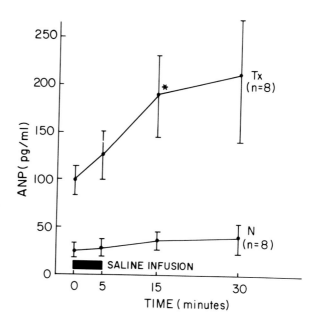

Figure 2–5. The response to a very rapid (5-minute) infusion of a liter of normal saline solution to a group of transplant patients (n = 8) and normal subjects (n = 8). Note the higher baseline level of ANP in transplant patients and the comparable increase of ANP to volume loading.

2–5).[97] Thus, the transplanted heart appears to maintain its ability to secrete ANP at rest and in response to appropriate physiologic stimulation.

HETEROTOPIC HEART TRANSPLANT

An absolute contraindication to orthotopic heart transplantation is said to be very elevated pulmonary artery resistance and pressure,[101] which would predispose to postoperative donor right ventricular failure from high right-sided afterload. Grover and coworkers[102] have pointed out the variability of pulmonary reactivity. Such variability appears to exist in the heart failure group undergoing transplant, a subgroup of whom have particularly high pulmonary arteriolar resistance. The reason for these vascular differences is not clear, although the duration of heart failure may play a role.[103] Barnard and Losman[104] described the use of heterotopic heart transplantation as an alternative to orthotopic heart transplantation in this setting. The technique of two hearts beating in parallel has been advocated as a means of allowing the native right ventricle to be used as the primary right-sided pump particularly in the immediate postoperative period.

Theoretically, both ventricles will eject a certain percentage of the cardiac output based on their contractile properties. Inflow into each ventricle will be determined by the relative compliance of each ventricle. In theory, failure of the donor heart by rejection or other process will be easier to handle inasmuch as the native heart will be available for pumping.[104–106]

Empiric descriptions of the physiology of the heterotopic heart transplantation are quite limited. One question that remains largely unanswered is whether the native left ventricle can continue to work as an effective pump in the long term. In theory, there are reasons to think that in this setting the native left ventricle may actually deteriorate. With the improved performance of the donor left ventricle, blood pressure may improve. This change may be further enhanced by the immunosuppressive agent cyclosporine. Thus, systolic and diastolic pressures, reflections of left ventricular afterload, may increase, which may further impair native left ventricular performance. Second, if the donor left ventricle is able to eject an adequate stroke volume with a relatively low filling pressure, such a decrease in filling will be reflected in the native left ventricle because these two hearts are connected. Thus, the native ventricle will be relatively understretched, further reducing its own performance.

In Barnard's original paper, a patient was described whose native heart developed ventricular fibrillation while the patient was eating supper.[104] The patient was undisturbed by the event. Thus, it is clear that the native left ventricle or right ventricle does not need to work if the patient does not require the native right ventricle as an auxillary pump. Beck and Gersh[107] described a patient who utilized the right ventricle for pulmonary flow. Melvin and associates[108] described a single patient in whom the left ventricle worsened postoperatively (left ventricular ejection fraction 19 to 9 percent). By Doppler technique, blood did not flow through the aortic valve but did flow through the mitral valve, eventually ejecting from the donor left ventricle. Thus, case reports have demonstrated in long-term observations both ventricular fibrillation and insufficient pumping in the native left ventricle to open the aortic valve. We have made the same observations (Fig. 2–6). Few if any data have been forthcoming to support the contention that the native left ventricle continues to act as a systemic pump in the long-term heter-

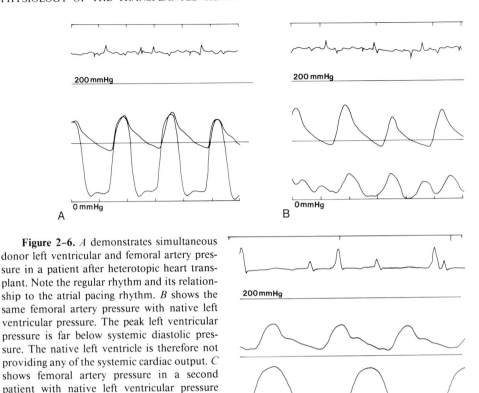

Figure 2–6. *A* demonstrates simultaneous donor left ventricular and femoral artery pressure in a patient after heterotopic heart transplant. Note the regular rhythm and its relationship to the atrial pacing rhythm. *B* shows the same femoral artery pressure with native left ventricular pressure. The peak left ventricular pressure is far below systemic diastolic pressure. The native left ventricle is therefore not providing any of the systemic cardiac output. *C* shows femoral artery pressure in a second patient with native left ventricular pressure measured by a high fidelity micromanometer-tip (Millar) catheter. Because of the lack of filling during diastole, a more precise evaluation of ventricular relaxation may be observed. In this patient, it appears that relaxation is slow and that the minimal pressure is zero. At least in this one patient with a very poorly contracting and relaxing left ventricle, no evidence for diastolic suction can be shown.

otope. It would be of interest to determine whether the native ventricle that has been in chronic ventricular fibrillation—that is, in a sense chronically rested—would show improved function after being defibrillated. Because of the real concern for dislodging a clot from this stagnant reservoir, it is unlikely that such an experiment will easily be performed.[109]

We have recently described regression of pulmonary hypertension and elevated pulmonary vascular resistance in a group of heterotopic heart transplantation patients.[103] The fall in pressures and resistance (Fig. 2–7) is similar to that found in orthotopic heart transplantation by 6 weeks, but in the first and second weeks, these parameters remain quite elevated in the range in which the donor right ventricle might in fact fail from pressure overload. Thus, the use of a short-term auxillary right ventricular pump may be justified in some cases.

Several disadvantages of this procedure have been recognized, the most serious being embolic phenomenon from the poorly functioning native left ventricle.[106] At present it is clear that the pulmonary hypertension in these cases can be reversed postoperatively. Therefore, strategies that can reduce pulmonary hypertension preoperatively[109] may obviate the need for this more cumbersome procedure.

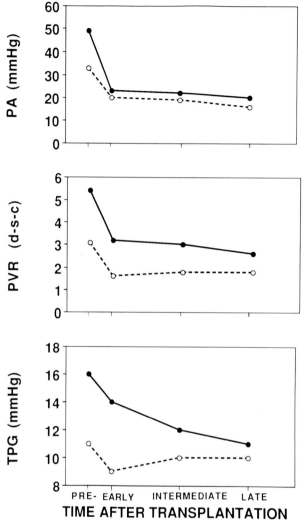

Figure 2–7. The time course of regression of pulmonary hypertension in a group of heterotopic (n = 5) and age and sex-matched orthotopic (n = 10) heart transplant controls is shown. Although the transpulmonary pressure gradient and resistance are similar in the groups at the intermediate timepoint, regression is somewhat slower in the heterotopic group. The solid circle (●) represents the heterotopic transplant group and the open circle (○) represents the orthotopic group. Early = <6 weeks after transplantation, intermediate = 6 weeks to 6 months, and late = >6 months.

FACTORS MODIFYING OR ENDANGERING FUNCTION OF THE TRANSPLANTED HEART

Acute Rejection

The rejecting myocardium profoundly affects cardiac function. Rejection ultimately causes the heart to stop functioning entirely.[1] It is interesting, however, that cardiac function tends to be preserved despite severe histologic rejection for rather long periods of time. In a dog study, Stinson and coworkers[7] showed that cardiac output did not fall until at least 24 to 48 hours of clearcut histologic evidence of tissue rejection. Blood pressure was maintained until shortly before death in this experimental study. Thus, studies reporting on the hemodynamic effects in a series of patients are unlikely to be affected by an occasional patient with severe rejection.[21,110] Conversely, although routine hemodynamic parameters are unlikely to detect early rejection (Fig. 2–8), severe hemodynamic abnormali-

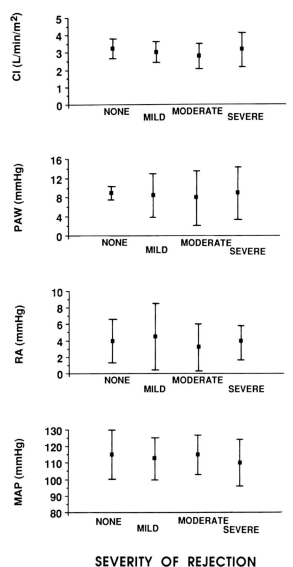

Figure 2-8. This diagram shows the results of histologic severity of rejection in 50 consecutive biopsies and relationship to hemodynamics. It is clear that severe rejection cannot be detected by routine hemodynamics.

SEVERITY OF REJECTION

ties, particularly in the early postoperative period (less than 6 months), should be taken as presumptive evidence of severe rejection (Table 2-1).

Repeated episodes of acute rejection that have been treated and healed culminating in a poorly contracting myocardium with multiple areas of scar is a theoretic possibility. Occasionally a patient has undergone retransplantation in this setting in which hemodynamic abnormalities, a diffusely scarred myocardium, and poor left ventricular function suggest repeated subclinical rejection episodes (Fig. 2-9).

Hypertension

Cyclosporine induces systemic hypertension in the majority of patients undergoing heart transplantation.[111] It also produces hypertension in patients

Table 2–1. Abnormal Hemodynamics in a Patient After Transplantation with Severe Rejection

	Removal of 300 ml pericardial fluid*				
Time (weeks) after Tx	2	2	12	56	68
RA (mmHg)	22	18	2	1	5
PA ($\overline{PA}$) (mmHg)	46/22 (36)	46/22 (36)	34/28 (24)	32/20 (26)	36/20 (23)
PAW (mmHg)	22	22	14	8	7
BP (MAP) (mmHg)	100/60 (75)	115/80 (95)	140/110 (125)	160/130 (145)	148/102 (128)
Pericardial (mmHg)	6	<0	—	—	—
CI (l/min/m²)	2.0	2.1	3.4	3.1	3.3
Bx histology	Severe rejection	—	Mild rejection	Mild rejection	Moderate rejection

Bx = biopsy, BP = systemic blood pressure, CI = cardiac index, MAP = mean arterial pressure, PA = pulmonary artery pressure, $\overline{PA}$ = mean pulmonary artery pressure, PAW = pulmonary artery wedge pressure, RA = right atrial pressure, Tx = transplantation.

The patient had very abnormal hemodynamics at 2 weeks after transplantation which were felt to be possibly related to delayed tamponade. After 300 ml of pericardial fluid were removed, hemodynamics were essentially unchanged, suggesting severe rejection. Intensive immunosuppressive therapy was immediately begun with resolution of abnormal histology and hemodynamics. Note that with moderate histologic rejection at 68 weeks, hemodynamics were not remarkable. This finding emphasizes that abnormalities in hemodynamics are an infrequent manifestation of rejection and are usually a late finding of severe rejection.

*Applies only to the first 2 columns.

undergoing other types of transplantation[112,113] and in nontransplantation situations as well.[114] The hypertension may become manifest as early as 7 days after beginning the drug.[115]

The hypertension is due at least in part to an elevated peripheral vascular resistance.[21] The mechanism by which an elevation in peripheral vascular resistance is produced is unknown. Bellet and associates[116] have shown that established hypertension is not dependent on activation of the renin-angiotensin system although cyclosporine has been shown to stimulate renin release in vitro.[117] Corcos and colleagues[110] have suggested that hypervolemia is a prominent factor in this form of hypertension, citing early data in experimental transplant studies *not* using cyclosporine for immunosuppression. If hypervolemia were the major mechanism, then hypertension would have been present frequently in patients on azathioprine/prednisone. In fact, hypertension is at least twice as common in cyclosporine- as in azathioprine-treated patients.[118]

It has been suggested that the hypertension is due to cyclosporine's inhibition of vascular endothelial prostacyclin synthesis, leading to arteriolar lesions and hypertension.[119] Additional support for this hypothesis has been provided by the reduction of prostacyclin synthesis factor, a lymphokine, demonstrated in cyclosporine-treated animals.[119] It is clear, however, that the development of cyclosporine nephrotoxicity does not necessarily produce hypertension, as shown in the rat.[120]

The concomitant use of steroids may increase the likelihood of the development of hypertension.[121] An association between cyclosporine-induced hypertension and hypomagnesemia has also been reported.[114] Additionally, hypertension appears to be dose-dependent (Fig. 2–10).[118]

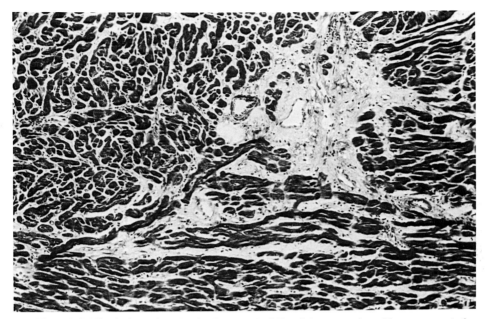

Figure 2–9. Histologic section showing large areas of fibrosis in a transplanted heart removed after 3 years because of poor contractile function. The large areas of fibrosis suggest areas of healed rejection.

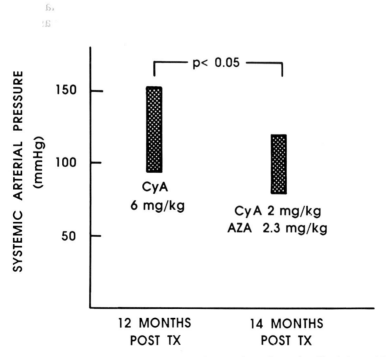

Figure 2–10. The blood pressure response to a decrease in cyclosporine (CyA) dose with addition of azathioprine (AZA) in a group of transplant patients is shown. These data suggest a dose-response relationship to the level of hypertension seen with cyclosporine.

We have recently shown that left ventricular hypertrophy accompanies cyclosporine-induced hypertension.[122] Left ventricular hypertrophy appears to be an independent risk factor for cardiac events.[123] Thus, when considering transplant as a viable life-long procedure, this issue should be considered. Very little has been written on effective therapy. It has been suggested that a multidrug regimen may be required for blood pressure control.[124] On the other hand, regression of left ventricular hypertrophy with good blood pressure control may be effected.[125]

It has been pointed out that patients with post-transplant hypertension do not show a fall in nocturnal blood pressure as encountered in those with essential hypertension.[126] Thus, the summated daily left ventricular afterload may be higher in post-transplant hypertension than in essential hypertension for any daily peak level of blood pressure. What is not known but is worthy of future study is whether nonhypertensive post–cardiac transplant patients show a fall in nocturnal blood pressure. It may be speculated that in the nonhypertensive cardiac transplant patient, particularly those *not* receiving cyclosporine, a decrease in sympathetic nervous system activity at night would decrease peripheral vascular resistance. On the other hand, cyclosporine may fix the level of peripheral resistance, possibly through continued central sympathetic activity. One may then expect blood pressure to remain elevated at night. Empiric observations are required to test this hypothesis. Furthermore, it would be of great interest to determine whether a nocturnal fall in blood pressure occurs in non-cardiac transplant, cyclosporine-treated patients (e.g., renal, bone marrow, or liver transplant patients).

Coronary Artery Disease

The development of coronary artery disease is a major long-term concern in the transplanted heart.[127,128] Surgeons have for some time classified coronary artery disease as a form of chronic rejection, although proof regarding the mechanism has not been forthcoming thus far (Fig. 2–11). The subject of coronary artery disease is covered elsewhere in this book, but it is mentioned here to emphasize that normal physiology can be impaired in at least two ways by this complication, and that coronary artery disease should be considered in the differential diagnosis of dyspnea occurring late after transplantation.

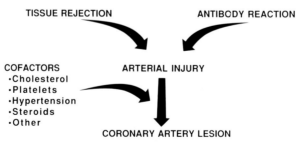

Figure 2–11. A proposed mechanism for the development of coronary artery disease after cardiac transplantation is shown. Vascular injury either secondary to circulating antibodies or tissue-based rejection begins the process. Cofactors that accelerate the injury and repair process may include hypertension, hypercholesterolemia, and steroids. Additionally, platelet interaction with the endothelial wall is probably involved. All of these cofactors and the immunologic process itself provide interventional strategies that may be evaluated to prevent this complication.

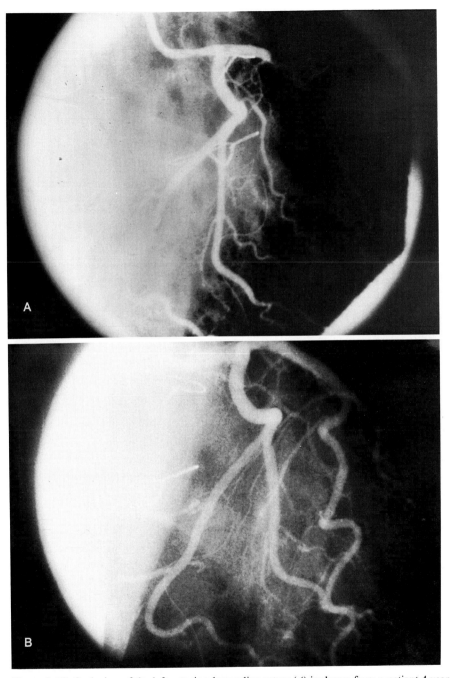

Figure 2–12. Occlusion of the left anterior descending artery (*A*) is shown from a patient 4 years after transplantation who presented with dyspnea (see Table 2–2). Postinfarction clinical status and hemodynamics approximated pretransplant status; the patient died 6 months after infarction. Left coronary arteriography at 3 years after transplantation with normal left anterior descending coronary artery is shown in *B* for comparison.

Table 2–2. Myocardial Infarction in a Patient After Cardiac Transplantation

Year after Tx	Pre-Tx	1	2	3	4 (after MI)
RA (mmHg)	11	4	4	2	16
PA ($\overline{PA}$) (mmHg)	75/38 (50)	26/16 (21)	28/20 (23)	26/14 (19)	60/36 (44)
PAW (mmHg)	35	15	6	36	—
LVEDP (mmHg)	42	20	22	8	36
BP (MAP) (mmHg)	100/68 (75)	184/110 (146)	170/103 (135)	150/100 (120)	140/90 (105)
CI (l/min/m^2)	2.9	2.3	2.3	2.7	1.5
EF (%)	10	59	51	73	17
NYHA Class	IV	I	I	I	IV

Abbreviations are the same as Table 2–1. Other abbreviations include AVO_2 = arteriovenous oxygen difference, EF = ejection fraction, LVEDP = left ventricular end diastolic pressure, MI = myocardial infarction, NYHA = New York Heart Association.

The patient was asymptomatic until 47 months after transplantation at which time he developed an acute anterior wall myocardial infarction. Hemodynamics after MI resembled those seen in patients with severe heart failure pretransplantation. In fact, the patient was dyspneic at rest despite maximal medical therapy and died 6 months after the fourth catheterization from terminal myocardial failure, 52 months after transplantation.

Coronary occlusion producing acute myocardial infarction is one syndrome produced by post-transplant coronary artery disease (Fig. 2–12, Table 2–2). Development of chronic left and right ventricular failure can be a sequel to this problem with hemodynamics mimicking congestive heart failure from other etiologies (Table 2–2). Additionally, acute myocardial ischemia can produce profound hemodynamic abnormalities, which in the denervated cardiac patient will be sensed as dyspnea. Although coronary artery disease is frequently diffuse, we have encountered three patients to date in whom the coronary artery disease was localized enough to perform angioplasty with reversal of symptoms (Fig. 2–13). This procedure in transplant coronary disease has been previously reported with success.[130–132]

Surgical Issues

In the first few years of our transplant program, we observed an occasional patient in the early (less than 6 weeks) period whose hemodynamic deterioration was on the basis of delayed cardiac tamponade, from slow bleeding into the pericardial space (Fig. 2–14). To minimize this complication, at our institution the parietal pericardium is currently left open, and with this approach no episodes of tamponade have occurred (personal communication, Dr. Robert Hardesty). A single case of pericardiectomy for chronic constrictive pericarditis has been reported.[132] With improvements in cardiac preservation, the time between explantation and implantation of the donor heart has increased. At present, the limit is considered to be approximately four hours. Experimental studies have reported viable grafts with longer ischemia times.[133,134] Hemodynamic derangements related to donor ischemia seemed to be limited to short-term problems. Few data exist that associate abnormalities in long-term cardiac function with donor ischemia and preservation if early cardiac viability can be achieved.

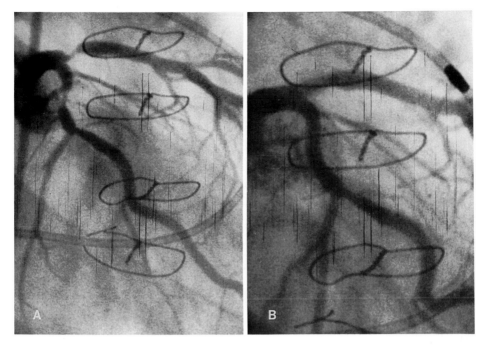

Figure 2–13. This patient had a markedly positive stress thallium study, with exercise-induced anterior lead ST segment depression, dyspnea, hypotension, and a reversible anterior wall thallium defect. Coronary arteriography showed high-grade lesions of the proximal circumflex and anterior descending arteries (*A*), which were successfully treated with angioplasty (*B*).

Dilated Cardiomyopathy

Occasionally, the post-transplant patient will develop a dilated cardiomyopathy not easily explainable by coronary artery disease, rejection, or other process. We have encountered this phenomenon occasionally at our institution (<1 percent). It has been assumed to be related to rejection, and in some cases there has been reasonable histologic evidence. It may be the case in all individuals but sometimes the left ventricular morphology has little evidence to suggest persistent rejection (Fig. 2–15).

Restrictive Cardiomyopathy

Resting hemodynamics in the routine post–cardiac transplant patient suggest that a mild element of chamber restriction occurs in the transplant population compared with a normal group. It has rarely been a clinical problem, however. Humen and coworkers[135] have presented data to suggest restrictive physiology in a few cases but their data suggesting an elevation in right atrial pressure during inspiration are as unconvincing as those of Young and associates.[20] We also have noted restrictive hemodynamics in some patients, which have resolved spontaneously. The etiology of this restrictive pattern is not clear. Karch and Billingham[136] suggested that cyclosporine produced progressive fine interstitial fibrosis, which could explain these hemodynamics. This finding has not been described by others and the amount of fibrosis noted on endomyocardial biopsy

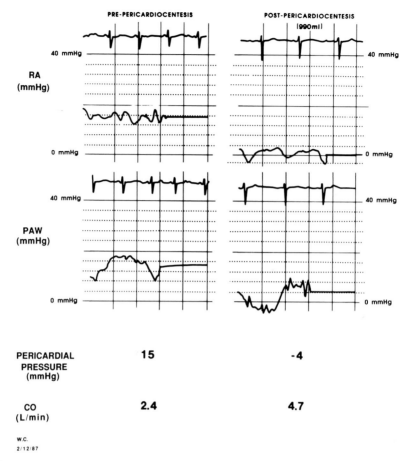

Figure 2-14. Abnormal hemodynamics in the early postoperative period related to delayed tamponade, and resolution with pericardiocentesis are shown. This problem has been minimized by leaving open the parietal pericardium at operation.

in patients with restrictive hemodynamics does not seem to be excessive enough to account for these findings.

Young and associates[20] showed that with rapid saline infusion right atrial and ventricular filling pressures rise rapidly and that a lack of right atrial pressure fall during inspiration suggests restrictive physiology. As in many other aspects of transplant physiology, the lack of normal control subjects makes their conclusion rather tenuous. Although a large amount of data is presently lacking, it may be that very rapid saline infusions in normal adults may cause similar findings (Fig. 2-16). In an early study, Willman and colleagues[14] rapidly infused fluid into a group of autotransplanted dogs and control subjects. Both groups showed a fivefold increase in right atrial pressure. These data suggest that once the elastic limits of filling during diastole occur, a so-called restrictive pattern may be found in innervated as well as transplanted denervated hearts.

It should be added, however, that a few symptomatic cases (<1 percent) of restrictive cardiomyopathy have been noted at our center. These cases are marked hemodynamically by normal systolic function, elevated diastolic ventric-

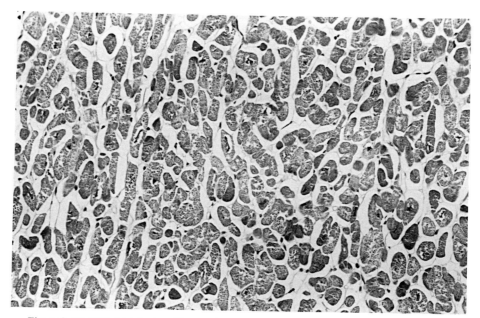

Figure 2–15. Little histologic evidence of persistent rejection or fibrosis was observed at the time of explantation in this patient, in whom a dilated cardiomyopathy developed 1 year after transplantation.

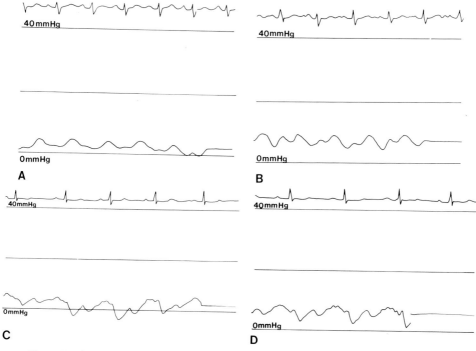

Figure 2–16. The response of right atrial pressure to rapid volume loading (1000 ml of normal saline) in a patient after transplantation (*A* and *B*) and in a normal individual (*C* and *D*). *A* and *C* are pre-saline infusion; *B* and *D*, at the end of infusion. Note a similar response in both patients, with similar increases in right atrial pressure and lack of phasic variation of pressure related to the respiratory cycle with volume loading. The reported restrictive pattern noted in transplant patients with volume loading may represent a universal phenomenon occurring when the elastic limits of the atrium have been reached.

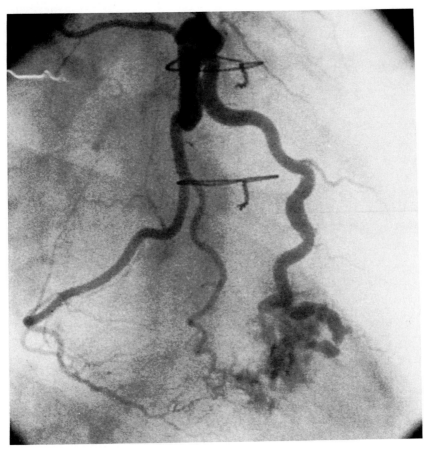

Figure 2-17. A coronary artery fistula of the right coronary artery in a transplant patient 1 year after operation is shown. It is suggested that this finding is a complication of endomyocardial biopsy.

ular pressure greater than one third of systolic pressure, and no evidence of pericardial constriction. The etiology of these cases remains unknown.

Coronary Artery Fistula

We have recently reported an inordinately high incidence (8 percent) of coronary artery fistula in post–cardiac transplant patients (Fig. 2–17). Although the origin of the fistula is distributed among all three coronary arteries, the drainage always goes to the right ventricle, which strongly suggests that the fistula is secondary to right ventricular endomyocardial biopsy. These fistulae tend to be small with minimal hemodynamic abnormalities, although cardiac output appears to be higher in this group compared with a control transplant group without fistula.[137] To date, they have not been associated with hemodynamic deterioration.

ACKNOWLEDGEMENT

I would like to thank Ms. Rhonda Oliver for her diligent efforts in preparing this manuscript. I would also like to thank Ms. Ann Lee for help in data retrieval.

Finally, my gratitude is extended to Mr. William McGowan for his willingness to write about his personal transplant experience.

REFERENCES

1. Mann, FC, Priestley, JT, Markowitz, J, et al: Transplantation of the intact mammalian heart. Arch Surg 26:219, 1933.
2. Dong, E, Jr, Hurley, EJ, Lower, RR, et al: Performance of the heart two years after autotransplantation. Surgery 56:270, 1964.
3. Willman, VL, Cooper, T, Cian, LG, et al: Autotransplantation of the canine heart. Surg Gynecol Obstet 115:299, 1962.
4. Willman, VL, Cooper, T, Cian, LG, et al: Neural responses following autotransplantation of the canine heart. Circulation 27:713, 1963.
5. Donald, DE and Shepherd, JT: Response to exercise in dogs with cardiac denervation. Am J Physiol 205:393, 1963.
6. Cooper, T, Gilbert, JW, Bloodwell, RD, et al: Chronic extrinsic cardiac denervation by regional neural ablation: Description of the operation, verification of the denervation, and its effects on myocardial catecholamines. Circ Res 11:275, 1961.
7. Stinson, EB, Tecklenberg, PL, Hollingsworth, JF, et al: Changes in left ventricular mechanical and hemodynamic function during acute rejection of the orthotopically transplanted heart in dogs. J Thorac Cardiovasc Surg 68:783, 1974.
8. Stinson, EB, Griepp, RB, Dong, E, et al: Results of human heart transplantation at Stanford University. Transplant Proc 3:337, 1971.
9. Dumont, L, Stanley, P, and Chartrand, C: Hemodynamic effects of hypertonic bicarbonate on denervated canine hearts. Heart Transpl 4:247, 1985.
10. Noble, MIM, Stubbs, J, Trenchard, D, et al: Left ventricular performance in the conscious dog with chronically denervated heart. Cardiovasc Res 6:457, 1972.
11. Donald, DE and Shepherd, JT: Sustained capacity for exercise in dogs after complete cardiac denervation. Am J Cardiol 14:853, 1964.
12. Willman, VL, Jellinek, M, Cooper, T, et al: Metabolism of the transplanted heart: Effect of excision and reimplantation on myocardial glycogen, hexokinase, and acetylcholine esterase. Surgery 56:266, 1964.
13. Daggett, WM, Willman, VL, Cooper, T, et al: Work capacity and efficiency of the autotransplanted heart. Circulation 35, 36 (Suppl I): 96, 1967.
13. Jellinek, M, Kaye, MP, Nigh, CA, et al: Alterations in chemical composition of canine heart after sympathetic denervation. Am J Physiol 206:971, 1964.
14. Willman, VL, Jerjavy, JP, Pennell, R, et al: Response of the autotransplanted heart to blood volume expansion. Ann Surg 166:513, 1967.
15. Dong, E, Jr, Angell, WW, Persson, LK, et al: Effect of cardiac transplantation on the homeostasis of blood volume. Circulation 35, 36 (Suppl II): 98, 1967.
16. Parent, R, Stanley, P, and Chartrand, C: Long-term daily study of blood volume in cardiac autotransplanted dogs. Eur Surg Res 19:193, 1987.
17. Gilmore, JP and Daggett, WM: Response of the chronic cardiac denervated dog to acute volume expansion. Am J Physiol 210:509, 1966.
18. Myers, BD, Peterson, C, Molina, C, et al: Role of cardiac atria in the human renal response to changing plasma volume. Am J Physiol 254 (Renal Fluid Electrolyte Physiol 23):F562, 1988.
19. Cooper, T, Willman, VL, Jellinek, M, et al: Heart transplantation: Effect on myocardial catecholamine and histamine. Science 138:40, 1962.
20. Young, JB, Leon, CA, Short, HD, et al: Evolution of hemodynamics after orthotopic heart and heart-lung transplantation: Early restrictive patterns persisting in occult fashion. J Heart Transplant 6:34, 1987.
21. Greenberg, M, Uretsky, BF, Reddy, PS, et al: Long-term hemodynamic follow-up of cardiac transplant patients treated with cyclosporine and prednisone. Circulation 71:487, 1985.
22. Stinson, EB, Caves, PK, Griepp, RB, et al: Hemodynamic observation in the early period after human heart transplantation. J Thorac Cardiovasc Surg 69:264, 1975.
23. Bhatia, SJS, Kirschenbaum, JM, Shemin, RJ, et al: Time course of resolution of pulmonary hypertension and right ventricular remodeling after orthotopic cardiac transplantation. Circulation 76:819, 1987.

24. Shaver, JR, Leon, DF, Gray, S, et al: Hemodynamic observations after cardiac transplantation. N Engl J Med 281:822, 1969.
25. Hallman, GL, Leatherman, LL, Leachman, RD, et al: Function of the transplanted human heart. J Thorac Cardiovasc Surg 58:318, 1969.
26. Carleton, RA, Heller, SJ, Najafi, H, et al: Hemodynamic performance of a transplanted human heart. Circulation 40:447, 1969.
27. Campeau, L, Pospisil, L, Grondin, P, et al: Cardiac catheterization findings at rest and after exercise in patients following cardiac transplantation. Am J Cardiol 25:523, 1970.
28. Stinson, EB, Griepp, RB, Schroeder, JS, et al: Hemodynamic observations one and two years after cardiac transplantation in man. Circulation 45:1183, 1972.
29. Pope, SE, Stinson, EB, Daughters, GT, II, et al: Exercise response of the denervated heart in long-term cardiac transplant recipients. Am J Cardiol 46:213, 1980.
30. Gaudiani, VA, Stinson, EB, Alderman, E, et al: Long-term survival and function after cardiac transplantation. Ann Surg 194:381, 1981.
31. Uretsky, BF, Bernardi, L, Greenberg, ML, et al: Diastolic dysfunction in long-term survivors of cardiac transplant. Circulation 70 (Suppl II):46, 1984.
32. Frist, W, Stinson, E, Oyer, P, et al: Long-term hemodynamic results after cardiac transplantation. J Thorac Cardiovasc Surg 94:685, 1987.
33. Murali, S, Uretsky, BF, Reddy, PS, et al: Hemodynamic abnormalities following cardiac transplantation in relationship to hypertension and survival. Am Heart J (in press).
34. Verani, M, George, SE, Leon, CA, et al: Systolic and diastolic ventricular performance at rest and during exercise in heart transplant recipients. J Heart Transplant 7:145, 1988.
35. Stinson, EB, Schroeder, JS, Griepp, RB, et al: Observations on the behavior of recipient atria after cardiac transplantation in man. Am J Cardiol 30:615, 1972.
36. Valantine, H, Appleton, C, Hatle, L, et al: Influence of recipient atrial contraction on left ventricular filling dynamics of the transplanted heart assessed by Doppler echocardiography. Am J Cardiol 59:1159, 1987.
37. Borow, KM, Neuman, A, Arensman, FW, et al: Left ventricular contractility and contractile reserve in humans after cardiac transplantation. Circulation 71:866, 1985.
38. Bernardi, L, Uretsky, BF, Reddy, PS, et al: Modeling the isovolumic relaxation period. Cath Cardiovasc Diagn 11:255, 1985.
39. Jose, A: Effect of combined sympathetic and parasympathetic blockade on heart rate and cardiac function in man. Am J Cardiol 18:476, 1966.
40. Thames, MD, Kontos, HA, and Lower, RR: Sinus arrhythmia in dogs after cardiac transplantation. Am J Cardiol 24:54, 1969.
41. Kavanaugh, T, Yacoub, M, Mertens, D, et al: Cardiorespiratory responses to exercise training after orthotopic cardiac transplantation. Circulation 77:162, 1988.
42. Alexopoulos, D, Yusuf, S, Johnston, JA, et al: The 24 hour heart rate behavior in long-term survivors of cardiac transplantation. Am J Cardiol 61:880, 1988.
43. Cannon, WB, Lewis, JT, and Britton, SW: A lasting preparation of the denervated heart for detecting internal secretion, with evidence from accesory accelerator fibers from the thoracic sympathetic chain. Am J Physiol 77:326, 1926.
44. Pflugfelder, PW, Purves, PD, McKenzie, FN, et al: Cardiac dynamics during supine exercise in cyclosporine-treated orthotopic heart transplant recipients: Assessment by radionuclide angiography. J Am Coll Cardiol 10:336, 1987.
45. Willman, VL, Cooper, T, and Hanlon, CR: Return of neural responses after autotransplantation of the heart. Am J Physiol 207:187, 1964.
46. Reitz, BA, Dong, E, and Stinson, EB: The Bainbridge reflex in canine cardiac autotransplants. Circulation 43/44 (Suppl I):136, 1971.
47. Donald, DE and Shepherd, JT: Changes in heart rate on intravenous infusion in dogs with chronic cardiac denervation. Proc Soc Exp Biol Med 113:315, 1963.
48. Donald, DE, Ferguson, DA, and Milburn, SE: Effect of beta adrenergic blockade on racing performance of greyhounds with normal and with denervated hearts. Circ Res 22:127, 1968.
49. Thomas, JA and Marks, BH: Plasma norepinephrine in congestive heart failure. Am J Cardiol 41:223, 1965.
50. Cannom, DS, Rider, AK, Stinson, EB, et al: Electrophysiologic studies in the denervated transplanted human heart. Am J Cardiol 36:859, 1975.
51. Brengelmann, GL: Circulatory adjustments to exercise and heat stress. Ann Rev Physiol 45:191, 1983.

52. Clark, DA, Schroeder, JS, Griepp, RB, et al: Cardiac transplantation in man. Am J Med 54:563, 1973.

53. Savin, WM, Alderman, EL, Haskell, WL, et al: Left ventricular response to isometric exercise in patients with denervated and innervated hearts. Circulation 61:897, 1980.

54. Donald, DE, Milburn, SE, and Shepherd, JT: Effect of cardiac denervation on the maximal capacity for exercise in the racing greyhound. J Appl Physiol 19:849, 1964.

55. Savin, WM, Haskell, WL, Schroeder, JS, et al: Cardiorespiratory responses of cardiac transplant patients to graded symptom-limited exercise. Circulation 61:897, 1980.

56. Bexton, RS, Milne, JR, Cory-Pearce, R, et al: Effect of beta blockade on exercise response after cardiac transplantation. Br Heart J 49:584, 1983.

57. McLaughlin, PR, Leiman, JH, Martin, RP, et al: The effect of exercise and atrial pacing on left ventricular volume and contractility in patients with innervated and denervated hearts. Circulation 61:897, 1980.

58. Yusuf, S, Theodoropoulos, S, Dhalia, N, et al: Effect of beta blockade on dynamic exercise in human heart transplant recipients. Heart Transplant 4:312, 1985.

59. Pearson, SB, Banks, DC, and Patrick, JM: The effect of beta-adrenoceptor blockade on factors affecting exercise in normal man. Br J Clin Pharmacol 8:143, 1979.

60. Epstein, SE, Robinson, BF, Kahler, RL, et al: Effects of beta-adrenergic blockade on the cardiac response to maximal and submaximal exercise in man. J Clin Invest 44:1745, 1965.

61. Mohanty, PK, Thomas, MD, Arrowood, JA, et al: Impairment of cardiopulmonary baroreflex after cardiac transplantation in humans. Circulation 75:914, 1987.

62. Schuler, S, Thomas, D, Thebken, M, et al: Endocrine response to exercise in cardiac transplant patients. Transplant Proc 19:2506, 1987.

63. Greenfield, LJ, Ebert, PA, Austen, WG, et al: The effect of total cardiac denervation on the cardiovascular responses to hypothermia and acute hemorrhage. Surgery 51:356, 1961.

64. Greenfield, LJ and Ebert, PA: Cardiac denervation effect in hypoxia and hypercapnia: Effect of total denervation on cardiovascular responses. Arch surg 87:29, 1963.

65. Tsakiris, AG, Donald, DE, Rutishauer, WJ, et al: Cardiovascular responses to hypertension and hypotension in dogs with denervated hearts. J Appl Physiol 27:817, 1969.

66. Donald, DE: Myocardial performance after excision of the extrinsic cardiac nerves in the dog. Circ Res 34:417, 1974.

67. Kontos, HA, Thames, MD, and Lower, RR: Responses to electrical and reflex autonomic stimulation in dogs with cardiac transplantation before and after reinnervation. J Thorac Cardiovasc Surg 59:382, 1970.

68. Cannom, DS, Graham, AF, and Harrison, DC: Electrophysiological studies in the denervated transplanted human heart. Circ Res 32:268, 1973.

69. Bexton, RS, Nathan, AW, Hellestrand, JK, et al: Sinoatrial function after cardiac transplantation. J Am Coll Cardiol 3:712, 1984.

70. Mackintosh, AF, Carmichael, DJ, Wren, C, et al: Sinus node function in first three weeks after cardiac transplantaton. Br Heart J 48:584, 1982.

71. Bexton, RS, Nathan, AW, Hellestrand, KJ, et al: Electrophysiological abnormalities in the transplanted human heart. Br Heart J 50:555, 1983.

72. Tuna, I, Barragry, T, Walker, M, et al: Effects of transplantation on atrioventricular nodal accommodation and hysteresis. Am J Physiol 87:1514, 1988.

73. Narula, OS and Runge, M: Accommodation of A-V nodal conduction and fatigue phenomenon in the His-Purkinje system. In Wellens, HJJ, Lie, KI, and Janse, MJ (eds): The Conduction System of the Heart: Structure, Function and Clinical Implications. Lea and Febiger, Philadelphia, 1976, pp 529–544.

74. Dempsey, PJ and Cooper, T: Supersensitivity of the chronically denervated feline heart. Am J Physiol 215:1245, 1968.

75. Lurie, K, Bristow, MR, Sageman, WS, et al: Increased β-adrenergic receptor density in cardiac transplants. Circulation 66 (Suppl II):72, 1982.

76. Lurie, KG, Bristow, MR, and Reitz, BA: Increased beta adrenergic receptor density in an experimental model of cardiac transplantation. J Thorac Cardiovasc Surg 86:195, 1983.

77. Donald, DE and Shepherd, JT: Supersensitivity to l-norepinephrine of the denervated sinoatrial node. Am J Physiol 208:255, 1965.

78. Ebert, PA: The effects of norepinephrine infusion on the denervated heart. Cardiovasc Surg 29:414, 1968.

79. Schaal, SF, Wallace, AG, and Sealy, WC: Protective influence of cardiac denervation against arrhythmias of myocardial infarction. Cardiovasc Res 3:241, 1969.

80. Mason, JW, Stinson, EB, and Harrison, DC: Autonomic nervous system and arrhythmias: Studies in the transplanted denervated human heart. Cardiology 61:75, 1967.
81. Alexopoulos, D, Yusuf, S, Bostock, J, et al: Ventricular arrhythmias in long term survivors of orthotopic and heterotopic heart transplantation. Br Heart J 59:648, 1988.
82. Goodman, DJ, Rossen, RM, Cannom, DS, et al: Effect of digoxin on atrioventricular conduction: Studies in patients with and without cardiac autonomic innervation. Circulation 51:251, 1975.
83. Leachman, RD, Cokkinos, DV, Cabrera, R, et al: Response of the transplanted, denervated human heart to cardiovascular drugs. Am J Cardiol 27:272, 1977.
84. Mason, JW, Winkle, RA, Rider, AK, et al: The electrophysiologic effects of quinidine in the transplanted human heart. J Clin Invest 59:481, 1977.
85. Bexton, RS, Hellestrand, KJ, Cory-Pearce, R, et al: The direct electrophysiologic effects of disopyramide phosphate in the transplanted human heart. Circulation 67:38, 1983.
86. Stemple, DR, Hall, RJC, Mason, JW, et al: Electrophysiological effects of edrophonium in the innervated and the transplanted denervated human heart. Br Heart J 40:644, 1978.
87. Bexton, RS, Cory-Pearce, R, Spurrell, RAJ, et al: Electrophysiological effects of nifedipine and verapamil in the transplanted human heart. Heart Transplant 3:97, 1984.
88. Gregg, DE, Khouri, EM, Donald, DE, et al: Coronary circulation in the conscious dog with cardiac neural ablation. Circ Res 31:129, 1972.
89. Nitenberg, A, Tavolaro, O, Loisance, D, et al: Dynamic evaluation of the coronary circulation in human orthotopic heart transplants. Transplant Proc 19:3772, 1987.
90. Lang, RE, Thalkenlt, Ganten, D, et al: Atrial natriuretic factor—a circulating hormone stimulated by volume loading. Nature 314:264, 1985.
91. Petterson, A, Hedner, J, Rieksten, SE, et al: Acute volume expansion as a physiologic stimulus for the release of atrial natriuretic peptides in the rat. Life Sci 38:1127, 1986.
92. Yamaji, T, Ishibashi, M, and Takaku, F: Atrial natriuretic factor in human blood. J Clin Invest 76:1705, 1985.
93. Anderson, JV, Millar, ND, O'Hare, JP, et al: Atrial natriuretic peptide: Physiologic release associated with natriuresis during water immersion in man. Clin Sci 71:319, 1986.
94. Richards, AM, Ikram, H, Yandle, TG, et al: Renal, hemodynamic, and hormonal effects of human alpha atrial natriuretic peptide in healthy volunteers. Lancet 1:545, 1985.
95. Biollaz, J, Nussberger, J, Porchet, M, et al: Four-hour infusion of synthetic atrial natriuretic peptide in normal volunteers. Hypertension 8 [Suppl]:II96, 1986.
96. Zimmerman, RS, Schirger, JA, Edwards, BS, et al: Cardiac-renal endocrine dynamics during stepwise infusion of physiologic and pharmacologic concentrations of atrial natriuretic factor in the dog. Circ Res 60:63, 1987.
97. Uretsky, BF, Murali, S, Valdes, AM, et al: Hypertension post-cardiac transplantation: Is atrial natriuretic peptide deficiency a factor in its development? J Am Coll Cardiol 9:241A, 1987.
98. Magovern, JA, Pennock, JL, Oaks, TE, et al: Atrial natriuretic peptide in recipients of human orthotopic heart transplants. J Heart Transplant 6:193, 1988.
99. Singer, DRJ, Buckley, MG, MacGregor, GA, et al: Increased concentrations of plasma atrial natriuretic peptides in cardiac transplant recipients. Br Med J 292:1391, 1986.
100. Day, ML, Schwartz, D, Weigard, RC, et al: Ventricular atriopeptin. Hypertension 9:485, 1987.
101. Griepp, RB, Stinson, EB, Dong, E, et al: Determinants of operative risk in human heart transplantation. Am J Surg 122:192, 1971.
102. Grover, RF, Vogel, JH, Averill, KH, et al: Pulmonary hypertension: Individual and species variability relative to vascular reactivity. Am Heart J 66:1, 1963.
103. Villanueva, FS, Murali, S, Uretsky, BF, et al: Resolution of pulmonary hypertension after cardiac transplantation: Comparison of orthotopic and heterotopic transplant. Circulation 78 (Suppl II):II-279, 1988.
104. Barnard, CN and Losman, JG: Left ventricular bypass. S Afr Med J 49:303, 1975.
105. Barnard, CN and Cooper, DKC: Heterotopic versus orthotopic heart transplantation. Transplant Proc 14:886, 1984.
106. Losman, JG and Barnard, CN: Heterotopic heart transplantation, a valid alternative to orthotopic transplantation: Results, advantages, and disadvantages. J Surg Res 32:297, 1982.
107. Beck, W and Gersh, BJ: Left ventricular bypass using a cardiac allograft: Hemodynamic studies. Am J Cardiol 37:1007, 1976.
108. Melvin, KR, Pollock, C, Hunt, SA, et al: Cardiovascular physiology in a case of heterotopic cardiac transplantation. Am J Cardiol 49:1301, 1982.

109. Murali, S, Reddy, PS, Armitage, JM, for the Heart Failure Study Group: The effect of prostaglandin E-1 on the transpulmonary gradient of heart transplant candidates. Circulation 78 (Suppl II):II-280, 1988.

110. Corcos, T, Tamburino, C, Leger, P, et al: Early and late hemodynamic evaluation after cardiac transplantation: A study of 28 cases. J Am Coll Cardiol 11:264, 1988.

111. Thompson, ME, Shapiro, AP, Johnsen, AM, et al: New onset of hypertension following cardiac transplantation: A preliminary report and analysis. Transplant Proc 15 (Suppl I):2573, 1983.

112. Barrett, AJ, Kendra, JR, Lucas, CF, et al: Cyclosporin A as prophylaxis against graft-versus-host disease in 36 patients. Br Med J 285:162, 1982.

113. Kahan, BD, Flechner, SM, Lorber, MI, et al: Complications of cyclosporine-prednisone immunosuppression in 402 renal allograft recipients exclusively followed at a single center from one to five years. Transplantation 43:197, 1987.

114. Palestine, AG, Nussenblatt, RB, and Chan, C: Side effects of systemic cyclosporine in patients not undergoing transplantation. Am J Med 77:652, 1984.

115. June, C, Thompson, C, Kennedy, M, et al: Correlation of hypomagnesemia with the onset of cyclosporine-associated hypertension in marrow transplant patients. Transplantation 41:47, 1986.

116. Bellet, M, Cabrol, C, Sassano, P, et al: Systemic hypertension after cardiac transplantation: Effect of cyclosporine on the renin-angiotensin-aldosterone system. Am J Cardiol 56:927, 1985.

117. Baxter, CR, Duggin, GG, Hall, BM, et al: Stimulation of renin release from rat renal cortical slices by cyclosporine A. Res Commun Chem Pathol Pharmacol 43:417, 1984.

118. Jarowenko, M, Flechner, S, Van Buren, C, et al: Influence of cyclosporine on post-transplant blood pressure response. Am J Kidney Dis 10:98, 1987.

119. Neild, GH, Rocchi, G, and Imberti, L: Effect of cyclosporine on prostacyclin synthesis by vascular tissue in rabbits. Transplant Proc 14:2398, 1985.

120. Kanchira, A, Shida, T, Nakamura, H, et al: Cyclosporine related hypertension and nephrotoxicity in rat heart transplantation. In Tanabe T, Hoak B, Endou, H (eds): Nephrotoxicity of Antibiotics and Immunosuppressants. Elsevier Science Publishers, 1986, pp 141–147.

121. Loughran, TP, Jr, Deeg, HJ, Dahlberg, MS, et al: Incidence of hypertension after marrow transplantation among 112 patients randomized to either cyclosporine or methotrexate as graft-versus-host disease prophylaxis. Br J Haematol 59:547, 1985.

122. McKoy, RC, Uretsky, BF, Kormos, R, et al: Left ventricular hypertrophy in cyclosporine induced systemic hypertension after cardiac transplantation. Am J Cardiol (in press).

123. Kannel, WB: Prevalance and natural history of electrocardiographic left ventricular hypertrophy. Am J Med 75 (Suppl 3):4, 1983.

124. Olivari, M-T, Antolick, A, and Ring, WS: Arterial hypertension after cardiac transplant with triple-drug immunosuppression therapy. J Am Coll Cardiol 11:150A, 1988.

125. Angermann, CE, Spes, CH, Hart, RJ, et al: Regression of ventricular hypertrophy in cardiac transplant recipients under effective antihypertensive therapy. J Am Coll Cardiol 11:151A, 1988.

126. Reeves, RA, Shapiro, AP, Thompson, ME, et al: Loss of nocturnal decline in blood pressure after cardiac transplantation. Circulation 73:401, 1986.

127. Hess, ML, Hastillo, A, Mohanakimar, T, et al: Accelerated atherosclerosis in cardiac transplantation: Role of cytotoxic B-cell antibodies and hyperlipidemia. Circulation 68 (Suppl II):II-94, 1983.

128. Uretsky, BF, Murali, S, Reddy, PS, et al: Development of coronary artery disease in cardiac transplant patients receiving immunosuppressive therapy with cyclosporine and prednisone. Circulation 76:827, 1987.

129. Hastillo, A, Cowley, MJ, Vetrovec, G, et al: Serial coronary angioplasty for atherosclerosis following heart transplantation. Heart Transplant 4:192, 1985.

130. Wohlgelernter, D, Stevenson, LW, and Brunbei, R: Reversal of ischemic myocardial dysfunction by PTCA in a cardiac transplant patient. Am Heart J 11:837, 1986.

131. Gammage, MD, Shis, MF, and English, TAH: Percutaneous coronary angioplasty in a cardiac transplant patient. Br Heart J 559:253, 1988.

132. Copeland, JG, Riley, JE, and Fuller, J: Pericardiectomy for effusive constrictive pericarditis after heart transplantation. J Heart Transplant 5:171, 1986.

133. Solis, E, Tago, M, and Kaye, MP: Cardiac function following prolonged preservation and orthotopic transplantation. J Heart Transplant 4:357, 1985.

134. Wicomb, WN, Rose, AG, Cooper, DKC, et al: Hemodynamic and myocardial histologic and

ultra structural studies on baboons from 3 to 27 months following autotransplantation of hearts stored by hypothermic perfusion for 24 or 48 hours. J Heart Transplant 5:122, 1986.

135. Humen, DP, McKenzie, FN, and Kostuk, WJ: Restricted myocardial compliance one year following cardiac transplantation. J Heart Transplant 3:341, 1984.

136. Karch, SB and Billingham ME: Cyclosporine induced myocardial fibrosis: A unique controlled case report. J Heart Transplant 4:210, 1985.

137. Sandhu, JS, Uretsky, BF, Zerbe, TR, et al: Coronary artery fistula in heart transplant patients: A potential complication of endomyocardial biopsy. Circulation 68 (Suppl II):II-253, 1989.

CHAPTER 3

Physiology of the Lung in Human Heart-Lung Transplantation*

James Theodore, M.D.

Since its successful clinical introduction in 1981,[1] combined heart-lung transplantation in humans has also served as a unique model for defining the physiology of the transplanted lung and respiratory system. Providing that no significant complications arise, it has become quite evident that the transplanted heart and lungs function sufficiently well to support the activities of normal life, despite cardiopulmonary denervation, the disruption of the pulmonary lymphatic and bronchial arterial systems, and transient ischemia of the allografts at the time of surgery. Long-term pulmonary function appears to be well preserved in the transplanted lung with the maintenance of essentially normal gas exchange for extended periods of time, which is now measurable in years. In general, the overall function of the respiratory system does not appear to be adversely affected by the extensive nature of combined heart-lung transplantation.[2-4]

Understanding the function of the uncomplicated transplanted lung is required for the proper management of patients with heart-lung, double lung, or unilateral single lung transplants. Such understanding is necessary for the early recognition of altered functions that are produced by disease and separate from alterations that are associated with the transplant process.

Although the physiology of the transplanted lung to be presented in this chapter is based primarily on studies performed on the human heart-lung transplant model, in general, most observations made on this model should be applicable to the lung function of single or double lung transplants, which do not include the heart.

*Supported by Program Project Grant HL13108 from the National Heart, Lung, and Blood Institute.

PULMONARY FUNCTION FOLLOWING HEART-LUNG TRANSPLANTATION

Volumes and Pulmonary Statics

The most significant alteration of pulmonary function that arises following heart-lung transplantation is the development of a mild to moderate restrictive ventilatory defect. This development is associated with significant reductions in all lung volumes, as compared with predicted normal values, with the exception of residual volume (RV) and functional residual capacity (FRC), which remain essentially normal.[2]

The reduction in volumes appears to be related primarily to a decrease in inspiratory capacity (IC) as a result of alterations of the chest wall produced at surgery. Under these conditions, determinations of the pressure-volume characteristics of the lung have indicated that the elastic properties of the transplanted lung are normal.[5] The reductions in total lung capacity (TLC) that are present correlate highly with reductions in maximum inspiratory pressure and transpulmonary pressure. These findings implicate chest wall factors as the source of the restrictive defect. In particular, they suggest reductions in the generation of inspiratory forces that could result from a variety of causes including postsurgical mechanical factors, alterations of length-tension relationships of the respiratory muscles due to geometric alterations of the chest wall, or muscular weakness per se, among others.[5]

Pulmonary Dynamics

Pulmonary dynamic function is essentially normal in the transplanted lung, although flow rates tend to be more variable than that ordinarily expected.

There are significant reductions in those variables, which are directly related to the reduction in vital capacity (i.e., forced vital capacity [FVC], forced expiratory volume in 1 second [FEV_1], and forced expiratory volume in 3 seconds [FEV_3]) and in those that are highly effort-dependent (peak expiratory flow rate [PEFR] and maximum expiratory flow rate [MEFR]). On the other hand, the FEV_1/FVC percent and FEV_3/FVC percent are usually increased in the early post-transplant period and are findings that are frequently present with restrictive defects.[2]

Effort-independent flow parameters that are volume related or volume corrected are usually normal. Any reductions in the effort-independent flow rates (i.e., forced expiratory flow between 25 percent and 75 percent of the FVC [FEF_{25-75}] and forced expiratory flow at 50 percent of the FVC [FEF_{50}]) can usually be directly related to decreased volumes. In this setting, if the FEF_{50} is expressed per FVC (i.e., FEF_{50}/FVC) to take into account the effects of the reduced FVC on this flow parameter,[6] flow is normal.[2] Measurements of airway resistance and specific airway conductance are also normal in the transplanted lung.[2]

Thus, although a number of patients showed reduced flow rates following heart-lung transplantation, these reductions in flow could be attributed to the reduced lung volumes without clearcut evidence of intrinsic airway obstruction in the uncomplicated lung.

The early recognition of discordant decreases in flow rates, which are not completely accounted for by reductions in volume, is imperative because this may be the first indication of obstructive airway disease. The most sensitive parameter in this respect is a decrease in the FEF_{25-75}. The early detection of obstructive airway disease is important because it may represent the first manifestation of obliterative bronchiolitis, the major complication of the long-term transplanted lung.[3,7,8]

The maximal voluntary ventilation (MVV) is well preserved following transplantation, with no significant differences found between pretransplant and post-transplant values for MVV. This finding clearly indicates that the ventilatory capacity of the respiratory system is not significantly altered as a result of transplantation. The MVV, usually found after transplant, reflects a ventilatory capacity that is more than adequate for meeting the ventilatory requirements of exercise.[2,4]

Distribution of Ventilation, Diffusing Capacity, and Arterial Blood Gases

In terms of standard measurements of pulmonary function at rest, gas exchange in the transplanted lung remains normal in the uncomplicated state. In this context, the distribution of ventilation within the lung, and the lung diffusing capacity for carbon monoxide (DCO) are also normal. In the early post-transplant period (i.e., within 3 months), DCO tends to be reduced toward borderline low-normal values, primarily as a result of low hemoglobin concentrations that are frequently present. DCO improves toward more normal values with the passage of time.[2]

The arterial blood gases confirm the ability of the transplanted lungs to sustain normal gas exchange. This is shown in Table 3–1, which contains serial pulmonary function data obtained over a 3-year period. The mean arterial Pao_2

Table 3–1. Pulmonary Function in Uncomplicated Heart-Lung Transplant Recipients*

Variable	Postop (n = 10)	First Annual Review (n = 9)	Second Annual Review (n = 6)	Third Annual Review (n = 4)
FVC	63·8 (17·1)	69·6 (14·3)	70·7 (10·0)	65·5 (13·5)
FEV_1	72·9 (17·8)	76·4 (15·3)	76·7 (7·4)	71·3 (13·6)
FEV_1/FVC(%)	88·2 (8·4)	87·7 (8·4)	84·7 (8·5)	84·0 (3·7)
FEF_{25-75}	83·9 (42·8)	84·2 (37·9)	88·7 (50·9)	74·0 (11·0)
FRC	85·7 (15·4)	79·9 (14·0)	81·2 (16·2)	66·8 (17·3)
TLC	73·3 (17·1)	75·0 (11·7)	79·3 (6·9)	71·0 (11·6)
sGAW	0·18 (0·07)	0·18 (8·05)	0·18 (0·08)	0·33 (0·19)
	n = 7	n = 7	n = 5	
DLCO	76·9 (25·5)	81·6 (20·2)	92·2 (12·8)	101·8 (6·4)
	n = 9	n = 8	n = 5	
Pao_2 (mmHg)	88·9 (7·8)	90·6 (7·6)	92·8 (6·6)	88·0 (7·0)
	n = 9	n = 8	n = 6	
$Paco_2$ (mmHg)	34·2 (3·5)	36·3 (2·6)	36·0 (2·1)	34·3 (3·0)
	n = 9	n = 8	n = 6	

*Results are means and standard deviations.
    FVC = forced vital capacity (% predicted); FEV_1 = forced expiratory vol, 1 s (% predicted); FEF = expiratory flow between 25% and 75% of FVC; FRC = functional residual capacity; TLC = total lung capacity; sGAW = specific airway conductance (normal range 0·112–0·4 l/s per cm H_2O per l); DLCO = CO diffusion capacity (% predicted).
    From Burke et al.,[3] with permission.

ranges between 88.0 and 92.8 torr, which are essentially normal values, over the period of time shown. Although the arterial Pa_{CO_2} findings indicate that mild alveolar hyperventilation is present, the calculated alveolar-arterial O_2 difference is within the normal range.[2,3]

Long-Term Pulmonary Function

Serial pulmonary function measurements from ten long-term survivors with heart-lung transplants, who remained free of complications and returned to normal life, are summarized in Table 3–1. The functional indices were obtained in the immediate post-transplant period and at yearly intervals up to the third annual review postoperatively. The mean postoperative period for the group is 22.6 months, with a range of 4 to 42 months. In the nine, six, and four patients studied at 1, 2, and 3 years, respectively, the functional indices are well preserved with time, and the values within the various time frames are not significantly different. The restrictive ventilatory defect (as judged by a TLC of less than 80 percent of predicted) present in the early postoperative period persists but shows no evidence of progression. All the other functional parameters remain essentially normal. These results demonstrate that the transplanted lung is capable of maintaining essentially normal function over a long period of time, provided that it remains free of complications.

DYNAMIC FUNCTIONS AT REST AND EXERCISE FOLLOWING HEART-LUNG TRANSPLANTATION

Post-transplant studies performed under dynamic conditions of exercise provide a more rigorous assessment of function than is possible from standard measurements of pulmonary function alone. Integrated functions of the heart and lungs can be maximally stressed under conditions of maximum exercise, which can be used to define any limitations that may exist.

Functional parameters assessing gas exchange, ventilation, and circulatory capacity were determined in 16 heart-lung–transplanted patients at rest and during increasing levels of constant work-rate treadmill exercise to tolerance. The results of these measurements obtained during rest and maximum exercise are summarized in the following sections and serve as the main source of the discussion here. In brief, as a preview, the transplanted lungs, together with the respiratory system, respond appropriately to the demands of increasing levels of exercise despite denervation of the cardiopulmonary axis. At maximum exercise, pulmonary gas exchange and ventilation are normal, and the limiting factors during exercise are not pulmonary, but circulatory in nature.[4] These are discussed in greater detail in the next sections.

Arterial Blood Gases

Post-transplant blood gas levels, obtained within 8 weeks of transplantation, showed normal oxygenation of arterial blood during both rest and exercise, with the maintenance of a mean arterial Pa_{O_2} of 98.9 ± 1.8 torr (mean $\pm$ SE) at maximum exercise with an A-a O_2 difference of 18.3 ± 1.7 torr. This was in marked contrast to pretransplant blood gas values in the same group of patients, which showed severe hypoxemia at rest (Pa_{O_2}:59.1 ± 5.4 torr) with an increased A-a O_2 difference of 53.8 ± 5.6 torr, and which became significantly worse during exercise.

Alveolar hyperventilation, as reflected by a reduction in arterial Pa_{CO_2}, which was present pretransplant persisted post-transplant with a Pa_{CO_2} of 32.1 ± 0.9 torr. Pa_{CO_2} at maximum exercise was slightly less and not significantly different than the resting value.[4]

Composition of the arterial blood gases during maximum exercise can be used as an index for determining the efficiency of pulmonary gas exchange. Under these conditions, the transplanted lungs are capable of essentially normal gas exchange. This finding would indicate that the integrating function required for matching ventilation and perfusion (i.e., maintenance of proper $\dot{V}/\dot{Q}$ relations) is intrapulmonary and autoregulatory in nature, and that an external nerve supply is not a crucial requirement for regulating gas exchange within the lung.

Ventilation

Post-transplant resting ventilation was mildly to moderately increased with increases in minute ventilation ($\dot{V}_E$), alveolar ventilation, dead space ventilation (VD/VT) and the ventilatory equivalents for CO_2 and O_2.

Minute ventilation ($\dot{V}_E$) increased appropriately with increasing levels of exercise. At maximum exercise, the ventilatory equivalents for CO_2 and O_2 were not significantly different from those values obtained at rest, despite being somewhat less, and closer to the expected normal values. VD/VT fell in the expected normal manner with increasing exercise. The rise in post-transplant $\dot{V}_E$ with maximum exercise over resting $\dot{V}_E$ was appropriate for the oxygen consumed and the increased work performed. This finding was in contrast with pretransplant responses in these same patients who had pulmonary hypertension (primary or congenital heart disease with Eisenmenger's physiology) prior to transplant. Before the transplant, the rise in $\dot{V}_E$ with exercise was excessive with respect to the oxygen consumed and the work performed. The post-transplant $\dot{V}_{E/MVV}$ ratio (i.e., $\dot{V}_{E/maximum\ voluntary\ ventilation}$) was 0.34 ± 0.04 (SE) during maximum exercise, which is well below the upper limit of 0.7, indicating that a substantial ventilatory reserve still remained.

The control of ventilation during exercise is also normal in heart-lung transplant recipients.[9] The ventilatory response to submaximal exercise, defined as the slope of minute ventilation over carbon dioxide production ($\dot{V}_E/\dot{V}_{CO_2}$), was determined in 12 normal subjects, 10 patients with pulmonary hypertension before and after heart-lung transplantation, and eight patients following heart transplantation. The results are summarized in Figure 3–1 and Table 3–2.

Before the transplant (pulmonary hypertension), the patients showed an augmented ventilatory response to submaximal exercise with a $\dot{V}_E/\dot{V}_{CO_2}$ slope value of 57.7 ± 6.8 (SE) ml/ml $\dot{V}_{CO_2}$ (line II), which is significantly greater than that present in normal subjects (22.3 ± 1.4 ml/ml $\dot{V}_{CO_2}$; $p < 0.001$) (line I). Following heart-lung transplantation, the slope of the $\dot{V}_E/\dot{V}_{CO_2}$ response in these same patients fell during exercise to a value of 24.7 ± 1.6 ml/ml $\dot{V}_{CO_2}$ (line III), which is not significantly different from that found in the normal controls. Patients after heart transplantation (line IV) show a mean slope value of 25.3 ± 1.3 ml/ml $\dot{V}_{CO_2}$, which is not significantly different than the normal value or the value found after heart-lung transplantation.[9]

Post-transplant ventilation appears to remain functionally normal without imposing any limitations on exercise capacity. Although limitations of this nature may have been a concern prior to human heart-lung transplantation,[10] the results of these studies indicate that this is not the case. At maximum constant work rate

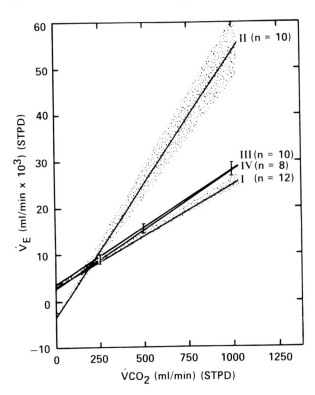

Figure 3–1. Relationship between $\dot{V}_E$ and $\dot{V}_{CO_2}$ during submaximal exercise for four groups. *Shaded areas* represent standard error of mean slope for normal group and groups with pulmonary hypertension. (From Theodore et al,[9] with permission.)

exercise, the $\dot{V}_{E/MVV}$ ratio remained well below 0.7, indicating that a sufficient ventilatory reserve remains and that ventilation is not a factor in limiting exercise.[4]

Despite cardiopulmonary denervation, ventilatory control during exercise also appears to be normal following heart-lung transplantation, as judged by the slope of the $\dot{V}_E/\dot{V}_{CO_2}$ response. The small standard error of the mean slope value present in normals suggests that the ventilatory response to exercise is narrowly regulated. Similarly, this narrow regulation of the ventilatory response to exercise is preserved in heart-lung transplant recipients who possess denervated lungs. This finding suggests that pulmonary neural afferents are not critical to the control of ventilation during exercise in normal subjects as well.[9]

Table 3–2. Slopes and Y Intercepts as Determined by Linear Regression for $\dot{V}_E/\dot{V}_{CO_2}$ during Submaximal Exercise*

Group	Slope	Y Intercept	r
1. Normal controls	22.3 ± 1.4	+2.8 ± 0.5	0.99 ± 0.005
2. Pulmonary hypertension before heart-lung transplant	57.7 ± 6.8	−3.5 ± 2.1	0.97 ± 0.019
3. After heart-lung transplant	24.7 ± 1.6	+3.5 ± 0.8	0.99 ± 0.003
4. After heart transplant	25.3 ± 1.3	+2.7 ± 0.8	0.99 ± 0.003

*Values represent means (±SE) of linear regressions obtained for each individual subject within respective group.

From Theodore et al.,[9] with permission.

After the transplant, VD/VT fell in a normal fashion during the transition from rest to maximum exercise. Despite this normal response, VD/VT still remained mildly elevated with respect to the predicted values given for maximal exercise. The reason for this finding is unclear, but the mild elevation of VD/VT does not appear to be of pathophysiologic significance.[4]

Circulatory Capacity

Cardiac and circulatory function associated with the denervated transplanted heart are well covered in other sections of the book and in this chapter, and will not be covered here in detail. In general, cardiac function in heart-lung transplants is not significantly different from that in heart transplants alone.

In exercise physiology, O_2 consumption ($\dot{V}O_2$), heart rate, O_2-pulse, and blood lactates are useful indices for approximating the limitations of the circulation in conjunction with defining exercise capacity. Measurements of these parameters at maximal exercise can be used to qualitatively estimate circulatory capacity.

Post-transplant resting parameters are not essentially different from what would ordinarily be expected, except for the modest increases in heart rate that are associated with cardiac denervation.[4]

Post-transplant exercise is significantly improved over pretransplant exercise, primarily as a result of an improved circulation, in patients who had undergone heart-lung transplantation for pulmonary hypertension. Although significantly improved, circulatory limitations may still persist after transplant, as judged by the $\dot{V}O_2$, heart rate, and O_2-pulse values that were attainable at maximum levels of exercise. At approximately 8 weeks after transplant, the $\dot{V}O_2$ was 39.3 ± 2.6 percent (SE); heart rate 68.1 ± 2.5 percent; and O_2-pulse rate 57.4 ± 2.5 percent of predicted values at maximum exercise. These values tend to be somewhat higher by 6 months after transplant (Tables 3–3 and 3–4). These limitations of exercise present in heart-lung transplanted patients are in keeping with previous observations made in heart transplanted subjects who were studied

Table 3–3. Comparison of $\dot{V}O_2$, Heart Rate, O_2-Pulse, Ventilation and Blood Gases Obtained at Maximum Tolerable Constant Work Rate Exercise as a Function of Time for 1 Year Post-Transplant (N = 10)

	Within 6 Months	1 Year	Paired t "p"
$\dot{V}O_2$ (ml/min/kg)	18.6 ± 1.8	19.4 ± 1.5	NS
$\dot{V}O_2$, % of max predicted	46.6 ± 4.1	49.3 ± 3.4	NS
Heart rate (beats/min)	136.8 ± 3.3	149.4 ± 4.1	<0.05
Heart rate, % of max predicted	73.0 ± 1.7	79.8 ± 1.7	<0.025
O_2-pulse (ml/kg/beat)	$0.134 \pm .010$	$0.130 \pm .009$	NS
O_2-pulse, % of max predicted	63.4 ± 4.5	62.2 ± 4.4	NS
$\dot{V}_E$ (l/min)	44.8 ± 5.9	46.7 ± 5.2	NS
VD/VT	$0.32 \pm .03$	$0.27 \pm .05$	NS
Pa_{O_2} (torr)	95.7 ± 3.5	92.0 ± 4.3	NS
Pa_{CO_2} (torr)	30.4 ± 1.4	30.1 ± 0.9	NS

Values are mean $\pm$ SE.
NS = not significantly different.
From Theodore et al.,[4] with permission.

Table 3–4. Comparison of $\dot{V}O_2$, Heart Rate, O_2-Pulse, Ventilation and Blood Gases Obtained at Maximum Tolerable Constant Work Rate Exercise as a Function of Time for 2 Years Post-Transplant (N = 6)

	Within 6 Months*	1 Year*	2 Years*
$\dot{V}O_2$ (ml/min/kg)	18.9 ± 2.8	19.6 ± 2.2	20.2 ± 2.3
$\dot{V}O_2$, % of max predicted	50.3 ± 5.6	52.8 ± 4.0	55.2 ± 5.2
Heart rate (beats/min)	134.3 ± 4.7	145.0 ± 5.6	142.0 ± 6.0
Heart rate, % of max predicted	72.7 ± 2.2	78.6 ± 2.7	77.4 ± 3.7
O_2-pulse (ml/kg/beat)	0.139 ± .015	0.134 ± .011	0.142 ± .014
O_2-pulse, % of max. predicted	68.6 ± 5.7	67.3 ± 4.5	71.0 ± 5.1
$\dot{V}_E$ (l/min)	44.2 ± 7.8	46.0 ± 5.2	46.7 ± 6.1
VD/VT	0.34 ± .05	0.25 ± .08	0.32 ± .05
Pa_{O_2} (torr)	93.6 ± 6.0	97.2 ± 3.5	92.8 ± 6.3
Pa_{CO_2} (torr)	30.4 ± 1.9	29.2 ± 1.4	29.6 ± 0.9
(mean ± SE)			

*The results in each time period are not significantly different when statistically compared to each other.

From Theodore et al.,[4] with permission.

hemodynamically by cardiac catheterization during supine exercise[11] and also by progressive incremental exercise to exhaustion on a bicycle.[12]

Long-Term Exercise

Tables 3–3 and 3–4 summarize mean data obtained from serial long-term followup exercise studies performed on heart-lung transplanted patients comparing the effects of time on maximal $\dot{V}O_2$, heart rate, O_2-pulse, ventilation, and arterial blood gases for periods of up to 2 years after transplantation.

Although the circulatory parameters tended to be somewhat greater at 6 months than at 8 weeks after transplant, the maximal values for all parameters were essentially unchanged for periods of time up to 2 years following transplantation.[4] In the group of 10 patients studied at 1 year (see Table 3–3), maximal heart rate was the only parameter that increased significantly over heart rate values that were obtained at less than 6 months after transplant. In the group of 6 patients studied over the 2 year period following transplantation (Table 3–4), the maximal values obtained were not significantly different for any of the time periods after transplantation.

In the absence of complications producing intrinsic graft injury, long-term cardiopulmonary dynamic function during exercise is well maintained for at least 2 years following heart-lung transplantation. Gas exchange and ventilation at maximum exercise are maintained at essentially normal levels. Circulatory limitations persist, but without significant trends in either direction, i.e., worsening or improving. However, a greater number of patients studied over longer periods of time would be required to firmly solidify this conclusion.

A number of factors are present in post-transplant patients that can limit exercise capacity and maximum $\dot{V}O_2$ and, as a result, directly influence qualitative estimates of circulatory capacity. These influences may lead to underestimates of "true" circulatory capacity by limiting exercise performance. Factors potentially limiting post-transplant exercise include cardiac denervation, chronic anemia, physical deconditioning, and, in a significant number of cases, systemic hypertension as a result of cyclosporine effects on the kidney. As a consequence of some of these limitations, it is possible that a number of the patients studied never achieved their actual maximum exercise capacity, thereby leading to an underestimation of the circulation.[4]

In summary, the results of studies described here clearly indicate that the integrated functions of the transplanted heart and lungs are well maintained with exercise. The dramatic clinical improvement observed in heart-lung transplanted patients is further substantiated by the increases in post-transplant exercise capacity. Although circulatory limitations may persist, the allografts perform sufficiently well to sustain the activities of normal life.

PHYSIOLOGIC ASPECTS OF THE DENERVATED HUMAN TRANSPLANTED LUNG

Studies aimed at defining the physiology of the denervated human lung are still in the preliminary stages, although a considerable amount of information from animal work has been available for years. Some newer insights into control mechanisms regulating airway function, the pulmonary circulation, and the control of ventilation have been derived from studies on the denervated lungs of heart-lung transplanted subjects. Some of the effects of lung denervation on respiratory function have already been discussed. Other aspects will be commented on here.

Airway Regulation in the Transplanted Lung

The central regulation of airway tone is primarily mediated via the broncho-constrictor activity of parasympathetic efferents on bronchial smooth muscle.[13] Despite denervation, however, airway tone and function in general do not appear to be particularly altered in the transplanted lung inasmuch as measurements of airway resistance, specific conductance, and dynamic function are essentially normal under baseline conditions.[2]

Under specific experimental conditions, however, new findings have been made in the transplanted human lung that may provide new insights into control mechanisms regulating airway responsiveness and function. These findings appear to be unqiue to the transplanted lung and, most likely, represent expressions of lung denervation.

The first finding is that the airways of the transplanted lungs are hyper-responsive to methacholine inhalation.[14] The degrees of bronchial hyper-responsiveness to methacholine are similar to those that are present in bronchial asthma. However, patients with heart-lung transplants do not have any of the clinical manifestations of bronchial asthma. It is speculated that post-transplant bronchial hyper-responsiveness could result from hypersensitive muscarinic receptors deprived of tonic vagal stimulation, or from a modification of the third nervous system (i.e., nonadrenergic, noncholinergic system), which normally inhibits bronchial smooth muscle tone.[14]

The second finding of significance is the absence of specific airway responses that are associated with respiratory maneuvers under highly specific conditions. The most notable of these affected responses is the loss of a specific airway reflex that is normally present, i.e., the bronchodilator response that is associated with deep inspiration immediately following induced bronchoconstriction is absent in the transplanted lung.[15]

Although the denervated lungs of heart-lung transplants show bronchial hyper-responsiveness, they react differently from the innervated lungs of patients with asthma, which similarly have bronchial hyper-responsiveness. Neither full inspirations, full expirations, nor vital capacity maneuvers significantly altered specific airway conductance in normal individuals or heart-lung transplant recipients under baseline conditions.[15] Such maneuvers result in significant decreases in specific airway conductance in individuals with asthma.[16-18] Following induced bronchoconstriction, single slow and rapid inspirations to total lung capacity transiently abolished or attenuated the bronchoconstriction in normal control subjects. This bronchodilatory effect was absent in the transplant recipients. Patients with asthma have a similar response as normal subjects, in terms of direction and time course, but to a lesser and more variable degree dependent upon the severity of their disease and bronchial hyper-responsiveness. It is likely that these phenomena are under neural modulation in the normal lung. The responses observed in the heart-lung transplant patients, therefore, may represent a result of persistent pulmonary denervation or selective and partial reinnervation.[14,15] However, a normal response has not been observed even at 4 years after heart-lung transplantation.[15] Thus, although some evidence suggested that pulmonary innervation may be reestablished 6 months after lung reimplantation in dogs,[19] the results in human heart-lung transplants suggests the persistence of long-term pulmonary denervation.

Pharmacologic Modulation of Airway Function

Studies with pharmacologic agents have been conducted to further investigate the nature of control mechanisms regulating airway responsiveness and function in the human denervated transplanted lung. These studies represent extensions of work described earlier.

MUSCARINIC CHOLINERGIC BLOCKADE

The prior inhalation of ipratropium bromide (atropine-like compound) inhibits the bronchoconstrictor response to the inhalation of methacholine in heart-lung transplanted subjects.[20] This finding provides evidence that the post-transplanted bronchial hyper-responsiveness to methacholine is mediated via muscarinic receptors inasmuch as ipratropium bromide exerts its inhibitory effect at the muscarinic receptor site. This indicates that the bronchial hyper-responsiveness to methacholine is not a nonspecific response in the transplanted lung. Ipratropium bromide also produces increases in specific airway conductance and FEV_1, indicating bronchodilation. This suggests the presence of some degree of "bronchial tone" in the airways of the transplanted lung despite denervation.

BETA ADRENERGIC BLOCKADE

The inhalation of propranolol, a beta adrenergic blocker, does not produce significant changes in airway conductance in the transplanted lung. This lack of response provides additional evidence that post-transplant bronchial hyper-responsiveness and the bronchial hyper-responsiveness associated with asthma are mechanistically different. Clinical asthma is frequently exacerbated with the use of beta blockers in asthmatic patients. Clinical asthma has not been a feature of the transplanted lung.[14,20]

BETA₂ ADRENERGIC AGONISTS

Salbutamol, a beta₂ agonist, produces a rise in FEV_1 and specific airway conductance, indicating a positive bronchodilator response when maximal doses are used.[20] Hyper-responsiveness to beta agonists has not been a feature of the human denervated transplanted lung.

Regulation of the Pulmonary Circulation in the Transplanted Lung

Heart-lung transplantation does not appear to adversely affect the pulmonary circulation. Pulmonary hemodynamics, at rest, remain normal for extended periods of time measurable in years after transplant.[21] Hypoxic pulmonary vasoconstriction persists in the transplanted lung, suggesting that this response does not depend on an intact neural supply to the pulmonary vasculature and is locally mediated within the lung vasculature itself.[22]

Neural Regulation of Ventilation

Overall, the control of ventilation appears to be virtually intact and normal in heart-lung transplanted subjects, despite lung denervation. As previously discussed, the ventilatory response to submaximal exercise in these patients is similar to that found in normal subjects.[9]

Overall Functional Effects of Lung Denervation in Heart-Lung Transplantation

The integrated functions of the respiratory system appear to be operationally intact and, at least grossly, unaffected by the denervation of the lungs. The integrated responses between the pulmonary and circulatory systems during exercise are grossly intact. The ventilatory response to increasing levels of exercise is normal, ventilation is not limiting to exercise with a sufficient ventilatory reserve at maximum exercise, and gas exchange is normal indicating that $\dot{V}/\dot{Q}$ relationships are well maintained during exercise. Thus, it is clear that the function of matching ventilation with perfusion for the purpose of optimizing gas exchange in the lung is not dependent upon an intact external nerve supply.

SUMMATION AND CONCLUDING REMARKS

The ability of the transplanted lung to maintain function during rest and exercise has a direct bearing on the clinical usefulness of heart-lung transplantation. Standard measurements of pulmonary function indicate that long-term function of the transplanted lung is well maintained, as are the integrated dynamic functions of the transplanted heart and lungs during exercise, for periods of time measurable in years. Gas exchange at rest and exercise remains essentially normal despite the persistence of a mild restrictive abnormality. The dramatic clinical improvement observed in patients with heart-lung transplant is further substantiated by increases in post-transplant exercise capacity. Although circulatory limitations of maximal exercise may persist, the transplanted heart and lungs perform sufficiently well to support normal life.

The denervated transplanted lung shows bronchial hyper-responsiveness to cholinergic stimulation (methacholine inhalation) and the loss of an "airway reflex," i.e., the absence of bronchodilation normally associated with deep inspiration following induced bronchoconstriction. Both of these changes may provide indices for lung denervation. The bronchial hyper-responsiveness may be related to muscarinic denervation hypersensitivity. Despite the existence of bronchial hyper-responsiveness, the transplanted lungs do not manifest clinical asthma. In general, however, lung denervation does not appear to adversely affect overall function of the respiratory system following heart-lung transplantation. From the standpoint of respiratory function, heart-lung transplantation appears to be an acceptable form of therapy in selected patients.

It is worthy of emphasis that the functional studies presented in this section represented post-transplant lung function at its best when the transplanted heart and lungs were essentially free of complications. Although the uncomplicated lungs function at essentially normal levels, it is important to note that late pulmonary complications have occurred in approximately 50 percent of the long-term survivors with heart-lung transplants. Obliterative bronchiolitis represents the pulmonary complication of most concern and, at present, is the greatest threat to long-term survival following transplantation. Severe obstructive airway disease rapidly develops with the onset of obliterative bronchiolitis in the transplanted lung, and if unchecked, can lead to a rapid and fatal downhill course.[3,7,8] Thus, careful observation of airway function is of the utmost importance in the management of heart-lung transplanted patients.

REFERENCES

1. Reitz, BA, Wallwork, JL, Hunt, SA, et al: Heart-lung transplantation: Successful therapy for patients with pulmonary vascular disease. N Engl J Med 306:557, 1982.
2. Theodore, J, Jamieson, SW, Burke, CM, et al: Physiologic aspects of human heart-lung transplantation: Pulmonary function status of the post-transplanted lung. Chest 89:349, 1984.
3. Burke, CM, Theodore, J, Baldwin, JC, et al: Twenty-eight cases of human heart-lung transplantation. Lancet 1:517, 1986.
4. Theodore, J, Morris, AJR, Burke, CM, et al: Cardiopulmonary function at maximum tolerable constant work rate exercise following human heart-lung transplantation. Chest 92:433, 1987.
5. Glanville, AR, Theodore, J, Harvey, J, et al: Elastic behavior of the transplanted lung: Exponential analysis of static pressure-volume relationships. Am Rev Respir Dis 137:308, 1988.
6. Knudson, RJ, Slatin, RC, Lebowitz, MD, et al: The maximal expiratory flow-volume curve. Normal standards, variability, and effects of age. Am Rev Respir Dis 113:587, 1976.
7. Burke, CM, Theodore, J, Dawkins, KD, et al: Post-transplant obliterative bronchiolitis and other late lung sequelae in human heart-lung transplantation. Chest 86:824, 1984.
8. Glanville, AR, Baldwin, JC, Burke, CM, et al: Obliterative bronchiolitis after heart-lung transplantation: Apparent arrest by augmented immunosuppression. Ann Intern Med 307:300, 1987.
9. Theodore, J, Robin, ED, Morris, AJR, et al: Augmented ventilatory response to exercise in pulmonary hypertension. Chest 89:39, 1986.
10. Nakae, S, Webb, WR, Theorides, T, et al: Respiratory function following cardiopulmonary denervation in dog, cat, and monkey. Surg Gynecol Obstet 125:1285, 1967.
11. Stinson, EB, Griepp, RB, Schroeder, JS, et al: Hemodynamic observations one and two years after cardiac transplantation in man. Circulation 45:1183, 1972.
12. Savin, WM, Haskell, WL, Schroeder, JS, et al: Cardiorespiratory responses of cardiac transplant patients to graded symptom-limited exercise. Circulation 62:55, 1980.
13. Nadel, JA: Autonomic regulation of airway smooth muscle. In Nadel, JA (ed): Physiology and Pharmacology of the Airways, Chapter 5, pp 215–257 (in Lenfant, C [ed]: Lung Biology in Health and Disease, Vol 15). Marcel Dekker, New York, 1980.
14. Glanville, AR, Burke, CM, Theodore, J, et al: Bronchial hyperresponsiveness after human cardiopulmonary transplantation. Clin Sci 73:299, 1987.
15. Glanville, AR, Yeend, RA, Theodore, J, et al: The effect of single respiratory maneuvers on specific airway conductance in heart-lung transplant recipients. Clin Sci 74:311, 1988.
16. Butler, J, Caro, CG, Alcala, R, et al: Physiological factors affecting airway resistance in normal subjects and in patients with obstructive respiratory disease. J Clin Invest 39:584, 1960.

17. Gayrard, P, Orebek, J, Grimaud, C, et al: Bronchoconstrictor effects of a deep inspiration in patients with asthma. Am Rev Respir Dis 111:433, 1975.
18. Simonsson, BG, Jacobs, FM, and Nadel, JA: Role of autonomic nervous system and cough reflex in the increased responsiveness of airways in patients with obstructive airway disease. J Clin Invest 46:1812, 1967.
19. Edmonds, LH, Graf, PD, and Nadel, JA: Reinnervation of the reimplanted canine lung. J Appl Physiol 31:722, 1971.
20. Glanville, AR, Theodore, J, Baldwin, JC, et al: Bronchial responsiveness after human cardiopulmonary transplantation. (In preparation for publication.)
21. Glanville, AR, Burke, CM, Hunt, SA, et al: Long-term pulmonary hemodynamics in human heart-lung transplant recipients. Chest 89 (Suppl):512s, 1986.
22. Robin, ED, Theodore, J, Burke, CM, et al: Hypoxic pulmonary vasoconstriction persists in the human transplanted lung. Clin Sci 72:283, 1987.

CHAPTER 4

Pathology of the Transplanted Heart and Lung

Margaret E. Billingham, M.B., B.S., F.R.C.Path.

The first successful clinical cardiac transplantation was performed by Christiaan Barnard in Capetown, South Africa, in 1968. Thereafter, cardiac transplantation was continued throughout the world at a slow rate until 1984. In 1984, cyclosporine became widely available for transplant centers and there was a resurgence of interest in cardiac transplantation, which was reflected in the 1988 International Society of Heart Transplantation Registry[1] showing more than 2200 cardiac transplant recipients in the previous year. Overall survival statistics, as calculated from actuarial tables, also continued to improve. For those patients treated with cyclosporine, the 1-year actuarial survival from the Registry is now 79 percent and the 5-year actuarial survival has increased to 78.3 percent. The longest heart transplant survivor is alive 19 years after transplantation. Many centers use different immunosuppressive protocols; some are now using monoclonal antibodies against cytotoxic cells (OKT3), and others are using different combinations of azathioprine, cyclosporine, and steroids. The latter protocols represent efforts to reduce some of the toxic effects of these drugs when taken in higher doses. As a consequence, there is a tendency in the pathology of rejection to revert toward that seen prior to the cyclosporine era. It is necessary therefore to describe a spectrum of pathology depending on the type of treatment used. The first part of this chapter will outline the temporal and sequential changes in cardiac pathology following cardiac allograft transplantation in the human. The pathology described is the same for heterotopic or "piggy-back" heart transplants. In 1986, more than 40 heterotopic heart transplantations were reported by the International Society of Heart Transplantation Registry.[1] Between 1974 and 1986, 165 heterotopic cardiac transplantations were reported.[1]

The type of patient most likely to benefit from cardiac transplantation is one who has end-stage dilated cardiomyopathy with a very poor prognosis,[2] but who otherwise has reversible organ damage elsewhere in the body. Cardiac transplantation is also performed for coronary artery disease, valvular disease, or any other end-stage cardiac disease. The primary cause of death in cardiac transplant

Table 4–1. Causes of Death (Stanford)

	First Postop Year Cyclosporine-Treated (N = 304)	>1 Year Postop Cyclosporine-Treated (N = 216)
1. Rejection	13	3
2. Infection	25	13
3. Graft vascular disease	1	14
4. Graft failure (non-specific)	5	—
5. Lymphoproliferative disease	2	3
6. Non-lymphoid malignancy	—	5
7. Pulmonary embolus	3	—
8. Pulmonary hypertension	2	—
9. CVA (cerebrovascular accident)	3	1
10. Other	5	4
Total Deaths	59	43

recipients is reflected in the Stanford experience and shown in Table 4–1, which is divided into the cause of death in the first year and in late survivors. It can be seen that infection and rejection are the most important problems, at least in the early postoperative period, and that it is important to make a correct diagnosis, because the treatment for infection and rejection are opposite. Although there are many noninvasive techniques being tested, some of which are listed in Table 4–2, at present the most reliable method of diagnosing acute rejection is by histologic diagnosis, obtaining the tissue by the invasive method of endomyocardial biopsy.

ENDOMYOCARDIAL BIOPSY

The endomyocardial biopsy that is in use today is a modification of the original Konno-Sakakibara bioptome.[3] Although there are several types of bioptomes, a shorter modification of the original is generally used,[4–6] which can be placed percutaneously through the internal jugular vein into the right ventricle; others prefer to use the long-sheath method from the femoral approach. These bioptomes and operative techniques have been well-described previously.[7,8] The

Table 4–2. Diagnosis of Rejection—Cardiac Transplantation

Noninvasive
  1. Clinical
  2. Electrocardiogram
  3. Impedance cardiography
  4. Radiologic
  5. Hemodynamics
  6. Echo-Doppler
  7. Serologic
  8. Immunologic
Invasive
  9. Endomyocardial biopsy

advantages of the percutaneous transjugular approach is that it is quicker, the patient does not need a general anesthetic, and it can be performed on an outpatient basis. Endomyocardial biopsy provides a safe, reliable morphologic index of acute rejection, and now plays an important role in the management of patients with cardiac transplantation. Repeated biopsies are well tolerated, permitting monitoring of acute rejection in cardiac transplant recipients. Some patients have undergone over 40 serial biopsies. Adequate sampling is crucial, however, and requires that at least four pieces of tissue, depending on the size of the bioptome, are obtained. If a 7 French bioptome size is used, four to six pieces are necessary to rule out a significant sampling problem. Based on the larger size 9 French bioptome, it has been shown that four pieces have a 2 percent false-negative error.[9] Hematoxylin eosin stains should be used to show the nuclear morphology and Masson's trichrome or other connective tissue stain to highlight early myocyte damage as well as fibrosis. Other stains should be used as required.

The tissue obtained should be fixed immediately in 10 percent formalin at room temperature (to lessen contraction artifact) unless it is being frozen for immunoperoxidase studies. After fixation and processing by embedding for either plastic or paraffin, the sections should be cut at not more than 4 microns thick and the blocks should be sampled at at least three levels. Some centers prefer to use immunoperoxidase staining to highlight the type of subpopulations of lymphocytes present; others believe that this is not particularly helpful in the management of rejection. Tissue can be fixed in the usual way for electron microscopy, if desired. Electron microscopy is thought by most people not to be useful for the day-to-day diagnosis of acute rejection, but it may be required for research or other purposes. Although some centers find that electron microscopy is useful,[10] in large centers where 15 to 20 endomyocardial biopsies are being performed daily, as at Stanford, electron microscopy becomes impractical for the immediate management of the patient.

The endomyocardial biopsy, therefore, can be used effectively and safely, even in very young children. In the Stanford experience of over 10,000 endomyocardial biopsies, there have been no deaths and the morbidity has been less than 0.3 percent.

THE PATHOLOGY OF CARDIAC TRANSPLANTATION

The pathology of cardiac transplantation can be divided into immediate perioperative changes, early postoperative changes (during the first 3 months following transplantation), and late changes in long-term survivors.

PERIOPERATIVE CHANGES IN CARDIAC TRANSPLANTATION

Sometimes, for reasons that are not entirely clear, the donor heart may not function at the time of transplantation. This may be due to a number of causes, some of which may be pulmonary hypertension in the recipient in which case the normal, nonhypertrophied right ventricle of the donor fails to support the circulation against the pulmonary resistance, or it may be due to overmedication of the donor, affecting the myocardium prior to organ donation. Very occasionally, hyperacute rejection due to ABO mismatch also will occur. In the case of hyperacute rejection, the myocardium shows marked hemorrhage, which is global, rather than focal, as seen in infarcts, and may show a neutrophilic infiltrate as well, if the heart is sustained for some while prior to retransplantation. Other changes that may be seen on a biopsy within the first 2 weeks following cardiac transplantation, are those of ischemia due to prolonged ischemic time of the donor heart prior to transplantation. This pathologic change is becoming more frequent, because owing to the donor shortage, many donor hearts have to be harvested distantly and may have ischemic times of up to or beyond 3 hours. Biopsies in the first or second week following transplantation often show the effects of reperfusion injury. Reperfusion injury, in contrast to acute rejection, shows more myocyte necrosis than is usually seen in moderate acute rejection and there is more myocyte damage than there is infiltrate, which may be minimal. Later on, the ischemic area is replaced with granulation tissue, which is also different from the monomorphous infiltrate of acute rejection and should not be confused with the latter. Other changes that may be seen in biopsies in the early postoperative period, are those of the characteristic focal necrosis encountered in catecholamine effect, especially where the donor or recipient have been on high "pressor" drugs.

Acute Cardiac Rejection

The sequential pathologic changes of the myocardium during acute cardiac rejection, modified by immunosuppressive treatment, have been worked out and described as a result of sequential endomyocardial biopsies in cardiac recipients.[11-14] There are now several new grading systems in use.[15,16] It is recommended that each center use a grading system of its own preference, but it is important that each center is consistent in its use and that different grading systems are not used by different people in the same center. For the purposes of this chapter, we will use a simple grading system, such as is used at Stanford, of mild, moderate, severe, and resolving acute rejection. The histopathologic changes using this grading and the comparative grading systems are summarized in Table 4–3.

Table 4–3. Grading of Acute Rejection by Endomyocardial Biopsy

1. Mild rejection	*	Perivascular lymphoblasts and/or sparse interstitial infiltrate.
0–4	†	
A1–A2	‡	
2. Moderate rejection	*	Increased perivascular or interstitial inflammatory infiltrate
4–9	†	with eosinophils. Subtle myocyte damage.
A3	‡	
3. Severe rejection	*	Florid interstitial infiltrate (mixed instead of monomorphous)
10	†	with hemorrhage, vasculitis and myocyte necrosis.
A4	‡	
4. Resolving	*	Decreased infiltrate of small lymphocytes, scar formation,
—	†	pigment, macrophages and scar.
A5a	‡	
5. Resolved	*	No evidence of infiltrate. Scar.
—	†	
A5b	‡	

*Stanford (Billingham) Heart Transplant 1:25, 1982.
†Texas (McAllister[16]).
‡Hannover (Kemnitz) Am J Surg Pathol 11(7):503, 1987.

THE PATHOLOGY OF EARLY OR MILD ACUTE REJECTION. This condition is characterized by plump mononuclear cells in a perivascular or endocardial position. Sometimes sparse cells may be seen in the interstitium, not directly abutting on adjacent myocytes and not causing myocyte damage. In most centers mild acute rejection is not treated, but because it is a harbinger of moderate acute rejection in approximately 30 percent of the cases, this diagnosis warrants a followup biopsy within 5 to 7 days. In some cases, the followup biopsy will be negative and it may be that the mild acute rejection seen earlier was a reflection of low cyclosporine levels in the patient at that time. In the case of a patient who is not being treated with cyclosporine but with the earlier conventional therapy (azathioprine and steroids), it is necessary to treat the patient much earlier because the development of a more severe rejection is much faster.

THE PATHOLOGY OF MODERATE ACUTE REJECTION. At this stage the mononuclear inflammatory infiltrates spread into the interstitium and become perimyocytic. The large plump mononuclear cells are seen to line-up alongside the myocytes, surround and overlap or indent them (Fig. 4–1). At this stage focal myocyte damage is frequently seen, although this may be quite subtle. The amount of inflammatory infiltrate is important whether or not myocyte damage can be seen. If there is a significant infiltrate in several of the biopsy pieces, it is important to treat the patient regardless of whether necrosis can be seen. The infiltrate of acute rejection has been shown to have a predilection for the conducting system[17] and, therefore, fatal arrythmias can occur even with a moderate infiltrate. In the case of cyclosporine treatment, eosinophils are commonly seen

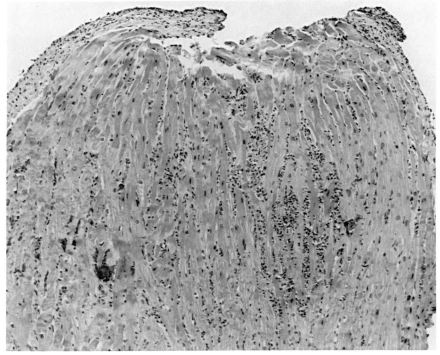

Figure 4–1. Biopsy showing moderate acute rejection with lymphocytes surrounding and in some cases replacing myocytes. Hematoxylin and eosin, magnification ×100.

at this stage of acute rejection. The presence of eosinophils in non–cyclosporine treated patients should alert the pathologist to the possibility of concomitant infection (e.g., toxoplasmosis). It is usual in most centers to treat a moderate acute rejection with augmentation of immunosuppression even though the patient may be hemodynamically stable, in order to prevent the accelerated vascular damage that is thought to be rejection-mediated. The infiltrate of moderate acute rejection following treatment usually will reverse within 10 days.

THE PATHOLOGY OF SEVERE ACUTE REJECTION. Severe acute rejection is characterized by a fairly dense interstitial and perivascular inflammatory infiltrate, which is now mixed rather than monomorphous and which may contain eosinophils and neutrophils as well as mononuclear cells (Fig. 4–2). In severe acute rejection, vasculitis will result in interstitial hemorrhage, which is an ominous sign. Myocyte necrosis also will be seen at this stage and is usually not so subtle. In severe acute rejection, an endocardial infiltrate is nearly always present, as seen and confirmed by autopsy specimens. Depending on the amount of previous treatment the patient may have had for ongoing acute rejection, the number of mononuclear cells may be suppressed as a result and there may be a preponderance of edema and hemorrhage rather than infiltrate. In the cyclosporine-treated patients, it is possible to more easily reverse a severe acute rejection.

THE PATHOLOGY OF RESOLVING ACUTE REJECTION. If the patient has been treated for acute rejection, the followup biopsies may show evidence of repair with fibroblast infiltration as well as pigment-laden macrophages and early fibrosis. Residual lymphocytes may be present, but following immunosuppressive

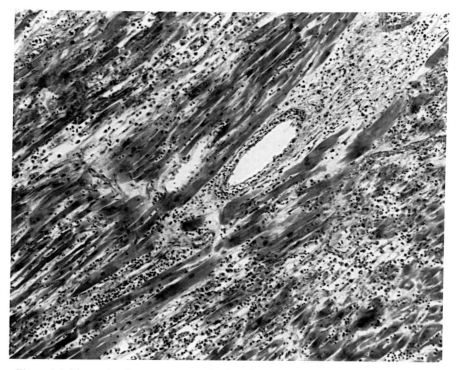

Figure 4–2. Biopsy showing severe acute rejection with a mixed inflammatory infiltrate and interstitial edema. Hematoxylin and eosin, magnification ×200.

therapy may be smaller and nonpyroninophilic. Resolved acute rejection results in a small focal scar that may retain trapped lymphocytes.

Pitfalls of Diagnosing Acute Rejection

The pathologist should be aware of several pitfalls in making the diagnosis of acute rejection. The first and most common pitfall is that of previous biopsy sites. These sites can usually be recognized inasmuch as they include part of the endocardium, they include fibrin if they are recent, and the base of the biopsy site shows marked myocyte disarray. Secondly, it is important to separate the inflammatory infiltrates of acute rejection from that of acute infectious myocarditis. In the immunosuppressed group of patients, it is not uncommon to have a superimposed infection that is discovered by endomyocardial biopsy. In general, protozoan infections, such as that due to Toxoplasma gondii, will induce a mixed inflammatory infiltrate, rather than the monomorphous type encountered in acute rejection (Fig. 4–3). The intact cysts should be looked for carefully inasmuch as they may not evoke an inflammatory infiltrate until ruptured.

Other organisms discovered in the endomyocardial biopsy include cytomegalic virus (CMV), which sometimes does not evoke an inflammatory reaction, although the inclusions can be seen within the myocyte nuclei. At other times the CMV will be accompanied with a mixed infiltrate as already described. A diagnosis of CMV has been known to have a deleterious effect on recipient survival.[18]

Another pitfall is the endocardial infiltrate or "Quilty" effect seen in approximately 5 to 9 percent of biopsies from patients treated with cyclosporine (Fig. 4–

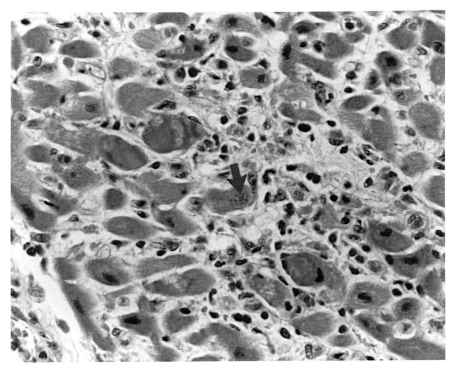

Figure 4–3. Biopsy showing a focus of mixed infiltrate around a myocyte with a cyst of Toxoplasma gondii (*arrow*). Hematoxylin and eosin, magnification ×400.

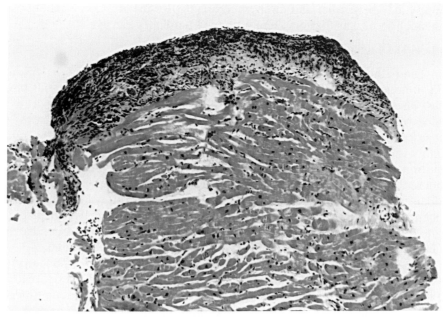

Figure 4–4. Biopsy showing "Quilty" effect of predominantly an endomyocardial infiltrate with vascular spaces. Hematoxylin and eosin, magnification ×100.

4). The endocardial infiltrate itself does not apparently cause any untoward reaction and is usually not treated. In some cases, acute rejection may occur in the biopsy concomitant with the "Quilty" effect, and in this case, of course, the rejection should be treated. The final pitfall has been alluded to previously and is that of ischemia or catecholamine effect rather than acute rejection.

The Pathology of Long-Term Cardiac Transplantation Survivors

In the late postoperative period, a number of complications can occur that may limit long-term survival. It should be remembered that acute cardiac rejection can still occur in long-term survivors. This may be due to a change in immunosuppressive regimen, either intentionally or unintentionally, such as might occur with marked weight gain. In some cases, the physicians change the treatment because of the development of unwanted side effects, such as hirsutism, nephrotoxicity,[19] hypertension, or osteoporosis. It is also known now that acute rejection may follow a CMV infection, and it should always be looked for in this setting. Acute rejection in the late postoperative period can be treated in the same way as in the early postoperative period and is usually more easily reversible. It is also true that infection may occur in the late postoperative period in cardiac recipients. The list of organisms responsible in immunosuppressed host is extensive and the infections in this group of patients may be seen in other organs of the body, including the brain and skin, which have been described previously[20] and will not be detailed in this chapter.

Accelerated Graft Vascular Disease

Acclerated graft vascular disease is encountered in heart allografts and in combined heart-lung allografts and has been described previously.[21,22] The term "chronic rejection" is sometimes used for this condition, but is best avoided as it causes a semantic confusion. The coronary circulation in the cardiac allograft is subject to the development of a rapidly progressive form of concentric intimal proliferation that eventually occludes the lumen of the coronary vessels. More insidious, however, is the fact that this same condition affects the entire length of the epicardial vessel including the small intramyocardial branches. In many cases, the small penetrating vessels are totally occluded before the epicardial vessels, and acute myocardial infarction may occur even though routine coronary arteriograms still show an adequate lumen. This vascular conditon may occur as rapidly as 3 to 9 months following cardiac transplantation, but it is more common after 3 years. The pathology of this condition differs from naturally occurring atherosclerosis in that the entire vessel length is often affected by the concentric intimal proliferation with an almost intact elastic lamina, in contrast to the focal asymmetric atherosclerotic plaques, frequently containing calcium, which tend to disrupt the underlying elastica. It is true that focal plaques may be found in heart recipients, and it is not clear whether these can occur independently in the graft vessels or whether they are acquired from the donor heart. Unfortunately, it appears that the condition of graft vascular disease occurs at the same rate in patients treated with cyclosporine as those treated with azathioprine. Accelerated graft vascular disease can now be detected in routine arteriograms in approximately 40 percent of cardiac transplant recipients by 2.5 years following cardiac transplantation.[23] Because the allografts are denervated, acute myocardial infarction resulting in sudden death can occur without the usual harbingers of angina or pain in the chest. An autopsy study on 100 recipient hearts at Stanford[24] and several other studies since then[25] have shown that the underlying accelerated coronary artery disease appears to have poor correlation with episodes of acute rejection, HLA mismatch, sex or age of the donor or recipient, and with many other risk factors, with the possible exception of hypercholesterolemia. In most centers, patients who have received cardiac allografts are monitored for the development of this disease with careful control of diet, blood sugar levels, and serum lipid profiles. In some centers, patients are routinely treated with aspirin or dipyridamole or similar antithrombotic agents. More recently, children who have received a cardiac allograft, have also been found to develop this condition. After 1 year survival, graft vascular disease becomes the most frequent cause of death in cardiac allograft recipients (see Table 4–1). This condition also accounts for the largest number of retransplantations in this group of patients.

INNERVATION OF THE TRANSPLANTED HEART

At the time of cardiac transplantation the heart is denervated. At autopsy, even many years following cardiac transplantation, intact viable ganglion cells can be seen in the atrioventricular groove. Although the preganglionic fibers are severed at operation the postganglionic fibers remain viable in the allograft. Recent studies have shown that significant reinnervation of the heart by sympathetic and sensory nerves apparently does not occur up to at least 10 years after cardiac transplantation.[26] There have been some unpublished reports of physiologic evidence of reinnervation,[27] but these have not yet been morphologically confirmed. It has been shown that the resting heart rate of the denervated heart is 110, plus or minus 10 beats per minute, and that this high rate reflects the absence of normal vagal tone. The heart rate in response to dynamic exercise tends to be slower and tends not to achieve peak levels during maximum exercise compared with age-matched normal controls.

SUMMARY

Cardiac transplantation offers an excellent chance of long-term survival and functional rehabilitation for the carefully selected patient with end-stage heart disease. At present, the role of the pathologist is still crucial in making the diagnosis of acute rejection by endomyocardial biopsy. Although many noninvasive tests are being tried out to reduce the number of endomyocardial biopsies (see Table 4–2), particularly in infants and children, none of these have so far been specific enough to use by themselves in patient management. It is possible that combinations of noninvasive tests used concomitantly may be able to guide management of the patients by indicating normal parameters so that the number of routine biopsies can be reduced.

THE PATHOLOGY OF COMBINED HEART-LUNG TRANSPLANTATION

For patients with end-stage lung disease and for those with end-stage heart disease resulting in severe pulmonary hypertension, combined heart-lung transplantation has now become a therapeutic option. At present, unilateral lung transplantation appears to be another therapeutic option for patients with end-stage pulmonary fibrosis, and double-lung transplantation for patients with obstructive lung disease or bilateral pulmonary disease such as fibrocystic disease. The first reported cardiopulmonary transplant was performed in an infant with severe congenital heart disease,[28] but the postoperative course was complicted by significant bleeding, and the patient died within 14 hours of transplantation. The second clinical case, reported by Lillehei and coworkers in 1970,[29] survived only a few days and died of infectious complications. The third patient to undergo combined heart-lung transplantation was reported by Barnard and associates in 1981,[30] but the patient died on the 23rd postoperative day of infectious complications.

Based on the encouraging results in the primate laboratory at Stanford and the successful introduction of cyclosporine therapy, a clinical program in heart-lung transplantation was begun again in March 1980. At the time of writing this chapter, 54 combined heart-lung transplants have been performed at Stanford, with an age range of 2 years to 45 years. Survival has paralleled cardiac transplantation, with the survival being approximately 10 percent less for each year of survival than in cardiac transplants until 4 years after heart-lung transplantation, at which time there has been a drop from 55 percent 4-year survival to 20 percent 6-year survival. Twenty-seven of the 54 patients are alive from 2 months to 6 years after transplantation, and there have been 13 hospital deaths and 12 late deaths in this group. The heart-lung transplantation actuarial survival curves in the Registry for the International Society of Heart Transplantation for patients operated from 1986 to 1987 worldwide showed a 62.45 percent survival at 1 year after transplant and 61.35 percent at 2 years.[1]

Since the initiation of human heart-lung transplant programs, significant advances have been made in defining the physiology of the respiratory system in the transplanted heart and lungs. Despite the ischemia of the graft at the time of transplantation and disruption of the cardiopulmonary nerves and lymphatics, as well as that of the bronchial arterial supply, it would appear that the transplanted heart and lungs function sufficiently well to support the activities of normal life for many of the recipients. From the standpoint of respiratory function, providing there are no significant complications, combined heart-lung transplantation appears to be an acceptable form of therapy in selected patients. At present, however, a greater clinical experience is required before a final determination can be made with regard to the long-term benefits of combined heart-lung transplantation. One of the major difficulties in the management of combined heart and lung tranplantations has been the fact that there is no reliable method to determine acute rejection of the graft and to separate the findings from those of acute infection. At present, the concomitant roentgenographic findings and results of pulmonary function tests are used together with observation of the peripheral activated cells (cytologic immunologic monitoring) as well as bronchoalveolar lavage (BAL) studies. The invasive tests of transbronchial and open lung biopsy appear to be the most reliable; however, being invasive, they also put the immunosuppressed patient at risk.

The purpose of this portion of this chapter is to describe the pathologic changes in the bronchial and transbronchial biopsies and the end-stage autopsy changes of combined heart-lung transplantation. It should be noted that acute rejection in the heart, as seen by endomyocardial biopsy, does not necessarily reflect acute rejection in the lung portion of the graft, which frequently occurs earlier than in the heart. In fact, acute rejection of the myocardium is relatively rare in combined heart-lung transplantation.[31] It is thought that the maximum donor-recipient interface is within the lung tissue and, therefore, rejection occurs there first. There is some question that there might also be a measure of graft-versus-host disease, given that normal lungs contain a large amount of peribronchial lymphocytes.

One of the unique problems of lung transplantation is the development of transient reversible defects in pulmonary gas exchange, compliance, and vascular resistance, coinciding with roentgenographic evidences of pulmonary edema in the early postoperative period. These phenomena develop early after transplantation, usually within the first 3 postoperative days, but they could remain a significant concern for at least 3 weeks postoperatively. This is known as the "reimplantation response"; however, many of the same changes also occur in acute lung rejection, making the diagnosis more difficult.

PATHOLOGY OF EARLY POSTOPERATIVE HEART-LUNG
TRANSPLANTATION

REIMPLANTATION EFFECT. At this stage there are perivascular and peribronchial edema-forming "halos" around vascular spaces. In addition, there is pulmonary edema, with alveoli filled with proteinaceous fluid and scanty inflammatory cells. If a bronchial biopsy is taken within 1 week of pulmonary transplantation, sparse collections of neutrophils also can be seen.

MILD ACUTE REJECTION. In this phase there is prominent "cuffing" of pyroninophilic mononuclear cells surrounding venules and arterioles (Fig. 4–5) as well as bronchioles. In the case of an open lung biopsy the venules may be seen coursing along the septa arising from the pleural surface. At this stage the perivascular

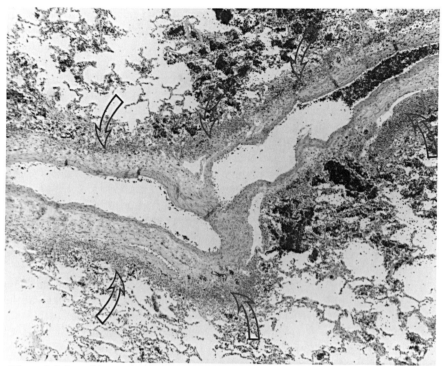

Figure 4–5. Lung biopsy showing vascular "cuffing" by lymphocytes *(arrows)*. Hematoxylin and eosin, magnification ×100.

and peribronchial cuffing are widespread and diffuse throughout the lungs, although the alveoli are clear of infiltrate or proteinaceous fluid. The lymphocytic infiltrate appears not to extend into the vessel walls, although it may be seen to extend into the alveoli and bronchial walls.

MODERATE ACUTE REJECTION. The perivascular infiltrate of pyroninophilic lymphocytes now extends into the alveoli walls, widening them. At this stage an acute bronchiolitis, with mononuclear cells extending into the bronchial wall, may also be seen. Pulmonary edema or scanty mononuclear cells within the alveoli may be seen at this stage.

SEVERE ACUTE REJECTION. At this stage, there is hemorrhage and a predominantly mononuclear infiltrate within the alveoli, with some necrosis of the alveola walls. Hemorrhage into the lung parenchyma is common. Bronchiolitis and sluffing of the bronchial epithelium is frequently seen. Grossly, at this stage a "hepatization" of the lungs occurs.

RESOLVING REJECTION WITHIN THE LUNG TISSUE. Resolving acute rejection manifests itself with plugs of granulation tissue filling the alveolar walls, and reparative changes of fibrosis and granulation tissue take place within the walls of damaged bronchioles.

PATHOLOGIC CHANGES IN LONG-TERM SURVIVORS OF HEART-LUNG TRANSPLANTATION

BRONCHIOLITIS OBLITERANS. Bronchiolitis obliterans has emerged as the single most significant long-term complication of human heart-lung transplantation.

This condition has been observed as early as 2 to 3 months after transplantation. Bronchiolitis obliterans can be seen in transbronchial biopsies, but the changes may be subtle and the elastic Van Giesen stains are useful in interpreting this lesion. Sequential transbronchial biopsies show that early damage to the bronchioles may be reflected by epithelial metaplasia, which is later followed by denudation of the ciliated respiratory epithelium. If the inflammatory infiltrate continues, this may lead to ulceration with sluffing of the bronchiolar walls into the lumen.[32] This in turn may progress to partial filling of the lumen with granulation tissue and fibrosis, ultimately leading to total obliteration or bronchiolitis obliterans. In time, only a small scar is left with residual fragments of smooth muscle and elastica (Fig. 4–6).

The bronchiolitis obliterans in heart-lung transplantation may be due to a number of factors; it may be caused by loss of bronchial circulation, denervation, or continued inflammatory infiltrate either by rejection and/or respiratory infection due to viral, bacterial or other pathogens. As pointed out by Yousem and associates,[32] chronic inflammation can result in squamous metaplasia with loss of surface cilia, which may lead to mucostasis and plugging, thus further increasing the risk of infection. Inflammation also may impair the secretion of IgA, an important opsonin in the protection of lung. With the loss of cough reflex from denervation of the transplanted lungs, not only is the propensity for infection increased, but also chronic aspiration may be a further factor causing inflammation of the bronchial tree.[32]

Approximately 50 percent of long-term survivors with heart-lung transplants

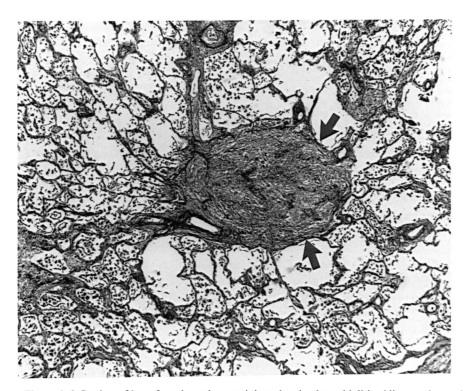

Figure 4–6. Section of lung from heart-lung recipient showing bronchiolitis obliterans *(arrows)*. Elastic van Gieson, magnification ×400.

have developed postoperative obliterative bronchiolitis in the Stanford series. It has been reversed on early detection with aggressive high-dose steroid therapy but has failed to respond in other cases in which steroids were administered relatively late in the course. The early diagnosis of bronchiolitis obliterans can be attempted with the use of pulmonary function tests showing a constrictive pattern.

PULMONARY INFECTION. This is also a severe cause of pathology and death in long-term survivors. The immunosuppressed patient is at risk for infections that may emanate from the donor lung or may be acquired. Almost any infection can be encountered in heart-lung transplantation; however, the most common ones are viral, particularly cytomegalic virus (CMV) and respiratory syncytial virus, adenovirus, or parainfluenza virus in children, and Hemophilus influenza, Legionella, and Mycoplasma viral infections in adults. Occasionally, recrudescence of unrecognized dormant granulomata may result in disseminated tuberculosis or coccidioidomycosis.

VASCULAR CHANGES. It has been shown earlier that acute rejection can affect venules as well as arterioles. In late heart-lung transplantation survivors, concentric intimal proliferation with sclerosis may be seen in both venules and arterioles. This change of accelerated intimal hyperplasia has been seen in both elastic and muscular arteries and arterioles in the lung grafts. Plexiform or angiomatoid lesions have not yet been recognized. It should be noted at this point that the coronary artery accelerated graft disease in combined heart-lung transplant is often worse than that in the lungs despite the fact that rejection tends to be less in the heart than in the lungs.[31]

FIBROSIS. All long-term heart-lung survivors have shown a marked increase in pleural thickening, often with extensive adhesions. In addition, there appears to be a definite increase in interstitial fibrosis of the alveolar walls. This may be due to cyclosporine, which has been shown to increase interstitial fibrosis in the kidney and heart, or it may be the result of ischemic damage at the time of transplantation, or again, it may be due to loss of bronchial and lymphatic circulation.

SUMMARY

Combined heart-lung transplantation is now being carried out in many centers around the world. Single-lung and double-lung transplantation are being done in only a few centers and are still considered to be experimental procedures. Combined heart-lung transplantation has been performed successfully in adults and in small children and offers a definite therapeutic alternative to such diseases as severe congenital heart disease with pulmonary hypertension, cystic fibrosis, and primary pulmonary hypertension. At present, the survival statistics for this procedure are similar to those for heart transplantation 15 years ago; it is hoped that, as with heart transplantation, survival rates will improve with better management and more reliable diagnosis of acute rejection, in order to prevent the insidious and relentless onset of obliterative bronchiolitis, which is now the most significant limiting factor to the success of long-term survival in heart-lung transplantation.

REFERENCES

1. Fragomeni, LS and Kay, MP: The Registry of the International Society for Heart Transplantation: Fifth Official Report—1988. J Heart Transplant 7:249, 1988.

2. Schroeder, JS and Hunt, SA: Cardiac transplantation: Where are we? Editorial. N Engl J Med 315:961, 1986.
3. Sakakibara, S and Konno, S: Endomyocardial biopsy. Jpn Heart J 3:537, 1962.
4. Caves, PK, Schultz, WP, Dong, D, Jr, et al: New instrument for transvenous cardiac biopsy. Am J Cardiol 33:264, 1974.
5. Caves, PK, Stinson, EB, Billingham, ME, et al: Percutaneous transvenous endomyocardial biopsy in human heart recipients. Ann Thorac Surg 16:325, 1975.
6. Caves, PK, Stinson, EB, Billingham, ME, et al: Serial transvenous biopsy of the transplanted human heart: Improved management of acute rejection episodes. Lancet 1:821, 1974.
7. Mason, JW: Techniques for right and left ventricular endomyocardial biopsy. Am J Cardiol 41:887, 1978.
8. Tilkian, AG and Daily, EK: Endomyocardial biopsy. In Tilkian, AG and Daily, EK (eds): Cardiovascular Procedures, Chapter 8. CV Mosby, St Louis, 1986, pp 180–203.
9. Spiegelhalter, DJ and Stovin, PGI: An analysis of repeated biopsies following cardiac transplantation. Stat Med 2:33, 1983.
10. Myles, JL, Ratliff, NB, McMahon, JT, et al: Reversibility of myocyte injury in moderate and severe acute rejection in cyclosporine-treated cardiac transplant patients. Arch Pathol Lab Med 111:947, 1987.
11. Billingham, ME: Some recent advances in cardiac pathology. Human Pathol 10:367, 1979.
12. Billingham, ME: The diagnostic criteria of myocarditis by endomyocardial biopsy. In Sekiguchi, Olsen, and Goodwin (eds): Myocarditis and Related Disorders. Springer-Verlag, 1985, pp 133–137.
13. Billingham, ME: Cardiac transplantation. In Waller (ed): Contemporary Issues in Cardiovascular Pathology. Cardiovascular Clinics, Vol 18(2). FA Davis, Philadelphia, 1987, pp 185–199.
14. Billingham, ME: The post-surgical heart: The pathology of cardiac transplantation. Am J Cardiovasc Pathol 1:319, 1988.
15. Kemnitz, J, Cohnert, T, Schafers, H-J, et al: A classification of cardiac allograft rejection. Am J Surg Pathol 11:503, 1987.
16. McAllister, HA, Schnee, MJ, Radovancevic, B, et al: A system for grading cardiac allograft rejection. Texas Heart Inst J 13:1, 1986.
17. Bieber, CP, Stinson, EB, Shumway, NE, et al: Cardiac transplantation in man. VII. Cardiac allograft pathology. Circulation 41:753, 1970.
18. Oyer, P: Heart, heart/lung transplantation. XII International Congress of the Transplantation Society. Book II. Sydney, Australia, August 14–19, 1988, (abstr).
19. Myers, BB: Cyclosporine nephrotoxicity. Kidney Int 30:1964, 1986.
20. Linder, J: Infections as a complication of heart transplantation. J Heart Transplant 7:390, 1988.
21. Billingham, ME: Diseases of the transplanted heart. In Symons, C and Wright-Bon, J (eds): Specific Heart Muscle Disease, Chapter 11. 1983, p 130.
22. Billingham, ME: Cardiac transplant atherosclerosis. Transplant Proc 19(Suppl 5):19, 1987.
23. Hunt, SA: Cardiac transplantation: Where do we stand? Post Grad Med 78:15, 1985.
24. Billingham, ME, Masek, MA, Khanna, K, et al: Long term cardiac allograft pathology in humans (abstr). Lab Invest 42:103, 1979.
25. Gao, SZ, Johnson, D, Schroeder, JS, et al: Transplant coronary artery disease: Histopathologic correlations with angiographic morphology (abstr). J Am Coll Cardiol, Feb 1988 (in press).
26. Rowan, R and Billingham, ME: Myocardial innervation in long-term cardiac transplant survivors: A quantitative ultrastructural survey. J Heart Transplant 1988 (in press).
27. Yacoub, M: Personal communication.
28. Cooley, DA, Bloodwel, RD, Hallman, GL, et al: Organ transplantation for advanced cardiopulmonary disease. Ann Thorac Surg 8:30, 1969.
29. Lillehei, CW, Wildevuur, CRH, and Benfield, JR: A review of 23 human lung transplantations by 20 surgeons. Ann Thorac Surg 9:489, 1970.
30. Barnard, CN and Cooper, DKC: Clinical transplantation of the heart: A review of 13 years personal experience. J Roy Soc Med 74:670, 1981.
31. Glanville, AR, Imoto, E, Billingham, M, et al: The role of right ventricular endomyocardial biopsy in the long-term management of heart-lung transplant recipients. J Heart Transplant 6:357, 1987.
32. Yousem, SA, Burke, CM, and Billingham, ME: Pathologic pulmonary alterations in long-term human heart-lung transplantation. Hum Pathol 16:911, 1985.

CHAPTER 5

Immunologic Mechanisms
of Cardiac Transplant Rejection*

René J. Duquesnoy, Ph.D.
Donald V. Cramer, D.V.M., Ph.D.

Cardiac transplantation has become an important therapeutic modality for patients with terminal heart disease. In recent years improved immunosuppressive strategies, largely based on cyclosporine, have dramatically increased the success of cardiac transplantation, and many centers now achieve 1-year patient survival rates of 80 percent or greater. Nevertheless, most transplant patients face a variety of postsurgical complications, including acute rejection, infection, cyclosporine toxicity, and accelerated arteriosclerotic disease. Thus, although short-term survival rates have improved dramatically, the late complications of cardiac transplantation have assumed a greater importance in the therapeutic management of these patients. In this chapter we examine the clinical and experimental data relevant to the immune mechanisms responsible for the rejection of cardiac allografts, initially by summarizing the information on the antigens that stimulate the immune response to the graft and then by examining the immunopathologic mechanisms responsible for the graft rejection.

One of the major problems in organ transplantation is the immune response of the recipient, which may lead to rejection of the donor allograft. This immune response is directed toward a variety of antigens collectively referred to as transplantation or histocompatibility antigens. Of primary importance are the transplantation antigens encoded by the major histocompatibility complex (MHC) (*HLA* in humans, *RT1* in rats, and *H-2* in mice)—a closely linked group of genes that are responsible for mediating a variety of immunologic functions and cell-to-cell interactions. Other genes outside of the MHC also can act as transplantation antigens. Although other antigen systems (such as ABO and Lewis blood groups, vascular endothelium cell [VEC], and tissue specific antigens) have been described, their role in human allograft rejection is less well documented. In both

---

*Supported by Grant AI-23467 from the National Institutes of Health.

rats and mice, these "minor" histocompatibility antigens can induce rejection of transplanted tissues, including hearts.

IMMUNOGENETICS OF THE HUMAN MHC

The human MHC consists of a series of genetic loci on the short arm of chromosome 6 that encode for two types of transplantation antigens (Fig. 5–1). The HLA-A, HLA-B, and HLA-C loci control the expression class I molecules, which consist of a 45 kd immunoglobulin-like glycopeptide (α chain) complexed with a 12 kd β2 microglobulin protein encoded for by a separate gene on chromosome 15.

Class I molecules exhibit extensive variations (polymorphism) of their antigenic structure, a physical characteristic that can be defined serologically by tissue typing methods using specific alloantisera and monoclonal antibodies. During the past 20 years, the definition of HLA antigens has been continually updated as the result of the efforts of many laboratories participating in histocompatibility workshops. As of the 10th International Workshop in 1987, 24 HLA-A, 50 HLA-B, and 11 HLA-C specificities have been recognized.[1]

In addition to the extensive polymorphism, one of the major characteristics of class I antigens is the high degree of cross-reactivity, which is due to structural similarity and the sharing of distinct antigens referred to as public epitopes.[2] With few exceptions, classical serology has largely ignored the definition of public determinants. However, many studies have now clearly established that class I molecules carry topologically distinct private and public antigens, both of which are involved in transplant immunity. Highly sensitized patients frequently show antibodies against public HLA antigens.

Class II HLA antigens are the second group of antigens encoded by the HLA-D region of the MHC (Fig. 5–1). This region has recently been divided into four subregions: HLA-DR, HLA-DQ, HLA-DP, and HLA-DO/DN.[1] Each subregion contains one or more genes encoding for transmembrane immunoglobulin-like glycoproteins that form dimeric molecules consisting of 33–35 kd (α) and 26–29

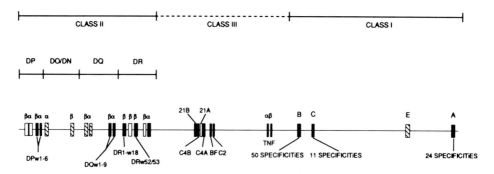

Expressed genes: black, pseudogenes: white, genes of undefined status: crosshatched

Figure 5–1. Genetic organization of the human major histocompatibility complex. Important in transplantation are class I HLA molecules, encoded by the HLA-A, HLA-B, and HLA-C loci and class II HLA molecules, encoded by loci in the HLA-D region. Between HLA-B and HLA-D are class III genes, whose products include complement components C2 and C4, factor B, 21-hydroxylase, and tumor necrosis factor.

kd (β) polypeptide chains. The degree of polymorphism differs for the α and β chains. For instance, DRα chains are nonpolymorphic, and DR polymorphism depends upon variations in the DRβ chains. On the other hand, both DQα and β chains carry antigenic determinants.[3] DP polymorphism is largely defined by the DPβ chain. Thus, at least four types of class II molecules have been identified on the cell membrane surface: DR (18 recognized specificities), the DRw52/53 system, DQ (9 specificities), and DP (6 specificities). Class II antigens are involved in the activation of T lymphocytes, primarily by virtue of their role in the presentation of foreign antigens, and they serve as a strong stimulus for allograft rejection.

HLA COMPATIBILITY AND CARDIAC TRANSPLANT SURVIVAL

The effect of HLA compatibility on transplant rejection has been most extensively studied with kidney allografts. In the early days, the superior survival rates of HLA-identical renal transplants exchanged between related donor-recipient pairs was clearly documented but the importance of HLA matching in unrelated cadaveric transplantation remained controversial. The introduction of more effective immunosuppression, particularly cyclosporine, has made it clear that HLA matching significantly improves cadaveric kidney transplant survival. This has been demonstrated not only for transplants followed over a relatively short period of time (i.e., 12 months), but more importantly, HLA matching also markedly improves long-term renal allograft survival rates.[4,5]

Although the human MHC encodes for multiple class I and class II molecules, many of them with considerable antigenic complexity, most analyses of the HLA effect on transplant outcome consider only HLA-A, HLA-B, and HLA-DR, and for these loci not all antigenic specificities are included. Nevertheless, these studies have shown that HLA antigen matching significantly improves renal transplant survival, with the strongest effect noted for HLA-DR, followed by HLA-B and HLA-A. The most convincing data have been obtained from multicenter studies because they generate a large data base, which yields sufficient numbers of transplant cases in the different match categories.

Until recently, there was little information about the effect of HLA compatibility on cardiac graft rejection. Most published reports, largely from single centers, must be considered inconclusive. Some studies showed a beneficial effect of HLA matching whereas others found no correlation.[6-8] On the other hand, HLA matching appears to be associated with a lower incidence of rejection as assessed by histologic examination of rejecting grafts.[9,10] The major problem in clearly establishing the importance of HLA for cardiac transplantation is due to the lack of prospective HLA typing and the small number of well-matched donor-recipient pairs. In contrast to kidneys, hearts are transplanted without previous consideration of HLA matching because of the time limitations for organ preservation. For cardiac transplantation, therefore, HLA matching is more a chance occurrence, and, because of polymorphism of HLA, the vast majority of cardiac allografts are mismatched for HLA. Opelz[11] recently analyzed data collected in the Collaborative Heart Transplant Study from 55 transplant centers worldwide. This retrospective analysis showed that transplants with 0 or 1 mismatch for HLA-A and HLA-B did better than transplants with a higher number of mismatched class

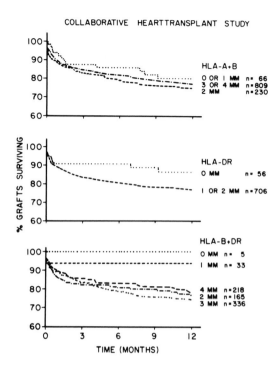

Figure 5–2. HLA mismatching and cardiac transplant survival in the collaborative heart transplant study (data kindly provided by G. Opelz), showing the effect of mismatching for HLA-A and HLA-B and the effect of mismatching for HLA-B + DR. For more details see reference 11.

I antigens (Fig. 5–2). Matching for HLA-DR antigens also is associated with improved cardiac graft survival (Fig. 5–2). Cardiac allografts with 0 and 1 mismatch for HLA-B + DR had comparatively good survival rates (Fig. 5–2). Because of the small numbers of patients, the HLA data still must be considered preliminary, and a larger series of well-matched transplants must be awaited for more definite conclusions about HLA compatibility.[11]

Humoral sensitization to HLA antigens of transplant candidates can be induced by transfusions, previous transplants, or pregnancy. The presence of humoral sensitization can be established by testing patient sera for lymphocytotoxic antibody activity against a panel of HLA-typed donors. The degree of sensitization expressed as percent panel reactive antibody (PRA) correlates with renal transplant survival. For heart transplant candidates the frequency of pretransplant sensitization is relatively low, and reduced survival of cardiac transplants has been observed for patients with PRA values of greater than 10 percent (Fig. 5–3).[11,12]

MHC COMPATIBILITY IN EXPERIMENTAL CARDIAC TRANSPLANT MODELS

The role of the MHC in cardiac transplant has been studied also in several experimental animal models, primarily inbred mice and rats (for review see reference 13). Initial studies in mice dealing with cardiac fragments transplanted into subcutaneous position in the ear showed that both class I (H-2D,K) and class II (H-21) antigens mediate cardiac allograft rejection.[14,15] These early experiments were repeated using intact, vascularized heart grafts in rats. It became evident that the response of the recipient to the vascularized graft was less vigorous than

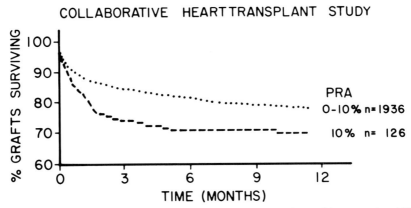

Figure 5–3. Reduced cardiac allograft survival in sensitized patients with greater than 10% panel reactive antibody. (Data kindly provided by G. Opelz, collaborative heart transplant study. For more details see reference 11.)

nonvascularized grafts, such as heart fragments or skin grafts.[16–18] This was observed for transplants across MHC barriers and in offspring to parent combinations in which there was no MHC incompatibility. These results suggest that the effect of either MHC or non-MHC histocompatibility loci on graft rejection is dampened by the presentation of the foreign heart graft as a vascularized organ. The rate of rejection depends on the donor-recipient strain combination and may not necessarily be correlated with the degree of incompatibility at the RT1 complex.[17–19]

Despite suggestions that the vascularized heart graft may be less sensitive to rejection because of differences in MHC antigens, it is clear that in both mice and rats, class I and class II antigens are capable of stimulating acute rejection. Differences in the rate of rejection of heart and skin grafts can be observed for strains that differ for individual MHC loci and/or groups of non-MHC differences (for review see references 20 and 21). Class I disparities are generally less stimulatory for cardiac rejection than class II differences between donor and recipient.[22–24] Selected class I MHC incompatibilities do not always cause rejection of heart allografts in the rat but do lead to rejection of skin grafts, indicating that class I antigens as a group may be less important than class II antigens for prospectively matching donor-recipient pairs.

It should be expected that the aforementioned rejection process is strongly influenced by a variety of poorly defined factors, some of which may include (1) immune response genes that influence the recognition and/or ability to respond to histocompatibility differences, (2) expression of tissue-specific antigens that are not identified by the traditional methods used experimentally or clinically to match donor-recipient pairs, (3) differences in the quantitative expression (modulation) of antigen expression in the graft following transplantation, and/or (4) differences in antigen recognition by the recipient as a function of the surgical placement of the graft. It is clear that until many of these variables have been defined, it will be difficult to accurately predict the outcome of a specific donor-recipient cardiac allograft exchange but that, in each individual case, the potential for an episode of acute rejection exists.[13]

ROLE OF NON-MHC ANTIGENS IN CARDIAC TRANSPLANTATION

In addition to MHC antigen systems that can be identified prospectively, either by tissue typing or by screening for lymphocytotoxic antibodies, there exist other histocompatibility systems that affect allograft survival. Some of these non-MHC antigens are collectively referred to as "minor" histocompatibility antigens by virtue of their comparison with similar loci in mice and rats, and they may include a wide variety of cell surface-associated macromolecules. Within the general category of non-MHC histocompatibility differences are blood group antigens, such as the ABO system, and other tissue-specific antigens such as the vascular endothelial cell (VEC)[25] and cardiac tissue–specific antigens.[26,40] At present, only matching for ABO blood group system is conducted before clinical cardiac transplantation because donor-specific ABO isoagglutinins may induce a hyperacute reaction of cardiac allografts.[27] In the experimental rat model, there are similar blood group systems, and the absence of the circulating isoagglutinins is associated with long-term cardiac graft survival.[20]

MECHANISMS OF ALLOGRAFT REJECTION

The general characteristics of the immune response responsible for rejection of foreign grafts, including the heart, are the recognition of donor histocompatibility differences by the recipient's immune system, followed by recruitment of activated lymphocytes, the development of immune effector mechanisms, and eventually, the destruction of the allograft. Both humoral (antibody-mediated) and cellular immune mechanisms may be involved in allograft rejection, depending primarily on the type of graft, the method of presentation, and the type of genetic disparities between donor and recipient. Allograft rejection may occur at any time following transplantation and, from a clinical standpoint, can be classified into three general categories: hyperacute rejection mediated by preformed donor-specific antibodies; cellular rejection induced by sensitized lymphocytes; and chronic rejection with the development of arteriosclerotic disease of the transplanted heart.

HYPERACUTE REJECTION

Preformed donor-specific antibodies in the recipient may cause hyperacute rejection of the allograft. This phenomenon has been studied extensively in experimental cardiac allograft models. In rats, ACI strain hearts transplanted into LEW recipients, previously sensitized with ACI skin grafts or infused with hyperimmune serum, show rapid functional rejection after less than 2 hours.[28,29] Hyperacute rejection is a vascular phenomenon and the target antigens are thought to be primarily the class I MHC antigens on the vascular endothelium, although additional non-MHC antigens might also be involved.[30,31] The early immunopathologic changes in hyperacute rejection involve deposits of immunoglobulin, complement components Clq and C3, and fibrinogen, damage to the endothelium, and aggregation of platelets in the microvasculature of the allograft.[32,33] Shortly thereafter, the affected tissues become heavily infiltrated with polymorphonuclear leukocytes, the microvascular system displays extensive damage, and there are confluent areas of myocardial necrosis.

Hyperacute rejection is caused primarily by complement-fixing antibodies, which bind to target antigens on the vascular endothelium. The antigen-antibody complexes activate the complement cascade, stimulate the generation of a variety of bioactive mediators that interact with the endothelium, thereby activating platelets, the coagulation cascade, and the attraction of polymorphonuclear leukocytes.

The presence of donor-specific cytotoxic antibodies may not always cause hyperacute rejection. Complement activation by antigen-antibody complexes requires a certain minimal density of target antigens on the cell surface.[34] The expression of class II MHC antigens is very low on normal vascular endothelium,[35,36] and class II specific antibodies are unlikely to mediate hyperacute rejection, even when they can fix complement. In certain cases, donor-specific antibodies have been shown to prolong survival of allografts.[37] Such antibodies can be identified in sera from recipients with well-established cardiac grafts and can, after transfer in a naive recipient, enhance allograft acceptance. This enhancement can be due to antihost antibodies that are capable of blocking, rather than initiating, immune damage to the graft or to anti-idiotype–specific antibodies that neutralize cytotoxic anti-HLA antibodies.[38]

In the clinical situation, preformed antibodies, either as naturally occurring ABO isohemagglutinins[27] or following sensitization of the recipient, are capable of inducing hyperacute rejection of the cardiac allograft. Cross-match testing of patient sera with donor cells may detect such preformed antibodies. Such tests, however, are not commonly performed because of the time limitations of donor heart preservation. Most patients do not show alloantibodies by lymphocytotoxicity screening, and a cross-match would likely to be negative. On the other hand, sensitized patients with greater than 10 to 15 percent PRA values are generally tested for donor-specific antibodies. A recent literature survey of eight heart transplant cases with donor-specific positive cross-matches showed only one definite and two possible hyperacute rejections.[39] However, many of these cardiac allografts failed during the first few months after transplant.[39,40]

Conversely, a negative cross-match does not preclude hyperacute rejection inasmuch as other non-MHC specific antibodies may be involved. Because the vascular endothelium is a primary target, it has been proposed that distinct VEC antigens may be recognized by such antibodies.[25,41,42] Passive transfer of HLA-specific antibodies via blood transfusions during transplant surgery might lead also to a hyperacute rejection of the cardiac allograft.[43]

T CELL ACTIVATION IN CELLULAR REJECTION

Cellular rejection is mediated by T cells that have undergone activation and functional differentiation after exposure to foreign transplantation antigens. Antigen-specific activation of lymphocytes is a two-signal process.[44] The first signal is T-cell receptor binding of antigen on the surface of an antigen-presenting cell (APC). The T cell actually recognizes a molecular complex made up of processed antigen and a self MHC molecule on the surface of the APC. This interaction induces the release of interleukin-1 (IL-1) from APC, which then, as a second signal, induces activation of the T cell. Activated T cells secrete interleukin-2 (IL-2), a lymphokine that induces further proliferation of activated T cells expressing IL-2 receptors on their surface. Other lymphokines are also produced, including B cell growth factor (interleukin-4)[45] and gamma-interferon, which regulate cell surface expression of MHC antigens.[46] T-cell activation following exposure to foreign transplantation antigens involves a similar two signal mechanism, with the exception that the T-cell receptor directly recognizes the alloantigenic determinants on foreign MHC molecules.

Two major subsets of T cells involved in graft rejection have been distinguished with monoclonal antibodies against T-cell differentiation markers.[47] Cells expressing the CD4 marker (the T helper/inducer subset) are generally reactive to or restricted by class II MHC antigens, whereas CD8+ cells (T cytotoxic/suppressor lymphocytes) are usually reactive to or restricted by class I MHC antigens. No specific function has been ascribed exclusively to these subsets; both CD4+ and CD8+ cells can produce IL-2 and other lymphokines, and both subsets can express cytolytic activity. Generally, cytotoxic CD8+ cells recognize class I MHC antigens whereas cytotoxic CD4+ cells are specific for class II MHC antigens.[48] Activated T cells of either subset may exhibit helper function, i.e., by release of lymphokines, they can induce differentiation of B cells into antibody-producing cells or expansion of other T cells to become effector cells mediating cellular immunity.[49]

Alloreactive effector cells may have cytotoxic activity and specifically kill target cells in the allograft or they could be responsible for damage via a delayed-type hypersensitivity (DTH) reaction.[50] In the latter, activated T cells, upon interaction with antigen, release lymphokines that attract and stimulate macrophages and monocytes to mediate tissue damage. In experimental models of cardiac rejection, both helper and cytotoxic T lymphocytes are involved in the rejection of the graft. Helper T cells are capable of stimulating acute rejection but complete restoration of the response depends upon both subsets and the presence of IL-2.[51]

The functions of T cells are determined to a large extent by their receptor specificity. The T-cell receptor (TCR) is a 90 kd heterodimer composed of two disulfide-linked glycoproteins containing variable and constant immunoglobulin-like domains.[52] TCR specificity is a result of gene rearrangements that control the interaction between these molecules. Two types of antigen-binding molecules expressed by T cells have been identified so far. The majority of circulating T cells express TCR of the α/β type whereas a small proportion recognize antigen via their γ/∂ receptors. Both types of TCR are associated in the T-cell membrane with a tripeptide CD3 molecule.[52] The CD3 component appears involved in signal transmission across the cell membrane after antigen binding.[53] Functional consequences of the antigen-binding to TCR-CD3 include the acquisition of responsiveness to IL-1 and IL-2.

In addition to the TCR-CD3 pathway of T cell activation, there is another pathway that involves CD2 (or T11) molecules expressed at the lymphocyte surface.[54] This alternate pathway of T-cell activation can occur in the absence of monocytes and IL-1.

INDUCTION OF CELLULAR IMMUNITY TO ALLOGRAFT

The immune response to an allograft consists of an afferent or sensitizing limb and an efferent or effector limb. Several mechanisms have been proposed for allograft sensitization; all deal with different forms of antigen presentation. The strongest effect appears to be mediated by donor-derived APC (passenger leukocytes), which migrate from the graft into the recipient lymphoid tissues where they induce activation and differentiation of recipient T cells.[44,55] These donor-derived APC could be leukocytes (e.g., monocytes) and tissue macrophages (Langerhans cells, dendritic cells). A second mechanism involves the release of soluble transplantation antigens from the allograft, which, via processing by recipient APC, induce subsequent T-cell activation in recipient lymphoid tissues. It should be noted that soluble MHC antigens by themselves are weakly immunogenic,[56] but in cooperation with APC are capable of producing a second signal for T lymphocyte alloactivation. A third mechanism involves recipient lymphocytes directly activated within the allograft itself.[57]

It is generally believed that the immune response to the transplant takes place primarily in the recipient's lymphoid tissues, which subsequently release alloreactive lymphocytes into the circulation. Accordingly, cellular rejection is caused by circulating lymphocytes, which must first interact with the microvascular endothelium, the central target of allograft destruction.[58] Endothelial damage permits infiltration of effector T lymphocytes and nonspecific inflammatory cells into the parenchymal tissues and subsequent injury to the myocardial fibers.

MECHANISMS OF CELLULAR INFILTRATION IN THE ALLOGRAFT

The early stages of allograft rejection depend on the specific recognition by circulating lymphocytes of target antigens at the surface of the microvascular endothelium. Under normal conditions, human vascular endothelium expresses class I MHC antigens but no or very few class II HLA antigens.[35,36] This restricted MHC antigen expression, which has been observed also in rats and mice,[59,60] implies that normal vascular endothelium might serve primarily as a target of class I specific cells. Indeed, during the early post-transplant period the alloreactivity of lymphocytes infiltrating the cardiac allograft tends to be more specific for class I than for class II HLA antigens of the donor.[61-63] On the other hand, MHC antigen expression on vascular endothelium is upregulated during rejection.[64,65] This could be mediated by gamma interferon released by activated T lymphocytes. This lymphokine is a potent inducer on class II HLA antigen expression by vascular endothelium.[66,67] Thus, an allograft may undergo a sequential infiltration of class I followed by class II specific cells.[62,63] Early rejection is mediated by class I specific cells, which, because of the ubiquitous expression of class I HLA antigens on the vascular endothelium, would lead to rather diffuse cellular infiltration (Fig. 5–4). Lymphokines released by class I specific cells would locally induce class II antigen expression on the vascular endothelium, and this could lead to focal infiltration of class II specific T cells. Recent in vitro studies have supported the role of specific class I and class II HLA antigens in the adherence of alloreactive lymphocytes to cultured human endothelium cell monolayers.[68] It also appears that CD4 and CD8 molecules are involved in this alloreactive lymphocyte adherence.

The sequential infiltration model is probably not the only mechanism to explain the infiltration of class II specific cells into the allograft. Other local processes, such as chronic inflammation and infection, might up-regulate class II antigen expression on vascular endothelium,[35,36] which then becomes a target of class II specific alloreactive cells.

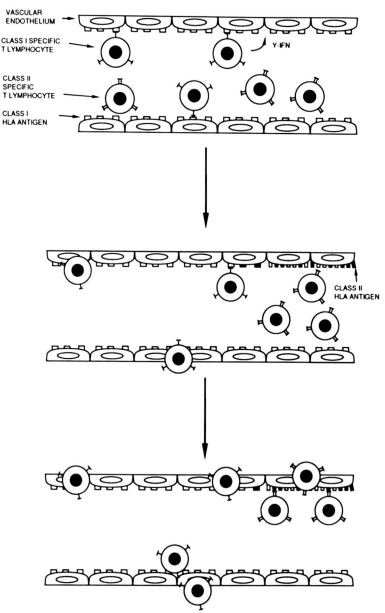

Figure 5–4. Model of sequential infiltration of allospecific lymphocytes. Resting endothelial cells bearing class I HLA antigens are recognized by only class I specific lymphocytes, which then infiltrate the graft. Upon specific binding, class I specific lymphocytes may also release lymphokines (gamma-interferon), which up-regulates class II antigen expression on vascular endothelium and then become a target of class II specific cells.

IMMUNOHISTOLOGY OF CARDIAC ALLOGRAFT REJECTION

Histologic examination of endomyocardial biopsies has become the "gold standard" used to diagnose cardiac allograft rejection in heart transplant patients.[69] Rejection is manifested by perivascular and endocardial infiltrates of mononuclear cells with extension during later phases to the interstitium and subsequent monocyte necrosis. Additional hemorrhage and infiltration of neutrophils with more extensive vascular damage may be encountered during severe rejection episodes. Immunohistologic staining of endomyocardial biopsies with T lymphocyte specific monoclonal antibodies has shown varying numbers of CD4+ and CD8+ T cells in cellular infiltrates.[70-73] Cyclosporine-treated human heart transplant recipients have mixtures of CD4+ and CD8+ cells in myocardial infiltrates, whereas in biopsies from azathioprine-treated patients, CD8+ cells are dominant.[72] Immunostaining for CD4+ and CD8+ cells and a determination of CD4/CD8 ratios, however, has been of limited prognostic value in cardiac transplant rejection.

Immunostaining has also been used to determine MHC antigen expression, especially on vascular endothelium and myocytes. Class I HLA antigens are readily detectable on vascular endothelium of normal cardiac tissue, but class II HLA antigens are absent or present in low quantities.[35,36] In transplanted hearts, endothelial expression of class I and especially class II antigen is frequently increased[74] but this expression does not correlate well with the histologic rejection grade nor with the phenotypes of T cells infiltrating the graft.[65] Sequential biopsy studies have indicated that in certain patients, increased HLA antigen expression may preceed increased histologic rejection grades.[75] Myocytes in normal cardiac tissue express very low levels of HLA antigens. In transplanted hearts, however, myocytes express class I antigens whereas conflicting reports have appeared about the expression of class II HLA antigens.[75-77] Recent studies have shown that during the early pretransplant period, increased class I antigen expression is followed by increased class II antigen expression.[78] These findings are compatible with our proposed model of sequential infiltration of class I followed by class II specific T cells in cardiac allografts.[62,63]

PROPAGATION OF LYMPHOCYTES FROM CARADIAC TRANSPLANT BIOPSIES

Recent methodologies to propagate lymphocytes from cardiac transplant biopsies have enabled additional characterization of T cell subsets involved in transplant immunity.[61] These methods are based on the concept that the graft is infiltrated by activated T lymphocytes, which can be expanded and characterized after exposure to IL-2, a potent lymphokine capable of inducing lymphocyte proliferation. The propagation of lymphocytes from heart transplant biopsies correlates with the histologic rejection grade (Fig. 5-5).[62,79] Biopsy-grown lymphocytes exhibit donor-specific alloreactivity as measured by secondary proliferation assays and cell-mediated lymphocytotoxicity.[61] This suggests that lymphocytes mediating rejection can be readily propagated from transplant biopsies containing cellular infiltrates. During the early post-transplant period, a significant number (about 30 percent) of biopsies with no or minimal cellular infiltration yield lymphocyte cultures—many with donor alloreactivity.[79] The outgrowth of cells from histologically negative cardiac biopsies is associated with a higher risk of subsequent rejection episode.[80] In our experience, biopsies from about 15 percent of cardiac transplant patients never yield lymphocyte cultures, and these patients experience a low frequency of clinical rejection episodes[80] (Fig. 5-6). Recent studies have shown a higher frequency of biopsy lymphocyte growth for heart transplant patients on OKT3 than RATG immunoprophylaxis.[81] These findings were

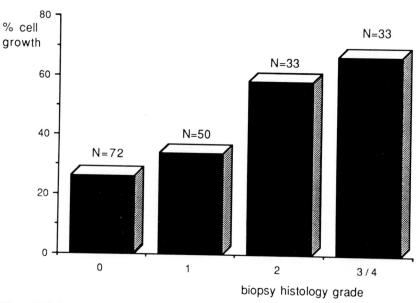

Figure 5–5. Correlation between histological rejection grade (according to Billingham[69]) and lymphocyte growth from endomyocardial biopsies cultured in vitro with interleukin-2.

consistent with observations of a higher incidence of rejection episodes in the OKT3 group.

Lymphocytes propagated from cardiac transplant biopsies generally exhibit more restricted allospecificity patterns when compared with lymphocyte cultures grown from peripheral blood. These restricted reactivity pattens may reflect a selection of cells infiltrating the allograft, perhaps related to HLA antigen expression on the vascular endothelium. Class I specific alloreactive lymphocytes have

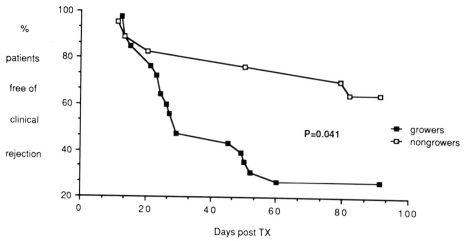

Figure 5–6. Percentage of patients free of clinical rejection with histologically negative biopsies that never yielded lymphocytes (nongrowers) or with lymphocyte growth (growers).

been propagated from biopsies obtained generally during the early post-transplant period and showing diffuse cellular infiltrates whereas class II specific cells are found in cultures from later biopsies with focal cellular infiltrates.[62,63]

CARDIAC TRANSPLANT ARTERIOSCLEROSIS

With improved therapy for rejection and infection, it has become apparent that accelerated arteriosclerotic disease has emerged as a major postsurgical complication affecting the long-term post-transplant survival of heart transplant patients. There is a 30 to 50 percent incidence of this disease 3 to 5 years after transplantation, and first evidence may be found as early as 3 months following transplant.[82–84] Pathologic changes show characteristic diffuse, concentric lesions affecting muscular arteries throughout the donor graft. There is myointimal proliferation with disruption of the internal elastic lamina. The penetrating intramyocardial branches are often occluded and this may cause an infarct before the larger pericardial arteries are affected.[83]

The etiology of cardiac transplant arteriosclerosis is unknown. Among those factors that have been suggested to be involved in the development of the disease are (1) prolonged treatment with drugs such as cyclosporine and corticosteroids that either directly or indirectly injure the graft vessels; (2) damage to the vascular endothelium, perhaps by viruses in an immunocompromised host, with acceleration of the more traditional nontransplant atherosclerosis of coronary vessels; or (3) immune damage as a result of low-grade chronic rejection. Cytotoxic antibodies directed to HLA-DR antigens on the vascular endothelium might be involved.[84] The occurrence of two or more previous rejection episodes appears associated with a higher incidence of accelerated arteriosclerosis.[85]

The appearance of arteriosclerotic lesions has been studied in several experimental models of long-term surviving heterotopic cardiac allografts (for review see reference 86). In most experimental models, prolonged graft survival was attained with immunosuppressive drug treatment. This has made it difficult to establish whether the development of arteriosclerotic lesions in these grafts was the result of immune damage secondary to rejection or was related to the toxic effects of immunosuppressive drugs.

Our understanding of the role of chronic rejection has increased through recent observations that the appearance of cardiac transplant arteriosclerosis can be stimulated by the exchanges of cardiac grafts between strains of rats differing for histocompatibility antigens that cause chronic rather than acute rejection of the graft.[86] These grafts do not require immunosuppression for long-term survival, eliminating the possible contribution of the immunosuppressive agents in the development of the lesions. The results of these studies demonstrate that weak histocompatibility antigens, both MHC and non-MHC, are capable of stimulating cardiac transplant arteriosclerosis. The possibility that transplantation across weak histocompatibility differences and/or inadequate control of graft rejection may stimulate graft arteriosclerosis suggests that improved immunosuppressive therapy may be important in preventing the development of this complication in human cardiac graft recipients. In a clinical setting, transplantation across weak histocompatibility barriers may allow for the long-term function of the graft but persistent weak episodes of graft rejection may be responsible for stimulating the arteriosclerosis.

SUMMARY

The successful application of cardiac transplantation as a useful therapeutic procedure has been the result of improved surgical techniques and the effective immunosuppression of cardiac rejection. Despite the improvements that have led to the successful application of cardiac transplantation, there are important limitations in our understanding and ability to manipulate the immune-mediated rejection of the donor heart by the host. Methods that allow for improved preservation of the donor heart are necessary to provide the opportunity to match more carefully the donor and recipient for histocompatibility antigens that stimulate rejection of the graft. Clinical data in humans and experimental studies in animals demonstrate that the rejection of the heart is stimulated by a wide variety of histocompatibility antigens, many of which may be neutralized by donor-recipient matching.

The immunologic mechanisms that influence the survival of the graft include (1) hyperacute rejection of the graft by recipient antibody directed against foreign antigens of the donor heart, (2) T lymphocyte-mediated acute cellular rejection of the graft, and (3) chronic rejection of the graft associated with the emergence of cardiac graft arteriosclerosis in otherwise successful long-term graft recipients. An increased understanding of these processes will provide opportunities to improve cardiac transplant outcome.

REFERENCES

1. Dupont, B (ed): Immunobiology of HLA. Proceedings of the Tenth International Histocompatibility Workshop, Springer-Verlag, 1988.
2. Rodey, GE and Fuller, TC: Public epitopes and the antigenic structure of the HLA molecules. CRC Crit Rev Immunol 7:229, 1987.
3. Trucco, M and Duquesnoy, RJ: Polymorphisms of the HLA-DQ subregion. Immunol Today 7:291, 1986.
4. Opelz, G: Effect of HLA matching in 10,000 cyclosporine-treated cadaver kidney transplants. Transplant Proc 19:641,646, 1987.
5. Takiff, H, Cook, DJ, Himaya, NS, et al: Dominant effect of histocompatibility on ten-year kidney transplant survival. Transplantation 45:410, 1988.
6. Stinson, EB, Griepp, RB, Payne, R, et al: Correlation of histocompatibility matching with graft rejection and survival after cardiac transplantation in man. Lancet 2:459, 1971.
7. Cooper, DKC, Boyd, ST, Lanza, RC, et al: Factors influencing survival following heart transplantation. Heart Transplant 3:86, 1983.
8. Yacoub, M. Festenstein, H, Doyle, P, et al: The influence of HLA matching in cardiac allograft recipients receiving cyclosporine and azathioprine. Transplant Proc 19:2487, 1987.
9. Zerbe, T, Arena, V, Kormos, R, et al: Role of major histocompatibility complex (HLA) matching in cardiac allograft rejection. Transplant Proc 20(Suppl 1):74, 1988.
10. Pfeffer, PF, Foerster, A, Froysaker, T, et al: Correlation between HLA-DR mismatch and rejection episodes in cardiac transplantation. Transplant Proc 19:691, 1987.
11. Opelz, G, Reichert, B, Mollner, H, et al: Preliminary results of the collaborative heart transplant study. In Reichert, B (ed): Recent Advances in Cardiovascular Surgery. Springer-Verlag, Heidelberg, 1989 (in press).
12. Kormos, RL, Colson, YL, Hardesty, RL, et al: Immunologic and blood group compatibility in cardiac transplantation. Transplant Proc 20(Suppl 1):741, 1988.
13. Cramer, DV: Cardiac transplantation: Immune mechanisms and alloantigens involved in graft rejection. CRC Crit Rev Immunol 7:1, 1987.
14. Huber, B, Demant, P, and Festenstein, H: Influence of M-locus (non-H-2 and K-end and D-end (H-2 region) incompatibility on heart muscle allograft survival time. Transplant Proc 5:1377, 1977.

15. Klein, J, Chaing, CL, Lofgreen, J, et al: Participation of H-2 regions in heart transplant rejection. Transplantation 22:384, 1976.
16. Bildsoe, P, Sorenson, SF, Pettirossi, O, et al: Heart and kidney transplantation from segregating hybrid to parental rats. Transplant Rev 3:36, 1969.
17. Barker, CF and Billingham, RE: Comparison of the fates of Ag-B locus compatible homografts of skin and hearts in inbred rats. Nature 225:851, 1970.
18. Bildsoe, P: Organ transplantation in the rat. The importance of the *Ag-B* or H-1 locus. Acta Microbiol Scand (Section B) 80:221, 1972.
19. Guttmann, RD, Forbes, RDC, Fuks, A, et al: Rejection and prolongation of rat cardiac allografts across intra-major histocompatibility complex (MHC) and non-MHC differences using congenic lines: Evidence for decreased class I immunogenicity. Transplant Proc 17:1911, 1985.
20. Katz, SM, Liebert, M, Gill, TJ, III, et al: The relative roles of MHC and non-MHC genes in heart and skin allograft survival. Transplantation 36:96, 1983.
21. Katz, SM, Cramer, DV, Kunz, HW, et al: Effect of MHC disparities on cardiac and   ft survival in the rat. Transplantation 36:463, 1983.
22. Peugh, WN, Superina, RA, Wood, KJ, et al: The role of H-2 and   -ii-2 antigens and genes in the rejection of murine cardiac allografts. Immunogenetics 23:30, 1986.
23. Burdick, JF and Clow, LW: Rejection of murine cardiac allografts. I. Relative roles of major and minor antigens. Transplantation 42:67, 1986.
24. Stepkowski, SM, Raza-Ahmad, A, and Duncan, WR: The role of class I and class II MHC antigens in the rejection of vascularized heart allografts in mice. Transplantation 44:753, 1987.
25. Cerilli, GJ and Brasile, L: Tissue specific antigens—a role in organ transplantation: A theory for the existence of tissue specific antigens *In* Cerilli, GJ (ed): Organ Transplantation and Replacement. JB Lippincott, Philadelphia, 1987, pp 208–222.
26. Harkiss, GD, Cave, P, and Brown, DL: Anti-heart antibodies in cardiac allograft recipients. Ind Arch Allerg Appl Immunol 73:19, 1984.
27. Weil, R, Clarke, DR, Iwaki, Y, et al: Hyperacute rejection of a transplanted human heart. Transplantation 323:71, 1981.
28. Guttmann, RD: Genetics of acute rejection of rat cardiac allografts and a model of hyperacute rejection. Transplantation 17:383, 1987.
29. Forbes, RDC, Guttmann, RD, and Pinto-Blonde, M: A passive transfer model of hyperacute rat cardiac allograft rejection. Lab Invest 41:348, 1979.
30. Guttmann, RD: A genetic survey of rat allograft rejection in presensitized recipients. Transplantation 22:583, 1976.
31. Guttmann, RD, Forbes, RDC, Cramer, DV, et al: Cardiac allograft rejection and enhancement in natural recombinant rat strains. Transplantation 30:216, 1980.
32. Forbes, RDC, Kuramochi, T, Guttmann, RD, et al: A controlled sequential morphologic study of hyperacute cardiac allograft rejection in the rat. Lab Invest 33:280, 1975.
33. Forbes, RDC and Guttmann, RD: Evidence for complement-induced endothelial injury *in vivo:* A comparative ultrastructural tracer study in a controlled model of hyperacute rat cardiac allograft rejection. Am J Pathol 106:378, 1982.
34. Linscott, W: The antigen density effect on the hemolytic efficiency of complement. J Immunol 104:1037, 1970.
35. Halloran, PF, Wadgymar, A, and Autenried, P: The regulation of expression of major histocompatibility complex products. Transplantation 41:413, 1986.
36. Forsum, U, Claesson, E, Hjelm, A, et al: Class II transplantation antigens: Distribution in tissues and involvement in disease. Scand J Immunol 21:389, 1985.
37. Hayry, P, Von Willebrand, E, and Parthensas, E: The inflammatory mechanisms of allograft rejection. Immunol Rev 77:85, 1984.
38. Suciu-Foca, N, Reemtsma, K, and King, DW: The significance of the idiotypic anti-idiotypic network in humans. Transplant Proc 18:230, 1986.
39. Braun, WE, Klingman, L, Steward, RW, et al: Two major serologic events in a successful cardiac transplant recipient—circumvention of hyperacute rejection despite a positive donor T lymphocyte crossmatch and late appearance of probably anti-idiotypic antibody. Transplantation 46:153, 1988.
40. Zerbe, TR, Berman, AB, Rabin, BS, et al: Cell mediated immunity to donor-specific antigen in heart transplantation. Transplant Proc 16:1514, 1984.
41. Brasile, L, Rabin, BS, Clarke, J, et al: The identification of antibody to vascular endothelial cells (VEC) in patients undergoing cardiac transplantation. Transplantation 40:672, 1985.

42. Trento, A, Hardesty, RL, Griffith, BP, et al: Role of the antibody to vascular endothelial cells in hyperacute rejection in patients undergoing cardiac transplantation. J Cardiovasc Surg 95:37, 1988.

43. Duquesnoy, RJ: A case of hyperacute rejection of a cardiac transplant. In Terasaki, P (ed): Visuals of the Clin. Histocomp. Workshop. One Lambda, Los Angeles, 1988, p 66.

44. Lafferty, KJ, Prowse, SJ, and Simeonovic, CJ: Immunobiology of tissue transplantation: A return of the passenger leukocyte concept. Am Rev Immunol 1:143, 1983.

45. Paul, WE and Ohara, J: B cell stimulatory factor -II Interleukin-4. Ann Rev Immunol 5:429, 1987.

46. Pober, J and Gimbrone, M: Expression of Ia-like antigens by human vascular endothelial cells is inducible in vitro: Demonstration by monoclonal antibody binding and immuno precipitation. Proc Natl Acad Sci 79:6441, 1982.

47. Ledbetter, JA, Evans, RL, Lipinski, M, et al: Evolutionary conservation of surface molecules that distinguish T lymphocyte helper/inducer and cytotoxic suppressor subpopulations in mouse and man. J Exp Med 153:310, 1981.

48. Swain, S: T cell subsets and the recognition of MHC class. Immunol Rev 74:129, 1983.

49. Andrus, L, Prowse, SJ, and Lafferty, KJ: Interleukin 2 production by both Lyt2$^+$ and Lyt2$^-$ T cell subsets. Scand J Immunol 13:297, 1981.

50. Mason, DW, Dallman, MJ, Arthur, RP, et al: Mechanisms of allograft rejection: The roles of cytotoxic T cells and delayed-type hypersensitivity. Immunol Rev 77:167, 1984.

51. Heidecke, CD, Kupiec-Weglinski, JW, Lear, PA, et al: Interactions between T-lymphocyte subsets supported in Interleukin-2-rich lymphokines produce acute rejection of vascularized cardiac allografts in T cell deprived rats. J Immunol 133:582, 1984.

52. Oettgen, HC and Terhorst, C: A review of the structure and function of the T-cell receptor-T3 complex. CRC Crit Rev Immunol 7:131, 1987.

53. Clever, H, Alarcon, B, Wileman, T, et al: The T cell receptor/CD3 complex: A dynamic protein ensemble. Ann Rev Immunol 6:629, 1988.

54. Meuer, S, Hussey, R, Fabbi, M, et al: An alternative pathway of T-cell activation: A functional role for the 50 kd T11 sheep erythrocyte receptor protein. Cell 36:897, 1984.

55. Tilney, NK and Bell, PRF: Studies on the enhancement of cardiac and renal allografts in the rat. Transplantation 18:31, 1974.

56. Batchelor, JR, Welsh, KI, and Burgos, H: Transplantation antigens per se are poor immunogens within a species. Nature 273:54, 1978.

57. Nembander, A, Soots, A, Von Willebrand, E, et al: Restriction of renal allograft responding leukocyte during rejection. J Exp Med 156:1087, 1982.

58. Forbes, RDC, Guttman, RD, Gomersall, M, et al: A controlled serial ultrastructural tracer study of first-set cardiac allograft rejection in the rat: Evidence that the microvasculature is the primary target of graft destruction. Am J Pathol 111:184, 1983.

59. Graziano, KD and Edidin, M: Serological quantitation of histocompatibility 2 antigens and the determination of H-2 in adult and fetal organs: Proceeding of the Symposium on Immunogenetics of the H-2 System. Karger, Basel, 1971, pp 251–256.

60. Milton, AD, Spencer, SC, and Fabre, J: The effects of cyclosporine on the induction of class I and class II MHC antigens in heart and kidney allografts in the rat. Transplantation 42:337, 1986.

61. Zeevi, A, Fung, J, Zerbe, TR, et al: Allospecificity of activated T cells grown from endomyocardial biopsies from heart transplant patients. Transplantation 41:620, 1986.

62. Fung, JJ, Zeevi, A, Markus, B, et al: Dynamics of allospecific T lymphocyte infiltration in vascularized human allografts. Immunol Res 5:149, 1986.

63. Duquesnoy, RJ, Zeevi, A, Fung, JJ, et al: Sequential infiltration of class I and class II specific alloreactive T cells in human cardiac allografts. Transplant Proc 19:1560, 1987.

64. Milton, AD, and Fabre, JW: Massive induction of donor type class I and class II major histocompatibility complex antigens in rejecting cardiac allografts in the rat. J Exp Med 161:98, 1985.

65. Singh, G, Rabin, BS, Griffith, B, et al: Post-transplant monitoring in cardiac allografts. Transplant Proc 15:1801, 1983.

66. Pober, JS, Collins, T, Gimbrone, MA, et al: Inducible expression of class II major histocompatibility antigens and the immunogenicity of vascular endothelium. Transplantation 41:141, 1986.

67. Markus, BH, Colson, YL, Fung, JJ, et al: HLA antigen expression on cultured human arterial endothelial cells. Tissue Antigens 32:241, 1988.

68. Colson, YL, Markus, BH, Zeevi, A, et al: Increased lymphocyte adherence to human arterial endothelial cell monolayers in the context of allorecognition (submitted).

69. Billingham, M: Diagnosis of cardiac rejection by endomyocardial biopsy. Heart Transplant 1:25, 1979.
70. Yacoub, MH, Gracie, JA, Rose, ML, et al: T cell characterization in human cardiac allografts. Transplantation 38:634, 1983.
71. Marboe, CC, Schierman, SW, Rose, E, et al: Characterization of mononuclear cell infiltrates in human cardiac allografts. Transplant Proc 16:1598, 1984.
72. Hoshinaga, K, Wolfgang, TC, Goldman, MH, et al: In situ identification of mononuclear cells in heart biopsies and correlation with allograft status. Transplant Proc 17:207, 1985.
73. Weintraub, D, Masek, M, and Billingham, ME: The lymphocyte subpopulations in cyclosporine-treated human heart rejection. Heart Transplant 4:213, 1985.
74. Milton, AD and Fabre, JW: Massive induction of donor-type class I and class II major histocompatibility complex antigens in rejecting allografts in the rat. J Exp Med 161:98, 1985.
75. Ahmed-Ansara, A, Radros, TS, Knopf, WD, et al: Major histocompatibility complex class I and class II expression by monocytes in cardiac biopsies post-transplantation. Transplantation 45:972, 1988.
76. Zerbe, T, White, L, Zeevi, A, et al: Tissue expression of major histocompatibility complex (HLA) antigens in cardiac allograft recipients. Transplant Proc 20:72, 1988.
77. Rose, ML, Coles, ML, Griffin, RJ, et al: Expression of class I and class II major histocompatibility antigens in normal and transplanted human heart. Transplantation 41:776, 1986.
78. Sell, KW, Tadros, T, Wang, YC, et al: Studies of MHC class I/II expression on sequential human cardiac biopsies post transplantation. Int J Heart Transplant (in press), 1988.
79. Weber, T, Kaufman, C, Zeevi, A, et al: Propagation of lymphocytes from human heart transplant biopsies: Methodologic considerations. Transplant Proc 20(Suppl 2):176, 1988.
80. Weber, T, Kaufman, C, Zeevi, A, et al: Lymphocyte growth from cardiac allograft biopsies with no or minimal cellular infiltrates: Association with subsequent rejection episode. Int J Heart Transplant (in press).
81. Kaufman, C, Zeevi, A, Weber, T, et al: Alloreactive lymphocyte propagation from endomyocardial biopsies from heart transplant patients on different immunoprophylactic protocols. In Dupont, B (ed): Immunobiology of HLA. (In press, 1988.)
82. Bieber, CP, Hunt, SA, Schwinn, DA, et al: Complications in long-term survivors of cardiac transplantation. Transplant Proc 13:207, 1981.
83. Billingham, ME: Cardiac transplant atherosclerosis. Transplant Proc 19:19, 1987.
84. Hess, ML, Hastillo, A, Mohanakumar, T, et al: Accelerated atherosclerosis in cardiac transplantation: Role of cytotoxic B-cell antibodies and hyperlipidemia. Circulation 68:94, 1983.
85. Uretsky, BF, Murali, S, Reddy, PS, et al: Development of coronary artery disease in cardiac transplant patients receiving immunosuppressive therapy with cyclosporine and prednisone. Circulation 76:827, 1987.
86. Cramer, DV, Qian, S, Harnaha, J, et al: Cardiac transplantation in the rat. I. The effect of histocompatibility differences on graft arteriosclerosis. Transplantation 47:414, 1989.

PART 3

Clinical Aspects

CHAPTER 6

Selection of Patients for Cardiac Transplantation

Andrea Hastillo, M.D.
Michael L. Hess, M.D.

Selection of recipients for cardiac transplantation is a complex process with dynamic criteria. Selection, and thus rejection, of candidates takes place because of limited donors for a growing and large group of excellent candidates, because of limited resources to care for the patients before and after transplantation, and because of other financial and economic constraints. Furthermore, as the transplant process taxes such vast and indepth resources, it is imperative that the candidates be as carefully selected as possible to survive the immediate postoperative period. The candidates also should be capable of working with the health care system to survive best long-term in a functional and socially rewarding fashion.[1,2]

Of some help to the selection process are the guidelines set forth by Medicare (Table 6–1). These guidelines, some of which will require further clarification, have changed even since published in 1987.[3]

Since cardiac transplantation first began in the United States in 1968, major changes in selection of candidates has occurred because of a change in the immunosuppressive regimen. Prior to the cyclosporine era, azathioprine and high-dose steroids were the mainstays of transplantation. Owing to major and multiple side effects of steroids, however, insulin-dependent diabetics were not considered appropriate candidates. The upper age limit for a recipient's candidacy was limited to 50 years of age, and the child who would fail to grow well on steroids was not considered an optimal candidate.

Following the introduction of cyclosporine, this major change in immunosuppressive therapy has altered candidate selection. There has been a decreasing need for high dose steroids and, in some instances, programs have even attempted to avoid maintenance prednisone.[4] With these steroid-sparing regimens, diabetics have been considered[5] and older persons have been given transplants. In general, with improved patient survival the selection criteria for candidacy have been broadened to include less ill patients and to include patients with other than solely New York Heart Association class IV failure.

Table 6–1. Selection Factors for Cardiac Transplantation

Strongly adverse factors
    Pulmonary hypertension/increased pulmonary vascular resistance
    Pulmonary infarction
    Advancing age
    Cachexia
    Compliance problems
    Renal or hepatic dysfunction
    Acute severe hemodynamic compromise
    Symptomatic peripheral or cerebrovascular disease
    Chronic obstructive pulmonary disease/chronic bronchitis
    Active systemic infection
    Systemic hypertension
    Other systemic diseases
    Second organ transplant
Other adverse factors
    Insulin-dependent diabetes mellitus
    Asymptomatic severe peripheral or cerebrovascular disease
    Documented peptic ulcer disease
    Diverticulitis

EARLY SELECTION PROCESS

The selection process begins with referral of a patient to a transplant center. The majority of patients considered appropriate candidates include those demonstrating New York Heart Association class IV or occasionally class III status. Recognition of a potential for an abrupt change from a class III to a class IV status has increased referral of these less ill patients.

If accepted, timing of initiation of a donor search is another decision to be made by the selection team. It is not an easy decision. Early studies had indicated that candidates for cardiac transplantation had a terrible prognosis if a donor could not be found.[7] More recent data such as that provided by Stevenson and coworkers[6] indicate also that patients who were medically eligible for cardiac transplantation but who were denied transplantation for other criteria demonstrated a remarkably high mortality rate at one year. In their study, 1-year survival for patients not transplantated was 21 percent versus 86 percent for those patients who were given transplants. Inasmuch as this study took place during the era of vasodilators, it demonstrates a continued poor prognosis for those patients even with the most modern medical care. Patients accepted for cardiac transplantation who are placed on computer should have an anticipated mortality with transplantation that is clearly less than without transplantation. A restricted lifestyle is an important factor in timing of transplantation, but this consideration alone is not a stringent reason to proceed with transplantation.

Selection and timing of candidacy, as already stated, should lead to a better prognosis with transplantation than without. However, one does not wish to wait until the patient is too ill to anticipate successful transplantation (raising a question of donor use) nor does one wish to potentially shorten the individual's survival by transplantation (transplanted "too early"). Unfortunately, there is no method to determine exactly when to proceed.

Unverferth and associates[8] in 1984 attempted to determine survival parameters for patients with dilated cardiomyopathy. They found that poor predictors for 1-year survival included left ventricular conduction delay (QRS complex greater than 100 msec) and elevated pulmonary capillary wedge pressure (survivors = 18 ± 9 mmHg, nonsurvivors = 25 ± 7 mmHg). Other pertinent predictors of nonsurvival were ventricular dysrhythmias, with increasing frequency and the more complex dysrhythmias predicting a worse survival. Mean right atrial pressure elevation, a low angiographic ejection fraction, atrial fibrillation or flutter, and the presence of a ventricular gallop also predicted poor outcomes. Thus, evaluation of patients with dilated cardiomyopathy and their potential for survival have provided some guidelines based on scientific data. These authors developed an equation for probability for 1-year survival, which utilized only the presence of left ventricular conduction delay, mean right atrial pressure elevation, and ventricular arrhythmias. They were able to generate curves that had an excellent prognostication for survival; however, this equation is seldom used.

One can always hope that newer drugs may afford increased survival. Although institution of afterload reduction has clearly improved the quality of life in many patients, overall survival for an individual may not be predictable. Without a doubt, patients with unstable yet chronic heart failure may be stabilized with some of these newer agents. In a study by Weber and colleagues,[9] they determined that enoximone was helpful in stabilizing patients; however, survival in these patients was still quite poor and even a positive response to enoximone did not preclude the need for transplantation. Enalapril, a more commonly used drug for heart failure, also may improve the patient's quality of life and even their functional class. The CONSENSUS Trial Study Group prospectively studied patients with severe congestive heart failure (New York Heart Association class IV).[10] This study was able to demonstrate improvement in many of the patients receiving enalapril when compared with those receiving placebo. Mortality, a definitive endpoint, was reduced by 27 percent in the enalapril group at the end of the study. The reduction in mortality was not due to a decreased incidence of sudden cardiac death but instead was due to a decreased incidence of progressive heart failure. It is impressive that use of this vasodilator may improve survival. Unfortunately the patients in these two groups were quite similar and there was no mechanism to differentiate those patients who would die from those who would not. Hence, even though a patient's quality of life might be improved, one is still faced with the decision of when to initiate the transplant process in the individual patient.

Prior to proceeding with transplantation, one must make sure that nothing reversible or otherwise remedial escapes the selection group's surveillance. A full cardiac catheterization should always be performed prior to transplantation to make sure that routine cardiac surgery cannot be utilized to help the patient. Although experimental or investigational drugs may improve the quality of life and help stabilize these candidates as a group, one must constantly be aware that survival *for an individual* cannot always be predicted.

Selection of candidates has been extended to include patients with severe multivessel coronary artery disease with poor left ventricular function for whom survival is limited should further infarction take place. Also, a group of patients with life-threatening recurrent dysrhythmias who have no alternative to survival utilizing antiarrhythmic drugs or electrophysiologic surgery may be considered candidates.

Since the inception of cardiac transplantation, another small group of candidates have been created—patients who require retransplantation. These candidates may either be in the throes of acute rejection or demonstrate the coronary disease of chronic rejection that relentlessly destroys the myocardium. Both can be successfully retransplanted, although locating an appropriate donor within the limited time constraints, prior sensitization through transfusions, and a chronic immunosuppressive state may limit the overall success rate.

The underlying disease process leading to transplantation has been compiled by the Registry of the International Society for Heart Transplantation, and the 1987 report showed that the most common underlying disease was a cardiomyopathy followed by coronary artery disease and then valvular disease.[11] Survival for patients who undergo transplantation for idiopathic cardiomyopathies and coronary artery disease are approximately the same. The risk of a 30-day nonsurvival increases if transplantation takes place for valvular disease, graft rejection, or congenital disease.

Thus, the reason patients are selected is to optimize survival, and the selection is influenced by the supply-demand problem. Referral should optimally take place before the patient is moribund. Timing of the donor search is important and may not be based often on scientific data but is often influenced by prior experience. Hopefully, transplantation will not take place too early (leading to an earlier than expected death) nor too late wherein survival is impaired because of transplanting a patient who is "too sick."

GUIDELINES FOR SELECTION

When one uses the Medicare guidelines, each contraindication, whether absolute or relative, needs some review. What is influenced by prior experience? What is based on fact? What is changing?

STRONGLY ADVERSE FACTORS

Pulmonary Hypertension

Early work[12] indicated that severely elevated pulmonary vascular resistance was associated with an abysmally early prognosis. Twenty-six patients in the early Stanford experience were studied retrospectively and were divided into three groups based on survival. Three of these patients died in less than 72 hours following transplantation and were characterized as different from the remaining two groups because they had very high pulmonary vascular resistances (11.3 Wood units versus 3.7 and 4.1 Wood units).*

Based on these observations, it was recommended that patients should not be given transplants if their pulmonary vascular resistance was greater than 10 Wood units or if their pulmonary artery mean pressure was greater than 50 mmHg. An increased risk was encountered in those patients with pulmonary vascular resistances equal to or greater than 5 Wood units or in those in whom the pulmonary artery mean pressure was equal or greater than 40 mmHg. Early death

---

$$*\text{Wood Unit} = \frac{\text{Mean Pulmonary Artery Pressure} - \text{Pulmonary Capillary Wedge Pressure}}{\text{Cardiac Output}}$$

was due to acute right ventricular failure, as the donor heart was unable to accommodate such high pressures.

By 1978 the same group had decided that if the pulmonary vascular resistance was fixed (no significant response to vasodilators) and greater than 8 Wood units, this finding was a contraindication to orthotopic cardiac transplantation.[13] The Arizona group initially used 8 Wood units as an absolute contraindication to orthotopic transplantation. Their cutoff still exists.[5] Currently this group uses a pulmonary vascular resistance of less than 4 Wood units as an acceptable level for routine orthotopic cardiac transplantation and they do not change their donor matching unless the pulmonary vascular resistance increases to 4 to 8 Wood units, at which time an oversized donor heart is employed. Many programs subscribe to these guidelines.

Because of the great concern of early death owing to acute right heart failure in the presence of fixed severe pulmonary hypertension, many attempts have been undertaken to devise mechanisms by which to separate reversible from irreversible pulmonary hypertension. Use of a vasodilator such as nitroprusside has become fairly common, with some comfort afforded by a fall in the pulmonary vascular resistance to lower levels. However, as demonstrated by the Columbia group,[14] even patients whose pulmonary vascular resistance remained high (8.4 and 7.8 Wood units) were able to survive. Other centers, on the other hand, have demonstrated that the opposite may occur[15] or that such a finding is not helpful.[16]

Other variations occur. The Pittsburgh group retrospectively studied 187 orthotopic recipients and found that early survival (7 and 30 days) did not correlate best with a pulmonary vascular resistance of less than 6. In patients with pulmonary vascular resistances less than 6, 7- and 30-day survival was 88 and 85 percent, respectively; however, even if the pulmonary vascular resistance was greater or equal to 6 Wood units, respective survival was still 92 and 85 percent. This group discovered that a better predictor of survival was the transpulmonary gradient* (TPG). Patients with TPGs less than 10 had better survival rates than patients with TPGs between 10 and 15; survival was even worse if the transpulmonary gradient was greater than 15.[17]

Further work needs to be done to discern which patients absolutely demonstrate contraindications for orthotopic transplantation, which patients should be selected to receive heterotopic cardiac transplantation, and in which patients use of a large donor heart should be adequate to prevent early or fatal right heart failure. Reversibility of pulmonary hypertension as judged by nitroprusside infusion is continuously being studied, and calculations of a pulmonary vascular resistance index is being studied also.[18]

Until definitive guidelines are available, it would seem reasonable to restudy the patient with an elevated pulmonary vascular resistance if the wait is long, in order to avoid the finding of surprisingly high resistances in the operating room.[19] Also, one should consider larger donors for patients with pulmonary vascular resistances greater than 4 in whom orthotopic cardiac transplantation is being undertaken. Heterotopic transplantation is a consideration for patients with pulmonary vascular resistances greater than 8. No clear cutoff of a numerical pul-

---

*TPG = Mean Pulmonary Artery Pressure − Pulmonary Capillary Wedge Pressure

monary vascular resistance, however, has been documented as an absolute contraindication based on available data.

Pulmonary Infarction

Many statements are found in the literature that recent pulmonary infarction or unresolved pulmonary infarction is a contraindication to transplantation.[5] The reason offered has been that a nonhealed pulmonary infarction will increase the risk for pulmonary abscess formation and infection.[13] Exactly how long a pulmonary infarction is termed "fresh" is unknown, and some groups even suggest that infarction must reach the scar stage prior to transplantation consideration. On the other hand, Yacoub and his group believe that patients with both acute pulmonary infarction and acute transplantation can be managed.[20]

They have transplanted eight patients with evidence of acute preoperative pulmonary infarction. Of these, seven patients survived. Survival, however, was not easy. Four patients required surgical intervention, and one expired. The postoperative management consisted of continued antibiotics and anticoagulation plus increased attention to nutritional support in the face of an empyema. In those patients whose pulmonary infarction resolved without surgery, resolution appeared to be complete in as few as 2 weeks and in as many as 7 weeks after surgery. The longest acute postoperative hospitalization period was only 22 days. Of those patients requiring surgery, one expired 13 days after transplantation owing to sepsis. He had been very ill preoperatively with acute renal insufficiency and he developed an acute empyema 4 days after transplant. Of the three other patients who underwent surgery and survived, one was a heterotopic recipient who required a tube thoracostomy, rib resection, and open drainage. The second patient required a Monaldie drainage, and the third required a right thoracotomy and decortication.

Thus, in contrast to the usual rules, Yacoub and his colleagues are willing to perform transplantation on patients with acute pulmonary infarction; and they have had a reasonable success rate, although their patients' postoperative course was clearly more complex. Current general policies, however, still require a potential recipient with a recent pulmonary infarction to wait for some degree of time until a healing process begins.

Patients who have no clearcut pulmonary infarction or embolization but who have abnormal chest roentgenograms should be thoroughly evaluated before transplantation. Occasionally one will find a lung cancer, which obviously should preclude transplantation, or one may find an asymptomatic pulmonary infarction. Explanation of any pulmonary roentgenographic abnormalities should be complete prior to transplantation.

Advancing Age

In the precyclosporine era, patients over age 50 were often not considered candidates owing to major side effects and lower survival rates[13] encountered with the high-dose prednisone program. More recently, programs have extended the upper age limit as steroid-sparing protocols have been instituted. Even the Medicare document—stressing that advancing age is a strongly adverse factor—states that adequately young "physiologic" age and the absence of significant and coexisting disease may allow patients beyond the age of 50 years to be candidates.

It is not surprising that an increasing number of older patients have been transplanted beyond the age of 50. The Registry of the International Society of Heart Transplantation's fourth official report in 1987 indicated that more than one fourth of patients reported to have undergone cardiac transplantation were aged 50 or older;[11] 1194 patients in the 50+ age group have been given transplants, with six of these patients aged 65 to 69 years. Thirty-day survival based on age groups does not indicate any significant difference between patients in the older age group (50 years or greater) and patients in the younger adult group (ages 20 to 49). The mortality of the younger group at 30 days ranged from 9.67 to 16.74 percent, whereas that in the 50-year or older age group ranged from 9.41 to 16.67 percent. In fact, survival for those patients in the age group of 55 to 64, percentagewise, was better than most of the other age groups, although this difference was not statistically significant. It appears, therefore, that the older patient can be successfully transplanted but one should suspect that their survival, which remains no different than the younger age group, may in fact be the result of a more careful selection process.

On the other hand, survival in the pediatric population remains nearly the same as in the adult. In the past, fewer pediatric transplants were done owing to steroid growth retardation. With use of cyclosporine and use of lower amounts of steroids the pediatric population may expand considerably in the future. Many considerations exist concerning the candidacy of the newborn and the extremely young but this may not be based on medical issues. Thus, the age limitations formerly imposed have been rescinded in this newer era of low-dose steroids with excellent results—at least in the older population—but one must continue to review the older patient perhaps with more attention to the possibility of coexisting cerebrovascular and peripheral vascular disease.

Even the Arizona group, which has championed acceptance of the older patient, has indicated that age still remains a significant selection factor. Their data indicate that, of those individuals referred, the percentage accepted in the older age group is less than in the younger age group. Survival in their program for patients older than 50 years of age has not differed significantly from survival in the younger group.[21]

Cachexia

Surgeons and nutritionists have long been aware of the fact that a poor nutritional status may be predictive of a significant increase in mortality and morbidity.[22] Data specific to cardiac transplantation, however, are scant. One preliminary report specifically addressed nutritional management of the heart transplant recipient.[23] They were able to demonstrate clearly that utilizing the usual laboratory parameters* for nutrition they were able to predict a better or poorer outcome for a specific patient. Although their group was small they were able to show that 5 of 10 patients who had severely compromised nutrition died; 3 of 13 who were marginally compromised died but only 6 of 29 who had adequate nutrition expired. The point of their study was not to use poor nutrition as a contraindication to transplantation but instead to indicate which individuals would need a more concentrated perioperative and postoperative nutritional support. It is

---

*Albumin, transferrin, total lymphocyte count, glucose, cholesterol and triglycerides, BUN, creatinine, and potassium, combined with anthropometric parameters.

noteworthy that in those patients who did expire, infection was the most common cause of death. Although severe cachexia is listed as an adverse factor for transplantation, definition of cachexia may be quite difficult. By the time many patients are referred for transplantation they are severely ill with marked muscle mass loss. During the waiting process a marginally compromised patient may become a severely compromised patient. Thus, one must pay careful attention to the absolute parameters used to define nutritional status.[24] Effort is necessary to maintain nutrition in patients who are not compromised, and extra effort is necessary to improve the nutritional status of patients who are acceptable candidates but marginally so. As the wait for donors has become so extended, certainly time is now available to improve the nutritional status of patients, which may, in some instances, include total parenteral nutrition.[25] It is sometimes very difficult to maintain nutritional status just with oral supplements inasmuch as nausea, anorexia, and vomiting are common features of the patient with end-stage congestive failure and absorption may be hindered by bowel edema.

Compliance

There is a strong belief permeating the transplant community that strong family support and a strong urge to live will favorably influence transplant survival. The opposite, therefore, is considered detrimental.

In an attempt to find objective evidence for future commitment to excellent self-care, one often will look at demonstrated compliance to a medical regimen and avoidance of substance abuse. Early data such as those proposed by Cooper and colleagues[26] have indicated that failure of patients who have undergone heart transplantation to comply with their physician's wishes predicted a poor outcome. This group indicated that nine patients with noncompliant behavior (mostly relating to medications) had poor post-transplant outcomes. Their study has had a great impact on how one will currently evaluate patients. Definition of medical compliance is not an exact process, however, and often, especially when a young adult is stricken with an acute and galloping viral cardiomyopathy, such a parameter is not applicable. Then one may focus one's attention on how an individual is behaving during the acute situation in the hospital. At times there are no strong guidelines to help determine whether a patient will be able to comply with a future complex medical regimen. Of course, when dealing with the pediatric population one often must shift the focus to the parent or caretaker and away from the child.

Many factors are involved in a patient's "compliance." Even in the modern age of patient enlightenment, the physician may tell a patient to take drugs but give no clearcut explanation as to why. The patient may become somewhat confused because many different names may exist for one drug and because the patient may not understand that scheduling of drugs at home is often different from that in the hospital. Moreover, as we have encountered, patients may be given written prescriptions and the physician may not recognize the fact that the patient cannot read. Patients have been labeled noncompliant because of this. Thus, when one selects patients based predominantly on compliance, one must factor in how the patient has been taught about drugs and what learning disabilities may be present.

Compliance, of course, goes beyond taking certain drugs, taking drugs at a certain time, taking certain dosages, and avoiding those not prescribed. One must also be compliant in keeping a complex medical followup, avoiding or curtailing substance abuse, and keeping certain records. Unfortunately, the psychosocial evaluation is not standardized and the individual's reaction may fluctuate from day-to-day as to how he or she will interact with the interviewer. Additionally, one may change one's behavior pattern depending on the input from the caring medical team. A patient's compliance may improve in response to a change of medical teams, and, before totally abolishing a patient's candidacy based on psychosocial reasons (unless clearly obvious) one must give the patient a second chance.

The Utah Cardiac Transplant Program, which retrospectively studied patients referred for cardiac transplantation or for heart failure, demonstrated that psychosocial exclusions were neither static nor flawless.[27] Of 151 patients referred for transplant, 37 were not accepted—23 for medical reasons, 2 for definite psychosocial reasons, and 12 for possible psychosocial reasons.

Over time, 9 of the latter 12 were accepted and 7 were successfully transplanted. These patients had had no definite contraindication to transplantation but were borderline and thus were enrolled in a close followup program under investigational protocols. As the same physicians and staff were involved in both the transplant and investigational protocols, they were able to later determine that these individuals could demonstrate acceptable psychosocial parameters and they were later accepted into the transplant program. Thus, if time permits, more data can be provided with such a followup and more patients may be found to be acceptable candidates.

Of particular note in the study is that survival statistics indicated that of the seven patients accepted for transplantation that were initially deferred, all were alive. Of those 64 patients who were immediately accepted for transplantation, survival was 90 percent at the same time after transplantation.

What should one do about substance abuse? There are many patients who have had a problem with substance abuse but who have discontinued this habit and have proven themselves to be excellent candidates and survivors after transplantation.[28] However, patients who continue with active alcoholism jeopardize not only their current life but also their ability to reliably follow a complex medical regimen. Current drug abusers likewise jeopardize their ability to follow complex medical regimens and, if they use intravenous drugs, clearly increase their risk of infection. These subsets of patients do not appear to be good candidates.

Certain psychiatric diagnoses may present a more acceptable contraindication to transplantation although dissension still exists.[29,30] Depression itself must be scrutinized inasmuch as many patients have situational depression that may be managed successfully with psychiatric input. Patients who are considered for transplantation should be seen by the psychiatric team to evaluate their ability to deal with transplantation and to review them for possible contraindications. Presently, however, there appears to be no single test to determine which patient will be compliant in the future. Medical contraindications to transplantation are much more readily handled by the patient and their family than psychosocial contraindications and perhaps one has less firm ground to stand on when a patient is rejected for psychosocial reasons. Yet to be tested are the legal aspects of this form of patient selection.[31]

It has also been stated that a strong family support is necessary to the success of cardiac transplantation. With the exception of the pediatric population, it seems that many individuals, at least in our experience, who do not have strong family support are still excellent candidates. Many have demonstrated strong ability to cope with the stresses of waiting for transplantation, undergoing transplantation, and then facing the stresses of uncertainty after transplantation. Again, help from social services, psychiatry, and psychology coupled with the common sense of the other transplant team members can help define which patients may be better candidates when a strong family support system is lacking.

Psychosoical reasons for selection are more nebulous and they are the most difficult and intangible reasons currently utilized for selection. Longitudinal followup of some individuals who have initially been rejected should be offered, if possible, to see whether patients who have no definitive psychosocial contraindications but who are not clearcut candidates could eventually fall into one or the other groups. Psychiatry and psychology experts need to continue working with one another to help devise mechanisms and tests to separate a potentially compliant from a potentially noncompliant patient. Extra effort must be made by the transplant group to help support individuals who may not have strong family support systems, who demonstrate more anxiety, whose personality may require more exogenous input than others, and whose sophistication of medical matters or education may be potential problems.

Infection

Because immunosuppressive drugs will lower the patient's immunity, one must be careful not to give transplants to patients with currently active infections. Before transplantation, specific attention should be given to potential sources of infection including recent exacerbations of diverticulitis, recurrent cholecystitis, recurrent urinary tract infections, and bronchitis. One must also pay careful attention to a patient's dental status and should attempt to have patients seen by oral surgery consultants to avoid acute post-transplant dental emergencies. During the lengthy waiting period, we attempt to avoid Foley catheterization as long as possible. Avoidance of central lines, prevention of atelectasis, and meticulous attention to any intravenous site are emphasized.

Renal or Hepatic Dysfunction

Severe renal or hepatic dysfunction that is not secondary to heart failure and is not believed to be reversible may preclude transplantation. Use of cyclosporine—a well-known nephrotoxic agent—will be restricted in patients with severe renal insufficiency.

Acute Severe Hemodynamic Compromise

Some patients deteriorate during their long waiting periods and some patients, at the time of referral, are "too sick" to be transplanted. Although the Pittsburgh group demonstrated excellent graft survival in mortally ill patients,[32] donors at that time were more readily located and the recipients' waiting time much less. These mortally ill patients were on inotropic agents while waiting. Currently, however, with the severe donor restrictions, often the only patients who ascend the waiting list are those who are not only receiving inotropic drugs but also on mechanical assist devices. The formally "mortally" ill are now common status patients. What makes a patient truly moribund and clearly not a viable candidate most probably would be loss of cerebral function. It is often difficult to determine what is or is not reversible. It is also very difficult, if a patient reaches this hemodynamic status after a long wait, to tell the family that the patient is now "too sick" to proceed with transplantation.

Symptomatic Cerebrovascular and Peripheral Vascular Disease

Symptomatic cerebrovascular and peripheral vascular disease are adverse factors to transplantation. An increased risk for an intraoperative stroke exists if they have symptomatic cerebrovascular disease. Increased progression of peripheral vascular disease in patients on immunosuppressive agents, specifically steroids, is a problem with already symptomatic peripheral vascular disease. Inasmuch as one cannot determine before transplantation who will or will not require steroids, this exacerbation continues to be a concern. Palliative surgery in this group of patients is more risky owing to poor wound healing, increased risks of infection, and possible Addisonian crisis depending on the immunosuppressive regimen.

Chronic Obstructive Pulmonary Disease and Chronic Bronchitis

Chronic obstructive pulmonary disease and chronic bronchitis are actually different diseases in that the latter is a risk factor for chronic infection, which in the postoperative course could be fatal. The former, chronic obstructive pulmonary disease, could interfere seriously with the perioperative weaning and later could negatively affect the improvement in the functional status of the patient during the rehabilitative phase. No specific pulmonary function tests are available to delineate an acceptable from an unacceptable patient with chronic obstructive pulmonary disease. Patients who have smoked should be scrutinized for these problems before acceptance.

Active Systemic Infection

Active systemic infection has been a strong adverse factor to transplantation owing to the need for immunosuppressive agents. Currently, as steroid doses can be decreased, one might consider proceeding with caution earlier in some patients who are being treated for a formerly active systemic infection.

Systemic Hypertension

Systemic hypertension should be considered as a selection factor. Over 90 percent of the cardiac transplant recipients will develop hypertension[33] and, if they have a history of severe systemic hypertension requiring multiple drugs for control, one might consider this a reason not to offer transplantation.

Other Problems

Many other diseases may be considered contraindications to transplantation if they severely restrict the rehabilitative phase of the patient or if they would be fatal in themselves. Sarcoidosis at one time was a contraindication to transplantation; however, many such patients have been given successful transplants.[32,34] One needs to determine the activity of the sarcoidosis and the extent of this disease before these patients are rejected. Amyloid heart disease has been treated with transplantation but unfortunately the underlying disease may recur,[35] and currently patients with amyloid heart disease are not considered good candidates. When evaluating individuals with prior cancer, one must attempt to determine the survival statistics for the individual cancer and make a judgment based on the patient and the extent of the previous disease.[36,37] We have performed a transplant successfully in one patient with a prior renal cell carcinoma whose life at 20 months continues in a normal fashion.

Other Transplantation

Medicare standards currently will not permit payment for patients who have had previous transplantation of a different organ or who need other organ transplantation concomitantly. This is due to the complexity of the situation and the fact that overall survival for at least one of the organs may decrease survival for the other organ. Some centers, however, will perform multiple organ transplantations or sequential transplantations. Multiple organ transplants will need to be individualized and may be considered investigational.

OTHER POTENTIALLY ADVERSE BUT LESSER FACTORS

Diabetes Mellitus

During the history of cardiac transplantation, insulin-dependent diabetes mellitus was considered a contraindication to the procedure.[38] Our own experience at Medical College of Virginia (MCV) was that of a high incidence of steroid-induced insulin-requiring diabetes mellitus in the precyclosporine era. Thankfully the majority of these patients were able to be managed without insulin as prednisone was lowered. Moreover, one of our longest-living early survivors was a pretransplant non–insulin-dependent diabetic, and the MCV program had not excluded patients treated with diet or with oral hypoglycemic agents.

Though the majority of transplant programs currently will still not transplant insulin-dependent diabetics, once again deviations from the common rules are occurring.[39] As more and more transplant protocols are using low-dose or no-dose maintenance steroids, reconsideration has been given to transplanting the non-complicated diabetic on insulin who does not have evidence of other end-organ damage. Copeland[5] states that his group is willing to perform transplants for patients with insulin-requiring adult-onset diabetes. However, patients who have manifestations of target end-organ damage due to diabetes, who are "brittle" diabetics, or who are otherwise complicated diabetics would not be candidates. Thus, once again an absolute contraindication has become, in some institutions, a relative contraindication.

Asymptomatic Severe Peripheral Vascular/Cardiovascular Disease

As is true with symptomatic severe vascular disease, one worries about the potential of steroids to hasten the advancement of peripheral and cerebrovascular disease. As noted previously, surgical inpatients receiving chronic steroid therapy may be jeopardized by the potential for Addisonian crisis, poor wound healing, and increased infection.

Documented Peptic Ulcer

It is not uncommon that chronically ill patients have had gastrointestinal bleeding, usually of a gastritis or stress-induced nature. Inasmuch as peptic ulcer disease may be exacerbated or renewed in the postoperative period, at least patients with active or recent peptic ulcer disease are considered poor candidates. However, there have been many successfully transplanted patients who have had a distant history of peptic ulcer disease.

Diverticulitis

As the patient population becomes older, more patients with presumptive diverticular disease will be given transplants. Active diverticulitis is considered an adverse factor because of the possibility of sepsis and death. In our program we have encountered post-transplant patients with unsuspected diverticular disease who present with an acute febrile illness. Often their abdominal examinations are generally unremarkable, and only after an extensive search are they found to have diverticulitis. Diverting colostomies have been performed in a few of these patients. Hence, a recent or current history of diverticulitis should preclude cardiac transplantation at that time.

CONCLUSION

Selection of candidates for transplantation remains an important but difficult part of the transplant process. As transplantation continues to be offered to more patients and as the donor pool continues to lag behind the demand, the selection process may change even more. Is cigarette smoking to be considered an adverse factor? Is obesity a major concern? Should the patient with severe lipid abnormalities be rejected? Who should control the selection process, and why should a selection process take place will most probably be debated and contested as time passes.

Currently, the selection process is designed basically to match the donor gift to the individual who will offer the best survival. How this concept changes in the future will be greatly influenced by financial, ethical, judicial, and political considerations.

REFERENCES

1. Brennan, AF, Davis, MH, Buchholz, DJ, et al: Predictors of quality of life following cardiac transplantation. Psychosomatics 28:566, 1987.
2. Freeman, AM, III, Folks, DG, Sokol, RS, et al: Cardiac transplantation: Clinical correlates of psychiatric outcome. Psychosomatics 29:47, 1988.
3. Federal Register 52:10949, 1987.
4. Katz, MR, Barnhart, GR, Szentpetery, S, et al: Are steroids essential for successful maintenance of immunosuppression in heart transplantation? J Heart Transplant 6:293, 1987.
5. Copeland, JG: Cardiac Transplantation: Current Problems in Cardiology. Vol 13. Year Book Medical Publishers, Chicago, March 1988.
6. Stevenson, LW, Fowler, MB, Schroeder, JS, et al: Patients denied cardiac transplantation for non-medical criteria: A control group. J Am Coll Cardiol 7:9A, 1986.
7. Pennock, JL, Oyer, PE, Reitz, BA, et al: Cardiac transplantation in perspective for the future: Survival, complications, rehabilitation, and cost. J Thorac Cardiovasc Surg 83:168, 1982.
8. Unverferth, DV, Magorien, RD, Moeschberger, ML, et al: Factors influencing the one-year mortality of dilated cardiomyopathy. Am J Cardiol 54:147, 1984.
9. Weber, KT, Janicki, JS, and Jain, MC: Enoximone (MDL 17,043), a phosphodiesterase inhibitor, in the treatment of advanced, unstable chronic heart failure. J Heart Transplant 5:105, 1986.
10. The CONSENSUS Trial Study Group: Effects of enalapril on mortality in severe congestive heart failure: Results of the Cooperative North Scandinavian Enalapril Survival Study (CONSENSUS). N Engl J Med 316:1429, 1987.

11. Kaye, MP: The Registry of the International Society for Heart Transplantation: Fourth official report—1987. J Heart Transplant 6:63, 1987.
12. Griepp, RB, Stinson, EB, Dong, E, Jr, et al: Determinants of operative risk in human heart transplantation. Am J Surg 122:192, 1971.
13. Schroeder, JS: Current status of cardiac transplantation, 1978. JAMA 241:2069, 1979.
14. Addonizio, LJ, Robbins, RC, Reison, DS, et al: Transplantation in patients with high pulmonary vascular resistance. J Heart Transplant 5:394, 1986.
15. Dreyfus, G, Guillemain, R, Amrein, C, et al: The inability of pulmonary vascular resistance measurements to predict posttransplant right ventricular failure. J Heart Transplant 5:378, 1986.
16. Copeland, JG, Emery, RW, Levinson, MM, et al: Selection of patients for cardiac transplantation. Circulation 75:2, 1987.
17. Kormos, RL, Thompson, M, Hardesty, RL, et al: Utility of preoperative right heart catheterization data as a predictor of survival after heart transplantation. J Heart Transplant 5:391, 1986.
18. Kirklin, JK, Naftel, DC, Kirklin, JW, et al: Pulmonary vascular resistance and the risk of cardiac transplantation. J Heart Transplant 7:125, 1988.
19. Fonger, JD, Borkon, AM, Baumgartner, WA, et al: Acute right ventricular failure following heart transplantation: Improvement with prostaglandin E_1 and right ventricular assist. J Heart Transplant 5:317, 1986.
20. Young, JN, Yazbeck, J, Esposito, G, et al: The influence of acute preoperative pulmonary infarction on the results of heart transplantation. J Heart Transplant 5:20, 1986.
21. Carrier, M, Emery, RW, Riley, JE, et al: Cardiac transplantation in patients over 50 years of age. J Am Coll Cardiol 8:285, 1986.
22. Mullen, JL, Gertner, MH, Buzby, GP, et al: Implications of malnutrition in the surgical patient. Arch Surg 114:121, 1979.
23. Frazier, OH, Van Buren, CT, Poindexter, SM, et al: Nutritional management of the heart transplant recipient. Heart Transplant 4:450, 1985.
24. Jensen, TG, Englert, DM, and Dudrick, SJ: Interpretation of nutritional assessment data. Nutr Supp Serv 1:14, 1981.
25. Poindexter, SM, Dear, WE, and Dudrick, SJ: Nutrition in Congestive Heart Failure in Nutrition in Clinical Practice. Am Soc Parent Ent Nutr 1986.
26. Cooper, DKC, Lanza, RP, and Barnard, CN: Noncompliance in heart transplant recipients: The Cape Town experience. Heart Transplant 3:248, 1984.
27. Herrick, CM, Mealey, PC, Tischner, LL, et al: Combined heart failure transplant program: Advantages in assessing medical compliance. J Heart Transplant 6:141, 1987.
28. Holland, C, Hagan, M, Volkman, K, et al: Substance abuse: Does this warrant exclusion for transplant. J Heart Transplant 7:70, 1988.
29. Frierson, RL and Lippmann, SB: Heart transplant candidates rejected on psychiatric indications. Psychosomatics 28:347, 1987.
30. Kay, J and Bienenfeld, D: Psychiatric qualifiers for heart transplant candidates. Psychosomatics 29:143, 1988.
31. Merrikin, KJ and Overcast, TD: Patient selection for heart transplantation: When is a discriminating choice discrimination? Journal Health Politics, Policy and Law 10:7, 1985.
32. Hardesty, RL, Griffith, BP, Trento, A, et al: Mortally ill patients and excellent survival following cardiac transplantation. Ann Thorac Surg 41:126, 1986.
33. Olivari, M-T, Antolick, A, and Ring, WS: Arterial hypertension after cardiac transplant with triple-drug immunosuppression therapy. J Heart Transplant 7:71, 1988.
34. Valantine, HA, Tazelaar, HD, Macoviak, J, et al: Cardiac sarcoidosis: Response to steroids and transplantation. J Heart Transplant 6:244, 1987.
35. Conner, R, Hosenpud, JD, Norman, DJ, et al: Heart transplantation for cardiac amyloidosis: Successful one-year outcome despite recurrence of the disease. J Heart Transplant 7:165, 1988.
36. Penn, I: Problems of cancer in organ transplantation. Heart Transplant 2:71, 1988.
37. Penn, I: Renal transplantation in patients with preexisting malignancies. Transplant Proc 15:1079, 1983.
38. Baumgartner, WA, Borkon, AM, Achuff, SC, et al: Heart and heart-lung transplantation: Program, development, organization, and initiation. Heart Transplant 4:197, 1985.
39. McAleer-Rhenman, MJ, Rhenman, B, Icenogle, TB, et al: Diabetes mellitus in heart transplantation. J Heart Transplant 7:64, 1988.

CHAPTER 7

Donor Identification
and Organ Procurement
for Cardiac Transplantation

Luis Sergio Fragomeni, M.D.
Gayl Rogers, R.N., B.A.N., M.B.A.
Michael P. Kaye, M.D.

The overall picture of heart transplantation is much different from that of 20 years ago when the first transplant was performed at the Groote Schuur Hospital in South Africa.[1] With the initial enthusiasm, a widespread number of heart transplants were performed in 17 different countries until 1969. As a consequence of the initial poor results, clinical cardiac transplantation was subsequently confined to few centers, with Stanford being the most active. Their important continuing investigation established the criteria of donor and recipient selection, immunosuppression, diagnosis of rejection, control of infection, and understanding of long-term complications. Heart transplantation currently is an established form of treatment for end-stage heart disease. The Registry of the International Society for Heart Transplantation currently reports a worldwide 1 year survival of 86.4 percent, with 84 percent of these patients alive after 5 years.[2] With an increasing number of referrals of cardiac recipients and the present scarcity of donors, distant donor heart procurement has become a necessity. More than 100 cardiac units performing heart transplant at present in the United States are dependent on distant organ procurement. The current organization of Transplant Donor Services and the affiliated transplant centers with an Organ Donor Coordinator always available has allowed maximum cooperation and subsequent successful transplantation. Inasmuch as donor availability is the major limiting factor, it is critical that every referral is optimized and the organ successfully transplanted. Better donor selection, management, and organ preservation has resulted in good results following 4 hours of ischemia.[3,4] Expansion of the criteria for heart donors has also increased, to a small degree, the number of available organs. Despite the fact that the number of transplants has steadily increased in the United States (1436 in 1987), more patients die while on the waiting list than after the transplant. It has been estimated that annually 12,000 to 14,000 brain-dead patients would have an adequate heart for transplantation,[5] but, in fact, only about 10 percent become heart donors. Continuing education of the professionals and the public in this complex matter, with its medical, social and legal implications, will benefit a great number of patients by increasing organ donation.

DONOR IDENTIFICATION

The donation and procurement of organs and tissues is a complex process involving many people (Fig. 7-1). It requires trust and cooperation between the donor hospital and the transplant facility and careful coordination for efficient, optimal results.

The process begins in the hospital when a potential organ donor is identified. Federal legislation has been enacted and most states have implemented laws requiring that the family of the deceased be approached and given the option to donate organs and tissues upon any hospital death.

Early identification of the donor is essential to maximize the viability of the organs. The specific organs or tissues that can be donated are related to the circumstances of the death and the present function of the organs.

DONOR REFERRAL

In our area, Transplant Donor Services of the St. Paul Red Cross provides toll-free phone numbers (Twin Cities, Minnesota, continental United States) to receive referrals of potential organ/tissue donors. An organ donor coordinator receives the call and initiates the complex process of evaluation of the potential donor and the procurement of a viable heart for transplant.

In general, it is useful for the organ donor coordinator to obtain the following information with the initial donor referral call: (1) the patient's name, age, weight, height, and sex; (2) blood type; (3) brain-death status; (4) whether the family has been approached for consent; (5) laboratory values from admission date and currently; (6) medications; (7) vital signs; (8) urine output; and (9) a short patient history and cause of death.

DONOR CONSENT

The request of organ donation is of utmost importance and should be handled with empathy, sensitivity, and honesty. The family should be presented with the "option" to donate and never pressured into a decision about which they are uncomfortable. Organ donation is an opportunity to make a positive, valuable contribution following an unexpected death. Most donor families feel comfort in the recognition that their gift helped others to live and to lead healthier lives.

In 1970 the Uniform Anatomical Gift Act was passed in the United States. Under this bill, any person has the legal right to donate all or part of his or her body after death, and the next of kin has the legal right to donate the loved one's organs should brain death occur. In practice, written consent is always obtained from the next of kin, even when there is a signed donor card.

Consent from the potential donor's family can be obtained by hospital staff or an organ donor coordinator. The family should not be approached about dona-

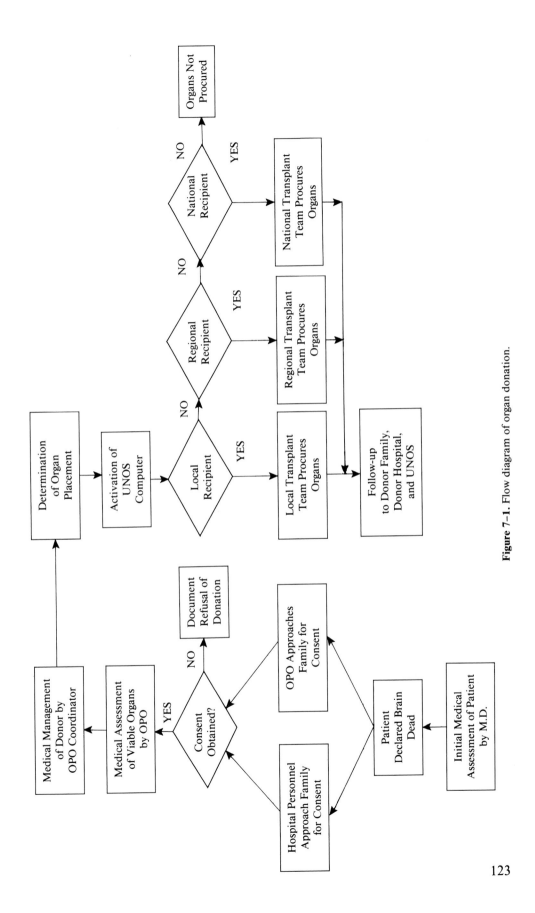

Figure 7–1. Flow diagram of organ donation.

123

tion until the attending physician has discussed the death or the imminent death with the family. The family should be allowed privacy for the discussion, and information should be presented about each organ/tissue for which consent is being obtained. Frequently asked questions include whether there is mutilation of the body, whether any costs will be incurred, and whether funeral plans will be delayed. The family is informed that organs are removed in the operating room under sterile conditions.

All medical and hospital costs incurred after the donor has been deemed an acceptable candidate until the body is transferred to the funeral home are the responsibility of the transplant center. Discussion of the family's funeral arrangement preferences allows the organ donor coordinator to give reasonable expectations as to the time the funeral director will receive the body.

The family members should receive a letter from the transplant hospital or organ procurement agency that will give them some information about the recipients of the donated organs and thanking them for the donation.

UNITED NETWORK FOR ORGAN SHARING

As part of the implementation of the National Transplantation Act, the United Network for Organ Sharing (UNOS) has divided the United States into regions (Fig. 7–2). It is also required that each waiting organ recipient be listed on the UNOS computer located in Richmond, Virginia. Patients are ranked in descending order of acuity based on a point system. Factors such as medical

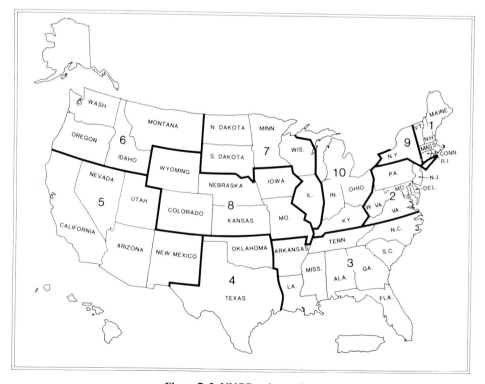

Figure 7–2. UNOS region codes.

Table 7-1. Medical Urgency Code

1. Working, in school, growing infant
2. Confined in home, self-care, infant not thriving but stable
3. At home, requiring professional care, infant losing development ground
4. Hospital bound, not in ICU
5. Hospital bound, ICU, cardiac patient requiring intravenous inotropic drugs
6. Mechanical assistance devices required for survival
7. Recipient temporarily inactive

urgency, represented by the status code in the recipient data base, which is defined as ranging from 1 to 7 and is specified in Table 7-1, time of waiting on the recipient list, and ABO compatibility are factors used in determining the point value. A notation is made for highly sensitized potential heart recipients who require a prior crossmatch because of the presence of cytotoxic antibodies.

The Organ Procurement Organization (OPO) must access the UNOS computer for each organ donor. The allocation of an extrarenal organ is first made to local institutions that are served by the designated local OPO. If no suitable recipient is identified locally, the organ is then offered to transplant centers with an identified waiting recipient within the region. Finally, national programs are screened for recipients outside the local or regional area. Local recipients are always given priority for the local organ. If a transplant center chooses, the organ may be offered to the sickest patient in the region or country.

GENERAL CRITERIA FOR DONORS

Brain Death

Head injuries due to motor vehicle accident, intracerebral hemorrhage, suicide, and brain tumors are the most common causes of brain death leading to potential organ donation for transplantation. Transplant programs in the United States have become dependent on national legislation for the definition and acceptance of brain death. Inasmuch as brain death is the first criteria for solid organ donation, nationwide standards and guidelines for the determination of death were released in 1981 in the Report of the Medical Consultants on the Diagnosis of Death to the President's Commission for the Study of Ethical Problems in Medicine and Biomedical and Behavioral Research.[6] Each state and all medical associations have adopted their own criteria based on these guidelines. The Ad Hoc Committee on Death of the Minnesota Medical Association adopted its criteria of brain death in November 1976 and requires an attending physician other than one involved in donor procurement to make the diagnosis of brain death. Based on the clinical examination and, if necessary, other complementary procedures, the diagnosis of brain death is established. When analyzing any case of irreversible brain damage, the following five points are to be satisfied:

1. Cerebral irresponsivity, i.e., absence of verbal or motor response on stimulation, deep coma with total unawareness, and unresponsiveness. Neither spontaneous movements nor involuntary posturing should be present with the exception of spinal segmental responses.

2. Apnea. The patient should not demonstrate any spontaneous respiratory movement over a minimum period of 3 minutes.
3. Absent main stem reflexes. Pupils should be fixed and in midposition (at least 50 mm in diameter). All brainstem reflexes are to be absent including oculocephalic, oculovestibular, corneal, gag, cough, swallowing, and decorticate or decerebrate posturing. Deep tendon reflexes and triple flexion responses may be present inasmuch as these are only indicative of a viable spinal cord and are not incompatible with irreversible cessation of brain function.
4. Observation over 12 hours. At least two examinations are to be performed in a 12-hour period to confirm the initial findings.
5. Irreversibility. Any reasonable possibility of a reversible central nervous system dysfunction should be excluded. The presence of hypothermia (below 32.2°C, 90°F core temperature), or sedative or anesthetic drugs such as barbiturates, benzodiazepines, meprobramate, methaqualone, or trichloroethylene could be misleading in the correct diagnosis of brain death. Patients in shock or younger than 5 years of age must receive special consideration.

Confirmatory tests are not essential because usually the clinical criteria can establish the diagnosis of death. The EEG is an objective documentation to substantiate clinical findings once intoxication, young age, or hypothermia are excluded. Electrocerebral silence confirms irreversible loss of cortical functions. Intracranial angiography showing no cerebral blood flow and other techniques can also be applied in selected cases or whenever the attending physician believes such studies are necessary.

Donor Evaluation

The availability of donors, although improved in recent years, is still the major limiting factor of organ transplantation. General public information by the media explaining the necessity for and the results of organ transplantation has increased the number of organ donors; yet only about 10 to 20 percent of potential donors are obtained. Further education not only of the public but also of the medical professionals may lead to more effective use of this potential donor pool.

During the early experience of heart transplantation, the donor and recipient had to be at the same hospital for the procedure. With scarcity of donors, it soon became evident that in order to be active, any transplant program had to spread its area of donor referrals. Stanford[4] started distant organ procurement in 1973 and established it as routine practice in mid-1977. It is now generally accepted that up to 4 hours is a safe period of myocardial ischemia and that this interval should not affect cardiac performance.[3,7-9] Nevertheless, histology of biopsy specimens has shown evidence of capillary endothelial damage in hearts that have been procured in distant locations when compared with those procured locally with shorter ischemic periods. Endomyocardial biopsies performed one year following transplantation have also shown increased vascular changes in hearts obtained from distant sites.[7] The Registry of the International Society for heart transplantation[2] documented increasing 30-day mortality with increasing ischemic times. It seems evident that although distant procurement cannot generally be avoided, maximum efforts must be made to reduce ischemic time to a minimum.

Ideally, a heart donor candidate should be less than 35 years of age. With an ordinary donor who is young, has sustained no chest injury, and has no family or previous history of heart disease, not much needs to be done in terms of preoperative investigation. A simple chest roentgenogram, a 12-lead ECG, and routine blood tests including basic serology (HBsAg, VDRL, HIV III) are usually enough to consider the donor's acceptance for heart transplantation. Nevertheless, we frequently have to exclude potential problems in a special group of donors. We have evaluated and transplanted hearts of donors up to 51 years of age. With referrals in which older age, previous cardiac arrest, or chest trauma need to be considered, complete investigation must be undertaken. Cardiac catheterization can exclude coronary atherosclerosis and assess left ventricular function. Echocardiogram also can add or confirm important information. Laboratory tests may include measurements of creatine phosphokinase (CPK MB band), LDH, PT, PTT, and arterial blood gases.

Potential recipients are matched regarding height and weight. It is possible to use heavier donors (30 percent) because of the recipient's dilated pericardial cavity. If the recipient has elevated pulmonary vascular resistance, we prefer not to use hearts from female donors in males of similar weight and size. Usually the female heart is smaller and may result in right ventricular failure in the early postoperative period. Following the aforementioned assessment, the heart is not accepted for transplantation if there is any evidence of heart contusion, prolonged cardiac arrest, active infection, or history of previous cardiovascular disease. The ABO blood group must be compatible with the potential recipient, and retrospective recipient serum-donor lymphocyte cross-matching is performed for recipients without antileukocyte antibodies to pooled donor lymphocytes. Prospective cross-matching is reserved for antibody-positive recipients. Final acceptance of the donor organ occurs when the surgical team directly inspects the heart.

DONOR MANAGEMENT

Once a donor is initially accepted for transplantation, care must be taken to control the physiologic parameters as well as the special factors added by the presence of brain death. In order to be maintained in a stable condition, donors should be treated as any other intensive care unit patient. Availability of complete cardiac monitoring, ventilatory support with a volume-cycled respirator, and measurements of urine output, CVP, temperature, pulse, blood pressure, and accurate input and output are necessary. Cardiovascular instability will likely occur but can be controlled with proper care. Systemic blood pressure is preferably kept at a mean of 80 mmHg, and inotropic support added if necessary. Dopamine is the drug of choice to maintain the desired blood pressure if fluid replacement is not effective. This drug is administered preferably in a dose not higher than 10 ug/kg/min, mixing 200 to 400 mg/250 ml of 5 percent dextrose. Isoprenaline is the second drug of choice, whereas adrenaline should be generally avoided. Whenever possible, inotropic support should be discontinued as soon as correction of volume deficits has achieved the desired blood pressure. Central venous pressure is kept at 10 to 12 cm H_2O; Ringer's lactate is generally infused to correct and maintain electrolytes and adequate urine output. Plasmamate or albumin may be required for volume expansion. Although we attempt to avoid blood transfusion, it is frequently necessary with multiple organ procurement. Whole blood or packed cells are given to replace blood loss and to keep the hemoglobin above 10 g/dl. Urine output should be maintained at about 100 ml/ hr (1 ml/kg/hr in pediatric patients); and if oliguria persists after adequate volume replacement, furosemide or mannitol, or both, are given intravenously. Because of their loss of thermal regulation, brain-dead patients rapidly become hypothermic, thus increasing the risk of dangerous cardiac arrhythmias and further cardiovascular deterioration. Severe hypothermia can usually be prevented with the use of electric blankets, warm environment, and infusion of warm fluids keeping the body temperature at about 36°C (97°F). Blood gases are kept in a normal range by increasing FiO_2 or by adding positive end-expiratory pressure (PEEP) if pulmonary edema develops.

Following brain death, there is depletion of myocardial energy stores as well as circulating thyroxine, cortisol, insulin, glucagon and antidiuretic hormone (ADH).[10] If diabetes insipidus is present, a massive urine output may occur and hypernatremia and hypokalemia will develop if not promptly corrected. If the administration of ADH (vasopressin) is desired, 0.1 to 0.25 U/kg is given intramuscularly or by means of intravenous infusion in a dose of 20 U/200 ml titrated as necessary.

The role of hormonal therapy is controversial and is currently under investigation. Novitzki and associates,[11] after inducing brain death in pigs, reported the potential value of hormonal therapy (T_3, insulin, and cortisol) in organ donors as a means of reducing anaerobic metabolism and improving myocardial function following brain death. Macoviak and coworkers[12] studied 22 organ donors referred to Stanford University who at the time of evaluation had low T_3 and T_4 levels. Although no thyroid hormone was given, normal graft function was observed after heart transplantation. They concluded that adequate general donor management with proper fluid, electrolyte, and glucose balance is generally acceptable, and at present there is no advantage to the addition of thyroid hormone therapy for maintenance of organ donors.

Because in most instances, organ procurement is carried out as soon as possible following the diagnosis of brain death, systemic replacement of primary neurohypophyseal secretions and their target hormones is probably not necessary. Nevertheless, investigations in this area should be continued to determine whether they will lead to any increase in donor supply.

DONOR OPERATION

The United Network for Organ Sharing today lists all vital organs that are available and required, so that multiple organ utilization is attempted for each available donor. As a general rule, different teams may procure heart, lungs, pancreas, liver, and kidneys at the same time. This imposes some complexities, and care must be taken to avoid any loss in communication or in continuity of donor management, thus leading to unnecessarily prolonged periods of ischemia.

The same care regarding donor management discussed earlier is carried out in the operating room. The anesthesiologist must be aware of fluid loss, electrolyte replacement, body temperature, blood pressure, filling pressures, and urine output. An arterial line is placed in the left radial artery and a central venous line in the right jugular vein. Sometimes we find it is helpful to have lines in the iliac vessels placed by the abdominal surgeons, so that fluid replacement can be easily accomplished. After the donor's monitoring lines are in place and preparation is completed, the operation is begun. A wide exposure is essential, and this is achieved by a midline thoracoabdominal incision. After median sternotomy, the heart is exposed by a longitudinal incision in the pericardium. The heart is inspected for any evidence of external damage due to trauma or any other morphological abnormality. The ascending aorta is mobilized, separating it from the pulmonary artery and exposing the innominate artery after mobilization of the innominate vein. The superior vena cava (SVC) is completely mobilized, opening the pericardial reflexion. The inferior vena cava (IVC) is also dissected close to the diaphragm so that a clamp may be placed just above the diaphragm. This technique prevents the spillage of warm IVC blood into the pericardium when the IVC is transsected.

Liver procurement teams working with us have generally found it adequate to vent the IVC from below. Consideration should be given to preserving as much suprahepatic vena cava as is possible for liver transplantation. The abdominal organs are dissected at the same time as the thoracic organs, and attention should be given to the prevention of hypothermia and hypotension during liver, pancreas

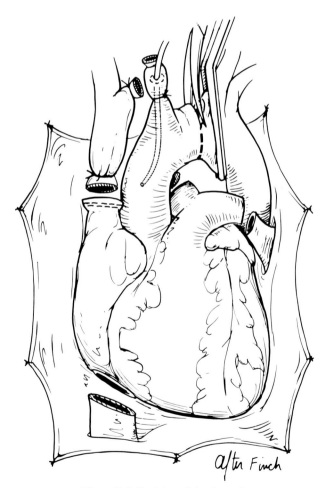

Figure 7–3. Excision of the donor heart.

or kidney dissection.[13] Warm air ventilation, warm intravenous fluids, and application of warm saline into the chest and abdominal cavities can help prevent low body temperature. In the abdomen, gentle mobilization of IVC and portal vein should be carried out, since even temporary partial occlusion can induce severe hypotension and jeopardize the heart. Severe hypotension can frequently be temporarily corrected by occlusion of the infrarenal aorta.

After all organs have been dissected up to the point of disconnection, 300 U of heparin/kg are given intravenously. The innominate vein is divided between ligatures exposing the innominate artery. At this point, all intravenous infusions on the left side are discontinued. A 14 F catheter is introduced into the innominate artery for rapid infusion of 1000 ml of 4°C cardioplegic solution (Plegisol, Abbott Laboratories). Any catheter in the SVC is removed at this point. The SVC is stapled and divided away from the right atrium, avoiding the SA node. The IVC is clamped and divided above the clamp. The heart is allowed to empty for 3 or 4 beats and the aorta is clamped above the innominate artery, at which point the cardioplegic infusion is started (Fig. 7–3). One pulmonary vein is usually cut to decompress the left side of the heart. Cold saline is poured into the pericardial cavity to cool the heart topically. Once the cardioplegic solution has been infused, the remaining pulmonary veins are cut and the aorta is divided as high as possible. The right and left pulmonary arteries are divided, and, after sharp dissection of mediastinal tissue posterior to the atria and the great vessels, the heart is removed from the pericardial cavity (Fig. 7–4). The heart is transferred to a sterile bowl containing cold saline solution. The left atrium is opened between the pulmonary veins and the mitral valve is inspected (Fig. 7–5). The atrial septum also is inspected, looking for the presence of any defects that must be corrected prior to reimplantation. After confirming normal internal anatomy, the heart is trans-

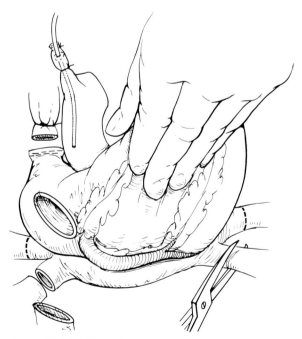

Figure 7–4. Division of the pulmonary veins.

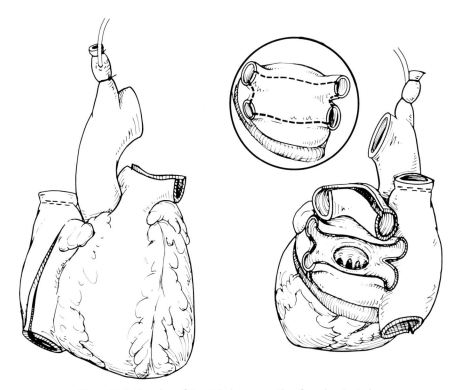

Figure 7-5. Opening of the atria in preparation for reimplantation.

ferred into an adjacent operating room or, in a case of distant procurement, placed in a plastic bag with cold saline, sealed in another sterile bag, and transferred in a container with ice.

Reducing ischemic time to its minimum is a major concern in any heart transplant program. Because distant procurement is the only way to increase donor availability, communication between donor and recipient teams is critical. Information must include time of cross-clamp and estimated time of transport to the recipient's hospital. In order to avoid unnecessary ischemia, the recipient's operation is begun before the arrival of the donor's heart, but excision of the recipient's heart is performed only when the new organ is actually in the operating room. If one considers the period of 4 hours to be a safe ischemic time for the heart, distant donors can be procured over a range of 1000 miles, thereby enhancing considerably the number of donors available.

Following the transplant, a report of the organ recipient's progress is sent to the donating hospital's personnel and to the donor's family. This procedure has proven to be effective in allowing family and staff to have better comprehension and understanding of an otherwise difficult situation.

REFERENCES

1. Barnard, CN: A human cardiac transplant: An interim report of a successful operation performed at Groot Shuur Hospital, Cape Town. S Afr Med J 41:1271, 1967.
2. Kaye, MP: Unpublished data, 1988.

 3. Thomas, FT, Szentpetery, SS, Mammana, RE, et al: Long distance transportation of human hearts for transplantation. Ann Thorac Surg 26:344, 1978.
 4. Watson, DC, Reitz, BA, Baumgartner, AB, et al: Distant heart procurement for transplantation. Surgery 86:56, 1979.
 5. Robertson, JA: Supply and distribution of hearts for transplantation: Legal, ethical and policy issues. Circulation 75:77, 1987.
 6. Medical Consultants on the Diagnosis of Death: Guidelines for the determination of death. JAMA 246:2184, 1981.
 7. Billingham, ME, Baumgartner, WA, Watson, DC, et al: Distant heart procurement for human transplantation: Ultrastructural studies. Circulation 62(Suppl 1):11, 1980.
 8. Mendez-Picon, GJ, Goldman, MH, Wolfgang, TC, et al: Long distance procurement and transportation of human hearts for transplantation. Heart Transplant 1:63, 1981.
 9. Emery, RW, Randall, CC, Levinson, MM, et al: The cardiac donor: A six year experience. Ann Thorac Surg 41:356, 1986.
10. Novitzky, D, Wicomb, WN, Cooper, DKC, et al: Electrocardiographic, haemodynamic and endocrine changes occurring during experimental brain death in the chacma baboon. Heart Transplant 4:63, 1984.
11. Novitzky, D, Wicomb, WN, Cooper, DKC, et al: Improved cardiac function following hormonal therapy in brain dead pigs: Relevance to organ donation. Cryobiology 24:1, 1987.
12. Macoviak, JA, Mc Dougall, IR, Bayer, MF, et al: Significance of thyroid dysfunction in human cardiac allograft procurement. Transplantation 43:824, 1987.
13. Rosenthal, JT, Shaw, BW, Hardesty, RL, et al: Principles of multiple organ procurement from cadaver donors. Ann Surg 198:617, 1983.

CHAPTER 8

Cardiac Transplantation: The Operative Technique

R. Morton Bolman III, M.D.

The operative procedure of cardiac transplantation is one of the three critical determinants of a successful outcome, the others being patient selection and postoperative management. Although the procedure as currently practiced is based upon the technique described by Lower and Shumway,[1] certain modifications have evolved which address the current patient population undergoing this procedure. In this chapter, I will review techniques of operative cardiac transplantation that have proven safe, reliable, and reproducible and that can be safely taught to surgical residents in training.

PREOPERATIVE PREPARATION OF THE TRANSPLANT RECIPIENT

When a cardiac donor becomes available, the recipient with an identical or compatible blood type on the local waiting list who is most critically ill is made ready for possible transplantation. Often, this individual will be in the hospital receiving intravenous pressor agents on mechanical support systems. The current status of this individual must be assessed to rule out intercurrent infections and to evaluate renal function and coagulation status, particularly if the patient has been receiving oral or intravenous anticoagulants. Table 8–1 outlines the immediate preoperative studies essential to the determination of a given recipient's readiness for transplantation.

TECHNIQUE OF CARDIAC TRANSPLANTATION

Intraoperative Monitoring

All recipients receive Swan-Ganz catheters introduced via the left internal jugular vein. This approach is chosen in order to preserve the right internal jugular route for postoperative endomyocardial biopsies. Radial arterial lines are routinely employed as in all cardiac surgery procedures. Parameters monitored

Table 8–1. Cardiac Recipient Final Pretransplant Assessment

1. Blood to HLA-laboratory for final cross-match
2. Complete blood count
3. BUN, creatinine, electrolytes
4. PT, PTT, TT
5. Urine, blood, throat swab for routine and viral culture
6. Serum for CMV, EBV, Herpes titers
7. Chest radiograph, PA and lateral
8. Type and cross-match
    8 units PRBC
    10 donor platelet concentrates
    10 units FFP
    —all above CMV negative for seronegative recipients
9. Discontinue heparin or Coumadin

via the Swan-Ganz catheter include core temperature, pulmonary artery pressures during anesthetic induction and mixed venous oxygen saturation. At the time of weaning from cardiopulmonary bypass, when the donor heart is initially assuming a workload, the Swan-Ganz catheter is most useful for assessment of central filling pressures including central venous pressure, pulmonary capillary wedge pressure, and pulmonary artery pressures. Periodic cardiac output determinations and on-line mixed venous oxygen saturation display also are of great assistance in the safe transition from cardiopulmonary bypass to complete circulation being provided by the donor heart.

Perioperative Infection Prophylaxis

All patients receive a second-generation cephalosporin while on call to the operating room and postoperatively until all drainage and monitoring lines have been removed. In addition, vancomycin is administered prior to surgery and for 48 hours postoperatively as prophylaxis against mediastinal sepsis. In the operating room, copious irrigation of the mediastinum is performed using a warm vancomycin solution following the termination of bypass. Patients seronegative for CMV pretransplant receive exclusively CMV negative blood and blood products throughout their hospital course. All recipients receive oral trimethoprim-sulfamethoxazole indefinitely as prophylaxis against Pneumocystis and Nocardia. Individuals treated for rejection with enhanced immunosuppression also receive acyclovir for 3 months for prophylaxis against viral infections[2] (Table 8–2).

EXCISION OF DISEASED RECIPIENT HEART

Incision

A midline sternotomy is performed in all recipients. In patients who have had one or more previous cardiac surgical procedures, particularly if the hemodynamic status is precarious, it is wise to isolate a femoral artery and vein such that rapid femoral-femoral bypass can be instituted should circulatory decompensation occur. Also in these individuals with greatly dilated myocardial chambers, it is possible to injure the right ventricle or aorta at the time of repeat sternotomy, and, in these situations, femoral-femoral bypass can be lifesaving.

Table 8–2. Perioperative Infection Prophylaxis

Antibiotics
    Cefazolin perioperatively and until all lines removed
    Vancomycin perioperatively for 48 hours
    Trimethoprim-sulfamethoxazole orally postoperatively indefinite
    Acyclovir if treated for rejection
Blood products
    CMV negative products if seronegative pretransplant

Mobilization of the Aorta and Right Atrium

In patients who have not had previous surgery, the pericardium is secured to the wound edges with sutures. The aorta and pulmonary artery are separated using electrocautery for subsequent placement of the aortic cross-clamp. The aorta often appears small in relation to the greatly dilated right atrium and pulmonary artery in patients with cardiomyopathy. In reoperative sternotomies, it is best to isolate the aorta and sufficient right atrium to permit venous cannulation. Often, because of unstable circulatory dynamics, further dissection will necessitate institution of cardiopulmonary bypass. The attempt is made in all cases to avoid systemic heparinization and the institution of cardiopulmonary bypass for as long as reasonably possible to lessen the period of bypass and attendant bleeding complications.

Cannulation for Cardiopulmonary Bypass

The ascending aorta is cannulated in routine fashion just proximal to the innominate artery. Venous cannulation differs from the method employed for routine cardiopulmonary bypass. In a patient with a dilated superior vena cava, commonly observed with cardiomyopathy, a venous return cannula is placed directly into the superior vena cava. In patients with ischemic heart disease and normal cavae, caval cannulae are inserted posteriorly in the right atrium near the orifices of the superior and inferior vena cava, respectively. In all cases we use right angle venous cannulae, 32 French for the superior vena cava and 36 French for the inferior vena cava. The cavae are then encircled with Rommel tourniquets to allow institution of total bypass. The caval cannulae are placed in the positions described to allow preservation of a generous cuff of posterior right atrium for anastomosis to the donor heart (Fig. 8–1).

Cardiopulmonary Bypass

When the donor heart has arrived safely on the ground and is being returned to the recipient hospital, the patient is placed on cardiopulmonary bypass and the body temperature is lowered to 28°C. The caval tourniquets are tightened to effect complete cardiopulmonary bypass and the aorta is cross-clamped. A vent catheter is introduced into the left ventricle via the right superior pulmonary vein and attached to cardiotomy suction to decompress the dilated recipient heart (Fig. 8–1).

Excision of the Recipient Heart

Removal of the diseased heart begins at the lateral right atrial wall. The heart is entered at the midpoint of the right atrium 2 to 3 cm anterior to the caval

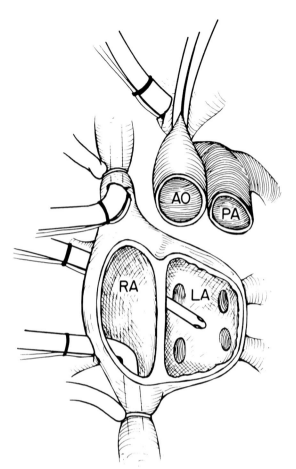

Figure 8–1. Appearance of the recipient mediastinum following excision of the diseased recipient heart. One can see the position of the arterial and venous cannulae for cardiopulmonary bypass as well as the left ventricular vent catheter passing via the right superior pulmonary vein. Posterior cuffs of left and right atrium, aorta, and pulmonary artery have been fashioned. (Adapted from Bolman et al.,[3] with permission.)

cannulae. This incision is extended around the superior aspect of the atrium and to the aortic root at the level of the noncoronary sinus. Inferiorly the atrial incision is carefully completed by incising 2 to 3 cm anterior to the inferior vena caval cannula. The coronary sinus is visualized on the interior aspect of the right atrium, and the atrial incision is carried into the coronary sinus near the atrioventricular (AV) groove. The aorta and pulmonary artery are then divided at the level of their respective semilunar valves. Retracting anteriorly on the aortic root, the roof of the left atrium is incised sharply just posterior to the aortic valve. The interatrial septum is then divided under direct vision leaving a generous portion of interatrial septum by incising near the AV groove. Superiorly the left atrial incision is extended between the left atrial appendage and the superior pulmonary vein. The heart is then retracted out of the pericardium to the right. The coronary sinus is incised and the left atrium is transected in the AV groove to leave a generous cuff of posterior left atrium about the pulmonary veins. The coronary sinus of the recipient organ can be used to bolster the left atrial suture line. This completes excision of the diseased organ (Fig. 8–1). The aorta and pulmonary artery are separated using electrocautery. Care must be taken to avoid injury to the right pulmonary artery during this maneuver.

Recipient Mediastinal Anatomy

Following removal of the diseased heart, the recipient mediastinum consists of left and right atrial remnants in addition to long cuffs of aorta and pulmonary artery. The atrial cuffs may be trimmed if necessary prior to implantation of the donor heart (Fig. 8–1).

Timing of Donor and Recipient Operations

The state of the art in cardiac transplantation is such that the donor heart will tolerate ex vivo cold preservation of 4 to 5 hours. Clearly, however, it is desirable to achieve reperfusion in the shortest reasonable time in which it can be accomplished. Particularly when the recipient has an elevated pulmonary vascular resistance, it is highly advantageous to achieve reperfusion in the shortest possible time to allow optimal right ventricular function. Coordination of donor and recipient operations is critical to the achievement of the goals of expeditious reperfusion and optimization of early postimplant function. Currently it is the rule rather than the exception that hearts are procured long distance or at least in a hospital separate from the recipient hospital. Once the donor heart has been visualized by the retrieving surgeon and found to be suitable for transplantation, preparation of the recipient can begin. The exact timing of recipient preparation is dictated by logistic factors including (1) anticipated time of arrival of the donor heart at the recipient hospital, (2) anticipated difficulty of monitoring line insertion and anesthetic induction, and (3) estimates of the time necessary for surgical preparation of the recipient, which obviously is much longer in patients who have had previous cardiac procedures. Within these confines, attempts are made to coordinate these procedures to allow minimal periods of waiting in the recipient operating theater and minimal periods of cardiopulmonary bypass. When the recipient has undergone previous cardiac procedures, extra time is allowed for mediastinal dissection to ensure that the transplant can proceed expeditiously once the donor heart arrives at the recipient hospital. It should be noted that no incision is made in the recipient until the retrieving surgeon is satisfied that the donor heart is indeed suitable for transplantation.

When the donor heart has safely arrived in the region of the transplant hospital, cardiopulmonary bypass is instituted and cardiectomy is performed, such that when the donor heart arrives in the operating theater, expeditious implantation can be performed.

IMPLANTATION OF THE DONOR HEART

The donor heart is removed from the sterile container and placed in a large basin containing sterile saline at 4°C. Using electrocautery, the aorta and pulmonary arteries of the donor heart are separated, taking care to avoid injury to either vessel. The posterior pulmonary artery attachments to the left atrium are divided using electrocautery. The superior vena caval orifice is oversewn with 4–0 Prolene suture. The cuffs of left and right atrium in the recipient mediastinum are visualized such that appropriately sized cuffs on the donor heart can be created. Beginning at the right inferior pulmonary vein, an incision is made in the left atrium creating a trap door of the posterior atrial wall by connecting incisions in the pulmonary veins. In this fashion, the posterior atrial wall can be excised and the remaining cuff of left atrium approximates the recipient atrium quite nicely. The fossa ovalis is inspected and if a septal defect or widely patent foramen ovale is encountered, this is oversewn with running monofilament suture. Right atrial incision is also performed at this time. The incision begins at the inferior vena caval orifice and extends toward the right atrial appendage taking great pains to avoid trauma to the area of the sinoatrial node, which is the pacemaker of the donor heart. This completes preparation of the donor heart for implantation.

Left Atrial Anastomosis

Implantation invariably begins with anastomosis of donor and recipient left atria. Anastomosis is effected using extra length 3–0 Prolene suture and beginning at a point approximating the base of the left atrial appendage near the left superior pulmonary vein. The initial sutures are placed with the heart resting on the chest wall. The heart is then lowered into the recipient mediastinum, and the left atrial anastomosis is completed by running the sutures inferiorly and superiorly until the atria are completely joined. This anastomosis is completed by joining the septal aspects of donor and recipient left atria (Fig. 8–2). At this point it is acceptable to insert an intravenous tubing into the left atrial appendange through which cold lactated Ringer's solution can be lavaged to cool the left heart and remove air. We have dispensed with this maneuver in the interest of a more expeditious implantation but it is certainly acceptable. During the period of implantation, frequent lavage of the donor heart with topical saline or lactated Ringer's at 4°C

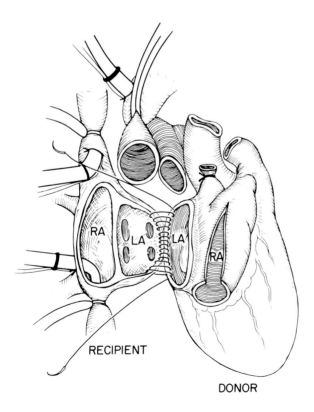

RA   LA   LA   RA

RECIPIENT

DONOR

Figure 8–2. The donor heart has been lowered into the operative field, and the lateral wall of the left atrial anastomosis is being fashioned. (Adapted from Bolman et al.,[3] with permission.)

is performed. Continuous pericardial lavage is also effective in myocardial protection, though somewhat more cumbersome to execute.

Timing of Implant Anastomoses

Whereas the left atrial anastomosis needs be performed as the initial procedure, the order of subsequent anastomoses is dictated by the ischemic time of the donor heart. From a technical standpoint, it is desirable to perform the pulmonary artery anastomosis as well as the portion of the right atrial anastomosis surrounding the coronary sinus prior to releasing the aortic cross-clamp. In patients with normal pulmonary vascular resistance with donor ischemic times within safe limits, this is the optimal sequence: left atrium, pulmonary artery, inferior right atrium, aorta, remainder of right atrium. This allows approximately 30 minutes of reperfusion for the donor heart while the right atrial anastomosis is being completed and the suture lines are being checked for hemostasis and reinforced where necessary. In situations in which the donor heart ischemic time is excessive, it is preferable to perform the left atrial anastomosis followed by the aortic anastomosis at which point the cross-clamp can be removed and perfusion restored to the donor heart.

Pulmonary Artery Anastomosis

Donor and recipient pulmonary arteries are trimmed substantially to prevent kinking of the pulmonary artery with restoration of right ventricular output. The donor pulmonary artery is transected 2 to 3 cm distal to the pulmonic valve. Donor and recipient pulmonary arteries are then joined using a running layer anastomosis with 4–0 Prolene (Fig. 8–3). Prior to completion of this anastomosis, the Swan-Ganz catheter, withdrawn from the right atrium at the time of cardiectomy, is carefully passed through the donor heart and placed into the recipient pulmonary artery. A Satinsky clamp is carefully passed retrograde through the pulmonic valve, right ventricle and tricuspid valve to grasp the Swan-Ganz catheter. This maneuver must be performed very carefully to avoid injury to the pulmonic or tricuspid valve. The pulmonary artery anastomosis is then completed.

Right Atrial Anastomosis

Anastomosis of donor and recipient right atria is initiated at the inferior septal level. The sutures are carried superiorly and inferiorly to complete the septal anastomosis, and then the lateral walls of the atrium are joined. Generally, a portion of this anastomosis is left to be accomplished following release of the aortic cross-clamp while reperfusion of the donor heart is occurring (Fig. 8–3). The anastomosis of the right atrium is completed by joining the lateral walls of the atrium. When this anastomosis is complete, if the cross-clamp is off, coronary sinus return will rapidly fill the atrium and the caval tourniquets must be removed at this point.

Aortic Anastomosis

Donor and recipient aortas are trimmed only slightly. It has proven advantageous to leave the aorta long to avoid tension on the anastomosis and to facilitate visualization of the left atrial suture line and posterior pulmonary artery suture line in case bleeding would occur following removal of the cross-clamps. The anastomosis is accomplished with the two layer technique, with an inner

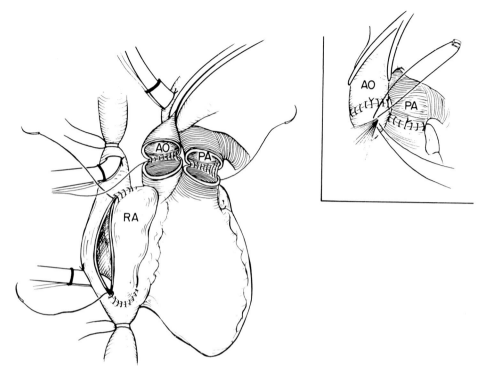

Figure 8–3. The medial aspect of the right atrial anastomosis has been completed, and the figure shows the methods of the anastomosis of the aorta and pulmonary artery. The insert demonstrates the technique of venting air from the ascending aorta as the aortic cross-clamp is released, restoring perfusion to the donor heart. (Adapted from Bolman et al.,[3] with permission.)

layer of horizontal mattress sutures and an outer layer of running sutures. Two 4–0 Prolene sutures reinforced with Teflon felt are placed as horizontal mattress sutures posteriorly and carried up each side of the aorta as an inner horizontal mattress and an outer running layer. Prior to release of the cross-clamp, the patient is placed in the Trendelenburg position and a stab wound is placed in the most anterior aspect of the ascending aorta to allow air to escape. The cardiopulmonary bypass flow is turned down and the cross clamp is removed, thus restoring perfusion to the donor heart (Fig. 8–3).

Completion of the Procedure

At least 30 minutes should be allowed for reperfusion of the donor heart to wash out the cardioplegia and allow thorough rewarming. Systemic rewarming of the patient is instituted at the beginning of the aortic anastomosis. Just prior to releasing the cross-clamp, 100 mg of lidocaine is instilled into the cardiopulmonary bypass circuit, and this effectively prevents fibrillation of the donor heart in most cases. During the period of reperfusion, the suture lines are checked for hemostasis. The left atrial suture line and posterior pulmonary artery suture line particularly are checked at this time inasmuch as these areas are very difficult to visualize once bypass is discontinued. When hemostasis is secured, and the patient is normothermic, temporary pacing wires are attached to the right atrium and right ventricle. An infusion of isoproterenol is instituted to achieve a heart rate of 100 to 120 beats per minute, and the patient is slowly separated from

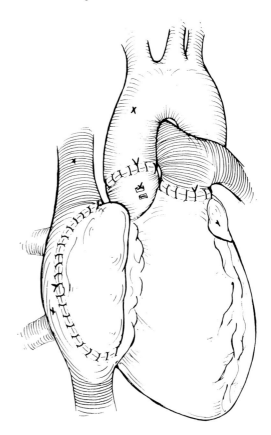

Figure 8–4. This is the completed preparation. Right atrial, aortic, and pulmonary suture lines are visible and the cardiopulmonary bypass cannulas have been extracted. (Adapted from Bolman et al.,[3] with permission.)

bypass. When the donor heart has assumed the circulation, the pump lines are removed and the mediastinum is copiously irrigated with a warm antibiotic solution (Fig. 8–4). Meticulous irrigation and hemostasis are critical to the prevention of postoperative infection and the need for re-exploration for bleeding.[3]

HETEROTOPIC HEART TRANSPLANTATION

General Considerations

In certain instances, it is advantageous to preserve the recipients' own ventricles when performing heart transplantation. These instances include (1) the recipient with elevation of the pulmonary vascular resistance that is fixed and cannot be reversed pharmacologically and (2) a situation in which only a small donor heart is available for a large recipient who is critically ill. Pulmonary vascular resistance elevation is a serious risk factor at the time of orthotopic cardiac transplantation and can be managed successfully with heterotopic transplantation.[4–7]

Excision and Preparation of the Donor Heart

Donor cardiectomy for heterotopic transplantation is similar to that for orthotopic transplantation, with the exception that the entire superior vena cava is removed. In addition, a longer segment of aorta than usual is removed to

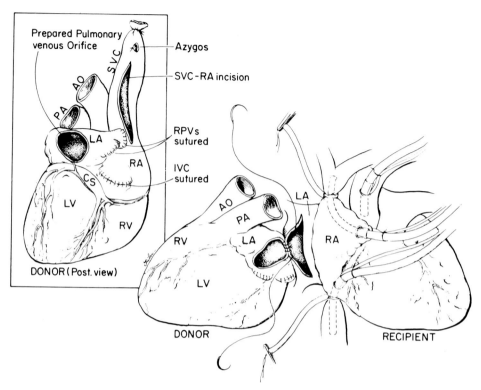

Figure 8–5. The inset reveals the donor heart in the posterior view. The long segment of superior vena cava is demonstrated with the posterior incision for subsequent anastomosis to the recipient right atrium. The right pulmonary veins and inferior vena cava are oversewn, and an opening has been created between the left pulmonary veins for anastomosis to the recipient left atrium. On the right is shown the recipient on bypass with the left atrial anastomosis being fashioned between donor and recipient hearts. (From Griffith et al.,[4] with permission.)

include the arch with ligated brachiocephalic vessels. Longer than normal segments of the superior vena cava and aorta are required because the technique of implantation necessitates that the right atrium of the recipient be anastomosed to the posterior wall of the superior vena cava. In addition, the long segment of donor aorta is necessary for end-to-side anastomosis to the recipient's ascending aorta.

Preparation of the donor heart for implantation requires several maneuvers that are unique to the heterotopic transplant. The left-sided pulmonary venous orifices are opened widely and united in preparation for future anastomosis with the left atrium of the donor. The right-sided pulmonary veins are oversewn. The inferior vena cava is closed at its atrial junction and the superior vena cava is ligated distally. The posterior portion of the superior vena cava is incised longitudinally, with the venotomy carried 3 to 4 cm onto the right atrial surface. This posterior position minimizes risk of injury to the sinus node (Fig. 8–5, inset).

Preparation of the Recipient

After a midline sternotomy, the pericardium is incised longitudinally in the midline and then laterally at the diaphragmatic level and also at the level of the great vessels to allow a flap to fall into the opened right pleural space. The inferior pulmonary ligament is mobilized on the right. Biatrial cannulation and routine aortic cannulation of the diseased recipient heart are performed and a vent catheter is placed in the apex of the left ventricle. When the donor heart has safely arrived in the area of the transplant hospital, the patient is placed on cardiopulmonary bypass and cooled to 28°C.

Atrial Anastomoses

With the patient on cardiopulmonary bypass, an incision is made in the recipient's left atrium in the interatrial groove similar to the approach for mitral valve surgery. The donor heart is positioned in the right chest anterior to the lung, and the created common orifice of the left pulmonary veins is anastomosed to the recipient left atrium (Fig. 8–5). Caval tourniquets are tightened around the vena caval cannulae following completion of the left atrial anastomosis, and a right lateral atriotomy of 5 to 6 cm is created in the recipient heart. A continuous anastomosis is created between the cavoatrial opening in the donor and the atriotomy of the recipient (Fig. 8–6). These atrial anastomoses are accomplished with running 4–0 Prolene.

Aortic Anastomosis

The aorta of the donor heart is left as long as possible and anastomosed end-to-side to the recipient ascending aorta, which is partially occluded with a side-

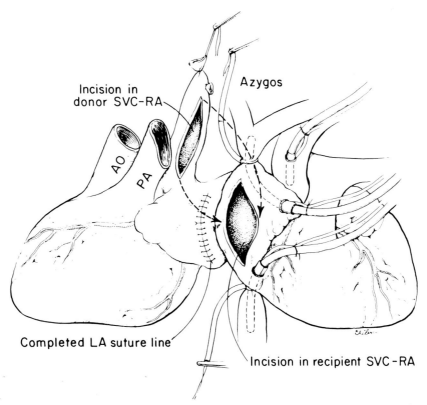

Figure 8–6. The posterior opening in the donor superior vena cava is anastomosed to the incised recipient right atrium as shown. (From Griffith et al.,[4] with permission.)

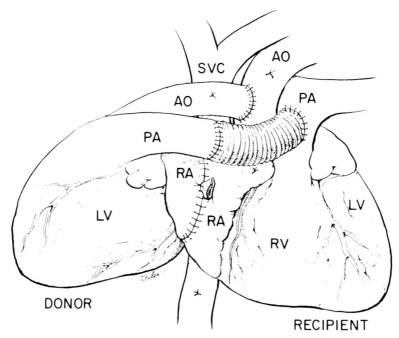

Figure 8–7. The great vessels have been connected. The donor aorta is anastomosed directly to the side of the recipient ascending aorta. The donor pulmonary artery and recipient pulmonary artery have been joined with an interposed Dacron graft. Alternatively, this may be accomplished with interposition of a segment of donor descending aorta. The right atrial suture line is visible, as is the final orientation of donor and recipient hearts. (From Griffith et al.,[4] with permission.)

biting vascular clamp (Fig. 8–7). The length of the donor aorta that is utilized is important in determining the position of the heterotopically transplanted heart. If the aorta is too long, the heart will fall too far into the right chest and compress the right lung. If the aorta is too short, the right atrial anastomosis will be somewhat distorted. Once reperfusion is accomplished in the donor heart, an air vent site is placed in the aorta of the donor heart to allow air to escape. During reperfusion the patient is returned to normal temperature.

Pulmonary Artery Anastomosis

The main pulmonary artery of the donor is generally of insufficient length to reach the recipient pulmonary artery. The right pulmonary artery of the donor can be used to bridge this gap. This can also be accomplished with a segment of donor aorta or a prosthetic graft that has been preclotted. Donor and recipient pulmonary arteries are joined using running 4–0 Prolene (Fig. 8–7).

Completion of the Procedure

Air is allowed to escape through the vent site in the aorta of the donor heart while the heart is reperfused and begins beating. When at least 30 minutes of reperfusion has been accomplished and the patient is normothermic, separation from bypass can ensue. Special attention is directed to ensuring complete inflation of the right lung and to positioning the heterotopically transplanted heart to avoid pulmonary atelectasis (Fig. 8–7).[4]

SUMMARY

The operative procedure of cardiac transplantation, whether orthotopic or heterotopic, must be performed with meticulous attention to technical detail and hemostasis. The price for technical misadventures and bleeding complications is high in terms of patient morbidity and mortality. Few cardiac surgical procedures are more straightforward than a heart transplant performed in a young individual who has not undergone previous cardiac surgery. Few greater technical challenges exist, however, than the patient in a state of precarious hemodynamic balance undergoing heart transplantation in the wake of one, two, or more previous cardiac surgical procedures. The principles outlined herein will serve as a foundation for the safe performance of cardiac transplantation regardless of the situation.

REFERENCES

1. Lower, RR and Shumway, NE: Studies on orthotopic transplantation of the canine heart. Surg Forum 11:18, 1960.
2. Bolman, RM, Cance, C, Spray, T, et al: The changing face of cardiac transplantation: Washington University program 1985–1987. Ann Thorac Surg 45:192, 1988.
3. Bolman, RM, Molina, JE and Anderson, RW: Heart Transplantation. In Simmons, RL, Fince, ME, Ascher, NL, and Najarian, JS (eds): Manual of Vascular Access, Organ Donation, and Transplantation. Springer-Verlag, New York, 1984, pp 209–231.
4. Griffith, BP, Kormos, RL, and Hardesty, RL: Hetertotopic cardiac transplantation: Current status. J Cardiac Surg 2:283, 1987.
5. Barnard, CN, Barnard, MS, Cooper, DKC, et al: The present status of heterotopic cardiac transplantation. J Thorac Cardiovasc Surg 81:433, 1981.
6. Losman, JG, Campbell, CD, and Replogle, RL: The advantages of heterotopic cardiac transplantation: Critical review of initial results. Heart Transplant 1:53, 1981.
7. Novitzky, D, Cooper, DKC, and Barnard, CN: The surgical technique of heterotopic heart transplantation. Ann Thorac Surg 36:476, 1983.

CHAPTER 9

Diagnosis and Treatment of Cardiac Allograft Rejection

John B. O'Connell, M.D.
Dale G. Renlund, M.D.

During the 20 years that followed the first operative survival of a cardiac transplant recipient, heart transplantation has evolved from an experimental curiosity to an accepted therapeutic modality for the treatment of end-stage heart disease. One-year survival has increased from 20 percent in 1968 to more than 80 percent in 1987. Although many scientific accomplishments were required before success of this magnitude could be realized, the two major achievements that have had the greatest impact on survival were the development of accurate techniques to detect cardiac allograft rejection in the absence of abnormalities of left ventricular function and specific and potent immunosuppressive agents designed to both prevent and treat allograft rejection. Despite these advances, the most common causes of death following cardiac transplantation continue to be rejection and infection.[1] Because the treatment of rejection requires intensification of immunosuppression, which in turn predisposes to infectious complications, the causes of death due to infection and rejection are closely intertwined. The purposes of this chapter are to describe the evolution of the diagnostic modalities used to diagnose rejection, to discuss the immunosuppressive agents used to prevent and/or treat rejection, and to describe agents that in the future may be applied to alter the rejection process in the cardiac allograft.

CLASSIFICATION OF REJECTION

The terminology describing the classification of rejection in cardiac transplantation has been modeled after the immunopathogenic events identified in renal transplantation.[2] Hyperacute rejection is defined by the presence of preformed antibodies in recipient serum that have specificity for donor HLA antigens and result from previous exposure to human antigens, usually through parity or previous blood transfusions. When the preformed antibodies are present in the serum in high titer, failure of the cardiac allograft in the operating room may result. Fortunately, it is unusual for a cardiac transplant recipient to be sensitized to donor antigens. Acute rejection is typically a T-lymphocyte–mediated response to the allograft that requires several days following transplantation to become firmly established. This acute reaction is the most common form of rejection, and most cardiac transplant recipients will experience one or more episodes during the first 3 months following the operation. Chronic rejection typically results from immune responses to vascular antigens, which result in a fibrointimal proliferation clinically manifested as coronary arteriosclerosis. The precise immunopathogenic events precipitating this reaction are poorly understood and will be discussed in another chapter in this book.[3] The following discussion will be limited to hyperacute and acute cardiac allograft rejection.

HYPERACUTE REJECTION

The identification of hyperacute cardiac allograft rejection has received little attention in the cardiac transplant literature, primarily because it presents nonspecifically with unexplained allograft dysfunction during or shortly following the surgery. Inasmuch as the pathology of the rejected allograft shows only myocyte destruction, with or without immunoglobulin deposition, accurate identification of the etiology of the cardiac dysfunction may not be proven although hyperacute rejection may be suspected.

Once the diagnosis of hyperacute rejection is suspected, the failing allograft must be supported hemodynamically with inotropic therapy, and early consideration for mechanical support should be given. In an allograft that fails as a consequence of hyperacute rejection, the ventricular dysfunction is likely to progress unabated until the immunopathogenic events are reversed and hence may necessitate retransplantation. If the rejection is not immediately life-threatening, therapy can be instituted to remove preformed antibodies using plasmapheresis. Plasmapheresis has been demonstrated to remove preformed antibodies in kidney transplant recipients but has not been studied extensively in cardiac transplant recipients.[4] Theoretically, the addition of immunosuppressive therapy that is highly selective for B cells, such as the substitution of cyclophosphamide for azathioprine, also may be warranted.[5] In general, the treatment of hyperacute cardiac allograft rejection has been disappointing and the likelihood of success is extremely poor once this form of rejection occurs.

In an attempt to avoid hyperacute rejection, patients being considered for cardiac transplantation undergo panel reactive antibody testing (PRA) in order to predict the likelihood of hyperacute rejection. Recipient serum is incubated in a microcytotoxicity assay with lymphocytes from a panel of individuals representing all HLA specificities. If recipient serum reacts to 5 to 10 percent of the cells in the random panel, the recipient may receive a randomly allocated donor organ to which there has been previous sensitization. As a result, most institutions routinely perform a prospective donor specific crossmatch on patients with a PRA greater than 5 to 10 percent in which specific donor lymphocytes are incubated with recipient serum and complement to identify the presence of preformed antibodies. Using this conservative approach, hyperacute rejection is unlikely because recipients prone to such a reaction are identified and precautions are taken to prevent the random allocation of a donor to which the recipient has antibody. It is not practical, however, to request specific crossmatches in all or

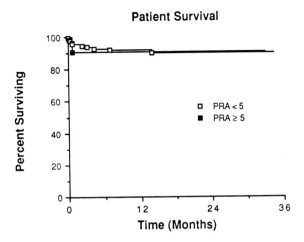

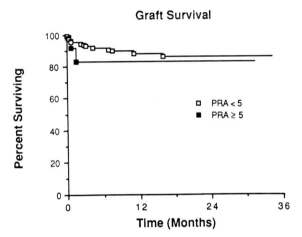

Figure 9-1. Patient and allo-graft survival comparing recipients with a reactive random panel (PRA ≥ 5%, n = 11) with those without presensitization (PRA < 5%, n = 107) without the benefit of a prospective cross-match. No difference in patient or allograft survival exists between the groups.

even most patients because of the logistical difficulty and time delay in obtaining a donor's blood and transferring it to the recipient institution where the cross-match, which requires 4 to 6 hours, is performed. As a result of the disadvantages of prospective cross-matching, some institutions no longer require a prospective cross-match even in highly sensitized recipients.[6]

In the UTAH Cardiac Transplant Program, 15 of 145 (10 percent) transplant recipients had a PRA greater than or equal to 5 percent.[7] Prospective cross-matching was not performed. Allograft and recipient survival (Fig. 9–1) and severity and incidence of rejection were not significantly different between the patients with reactive random panels and those without. Four patients had positive retrospective donor-specific cross-matches (Table 9–1). When the positive cross-match was reported, immunosuppression was modified by the introduction of plasmapheresis daily for 3 days, the substitution of cyclophosphamide for aza-thioprine, and the addition of high-dose corticosteroids. Both patients with a neg-ative PRA and a positive retrospective cross-match survived but had early and frequent rejection. One of two patients with a positive cross-match and a reactive

Table 9–1. Cross-Match Positive Recipients*

Age/Sex	Etiology	EF	PA$_s$	PCW	CI	PRA	Days to First Rejection	Rejection Episodes		Result
								1st 4 Months	1 Year	
1. 43/M	CAD	0.22	38	30	1.7	98%	15	5	8	Death—rejection 14 months
2. 52/M	CAD	0.16	—	25	1.7	0	3	4	6	Alive—749 days
3. 63/M	CAD	0.20	67	35	2.3	0	8	3	3	Alive—430 days
4. 59/F	CAD	0.28	33	11	2.8	20%	—	—	—	Death—intraoperatively hyperacute rejection

*Immunosuppression modified: plasmapheresis daily × 3, cyclosposphamide substituted for azathioprine, steroids maintained.

CAD = coronary artery disease; CI = cardiac index in 1/min/mm²; EF = ejection fraction; PA$_s$ = pulmonary artery systolic pressure in mmHg; PCW = pulmonary capillary wedge pressure in mmHg; PRA = panel reactive antibody.

PRA survived 14 months but died of rejection when attempts at corticosteroid dose reduction were made. The remaining patient died intraoperatively of hyperacute allograft rejection. Thus, the likelihood of a positive donor-specific cross-match in patients with a reactive PRA remains small (13 percent) and survival is feasible in patients with a positive donor-specific cross-match. In summary, hyperacute rejection is a rare condition in which therapeutic strategies are inadequate but may be successfully prevented. Conceivably, the development of immunosuppressive agents specifically directed against antibody-mediated myocardial injury may eliminate the necessity of a donor-specific cross-match.

ACUTE REJECTION

Diagnostic Techniques

The major limiting factor for survival following cardiac transplantation is the successful diagnosis, prevention, and treatment of acute cardiac allograft rejection. From the very beginning, the accurate diagnosis of rejection has alluded conventional noninvasive cardiac testing. Since nuclear and echocardiographic techniques had not been developed by 1967 when the first human cardiac transplant was performed, no techniques were available to serially follow cardiac function. As a result, the diagnosis of rejection included the development of symptoms of malaise and fever, congestive heart failure, a pericardial friction rub, enzyme leak of which the LDH isoenzymes were most sensitive, and electrocardiographic abnormalities.[8,9] Although each abnormality suggested rejection, none unequivocally could prove its occurrence, resulting in overimmunosuppression of patients by treating them for rejection when the accurate diagnosis could not be established. Of all the noninvasive markers of cardiac rejection previously used, the most sensitive were electrocardiographic changes—particularly, decreases in the amplitude of the QRS complex.[10,11] An unexplained decrease in QRS voltage was a presumptive indication of rejection, which prompted the intensification of immunosuppression.

The technique of endomyocardial biopsy developed at Stanford University allows for the precise diagnosis of cardiac allograft rejection.[12] Using a modification of the Konno-Sakakibara bioptome developed in Japan in the early 1960s,[13] Caves and coworkers[12] were able to insert the instrument through the internal jugular vein, allowing for the removal of tissue fragments from the apicoseptal portion of the right ventricle. The modification added safety so that the incidence of cardiac perforation and subsequent tamponade was less than 0.1 percent and the procedure could be performed in the outpatient setting. Clinical-pathologic correlation was completed at Stanford University, and Billingham established the most widely accepted system of grading acute rejection by endomyocardial biopsy.[14] For the first time, the concept of "surveillance" biopsy was established and signs of allograft dysfunction were not necessary to make the diagnosis of rejection. As a result, it is possible for immunosuppression to be intensified before irreversible damage occurs in the allograft, with long-term cardiac allograft function remaining normal.

Because episodes of acute cardiac allograft rejection occur at the highest frequency during the first 3 months after transplant, endomyocardial biopsies should be performed at short intervals during that time. Although acute rejection

Table 9–2. Limitations of Endomyocardial Biopsy as the
Diagnostic Standard for Rejection

1. Invasive nature of the procedure
2. Sampling error
3. Predisposition for sampling previous biopsy sites
4. No diagnostic standard for antibody-mediated rejection

is much less common after the first 6 months, histologic abnormalities may be detected for several years after transplant, necessitating surveillance endomyocardial biopsies at a low frequency for an indefinite period.

Although endomyocardial biopsy may establish the diagnosis of rejection without evidence of allograft dysfunction, it is not the perfect "gold standard" (Table 9–2). Although technically safe, endomyocardial biopsy is uncomfortable for the patient, costly because it requires fluoroscopic or echocardiographic guidance, and is associated with small but significant morbidity, particularly at the venous access site. Despite the high concentration of inflammatory cells in the right ventricle of primate models, there is variability in intensity of infiltrate from fragment to fragment, suggesting the possibility of sampling error, particularly when an adequate biopsy specimen is not obtained. Because the bioptome tends to follow the trabecular pattern of the right ventricle to a similar anatomic position with each pass, specimens frequently contain fibrous and granulation tissue representing old biopsy sites, which makes interpretation difficult if not impossible. As a result, what appears to be an adequate sample of four specimens may become a sample consisting of only one or two specimens; and a biopsy with less than three adequate specimens cannot be considered to be representative of the intensity of immunologic response to the allograft.[15] To complicate the matter further, the histologic diagnosis of rejection is predicated upon the hypothesis that acute cardiac allograft rejection is always a result of cell-mediated immune responses. The patient with unexplained cardiac dysfunction who has obvious myocytic abnormalities histologically but does not meet the conventional cellular criteria for rejection, creates a serious clinical problem. It is likely that some of these patients represent antibody-mediated rejection, for which there are no established pathologic standards.

It should be apparent from the aforementioned disadvantages that an accurate noninvasive technique is not only desirable but necessary to screen for acute rejection (Table 9–3). Electrocardiography was used with endomyocardial biopsy in the "precyclosporine" era to screen for cardiac allograft rejection. The correlation between reduction of electrocardiographic voltage and histologic evidence of cardiac allograft rejection was so close that most centers tattooed the location of the V leads of the electrocardiogram on the chest for each recipient so that daily electrocardiograms could be accurately compared.[8] If there was a reduction in electrocardiographic voltage by 10 to 15 percent, an endomyocardial biopsy would be performed. When similar correlations were attempted following the introduction of cyclosporine as a primary immunosuppressive agent, the close correlation no longer existed.[16] In fact, no correlation remains between a reduction of electrocardiographic voltage and the appearance of moderate cardiac allograft rejection histologically. In an effort to further explore the possibility of an electrocardiographic correlate to rejection, intramyocardial electrograms and signal averaged electrocardiography were compared with endomyocardial biopsy. In

Table 9–3. Proposed Noninvasive Adjuncts to Biopsy in Identifying Rejection

1. Electrocardiographic voltage changes
   Intramyocardial electrograms
   Signal averaged electrocardiography
2. Torsional deformation of surgically implanted intramyocardial markers
3. Gated blood pool imaging for alterations in left ventricular volume
4. Echocardiographic assessment of systolic and diastolic function with Doppler
5. Nuclear imaging with indium-111–labeled leukocytes and antimyosin Fab fragments
6. Magnetic resonance imaging detection of increase in the T2 relaxation time and intensity
7. Cytoimmunologic monitoring with a helper/suppression ratio greater than 1
8. Measurement of metabolic byproducts of lymphocyte activation
   Interleukin 1
   Transferrin receptor positive lymphocytes
   Urinary thromboxane excretion
   Prolactin

a preliminary report, intramyocardial electrocardiography transmitted by an implanted telemetric pacemaker using a voltage reduction more than 15 percent of control had 88 percent sensitivity and 96 percent specificity.[17] Unfortunately, this approach has been limited to small series and has yet to be confirmed by multiple institutions. Similarly, signal averaged electrocardiography improved the correlation between electrocardiographic changes and rejection when QRS duration, high-frequency voltage-amplitude of the total QRS complex and of its thirds, peak QRS voltage amplitude, and QRS integrated voltage time product were compared with biopsy.[18] However, signal averaged electrocardiography was incapable of detecting rejection in the early postoperative period, and detected rejection only when it had advanced beyond a mild degree of severity. These electrocardiographic techniques therefore can not be considered clinically applicable at this time.

When left ventricular function is examined, subclinical abnormalities in systolic and diastolic function may be present when there is evidence of rejection with myocyte necrosis. Hansen and colleagues[19] examined torsional deformation of the heart using surgically implanted intramyocardial markers and computer-aided analysis of cineradiographic images. When myocyte necrosis was present, left ventricular torsional deformation amplitude and peak rate of left ventricular systolic torsion decreased significantly compared with baseline. Radionuclide angiographic blood pool imaging was found to be predictive of a positive biopsy when parameters of left ventricular volume were examined; however, ejection fraction did not significantly correlate with rejection.[20] Echocardiographic analysis of systolic and diastolic function with the addition of Doppler echocardiography has identified changes in left ventricular filling dynamics as measured by isovolumetric relaxation time, the extent of which correlates with increasingly severe grades of rejection.[21,22] Although correlations may exist, the predictability of ventricular function techniques is not sufficient to obviate the necessity of repetitive endomyocardial biopsies. However, in the situation in which serial myocardial biopsy is not possible, such as transplantation in neonates, echocardiography may be the only potential noninvasive technique that is useful in suggesting cardiac allograft rejection.

Nuclear imaging with indium-111–labeled lymphocytes showed a close correlation with rejection in the experimental model;[23] however, when compared with endomyocardial biopsy in human cardiac allograft recipients using a leukocyte label, only a 58 percent sensitivity and 36 percent specificity occurred.[24] Preliminary studies with indium-111–antimyosin antibody imaging have shown a close correlation between rejection and uptake in the animal model[25] and a sensitivity and specificity of 80 percent in assessing the presence of human cardiac allograft rejection.[26] Large multicenter studies are necessary to confirm these optimistic preliminary reports before these radioisotopic techniques should be applied on a broad scale.

Magnetic resonance imaging of allografts yields an increase in the T2 (spin-spin) relaxation time and intensity values compared with nontransplanted hearts in the animal model.[27] A significant correlation exists between the severity of rejection and T2 relaxation times using this technique. However, evidence to date suggests that tissue characterization studies are only accurate for more severe degrees of rejection and that mild cardiac allograft rejection is not likely to significantly alter magnetic resonance-generated parameters.

Cytoimmunologic monitoring of changes in lymphocyte subpopulations, particularly an increase in the helper/suppressor ratio (CD4/CD8) to more than 1, has a sensitivity of 95 percent and a specificity of over 70 percent in establishing a diagnosis of cardiac allograft rejection.[28] Other variables, however, such as the intensity of immunosuppression and infections, particularly cytomegalovirus, also will alter the helper/suppressor ratios and decrease the specificity of using lymphocyte phenotypes to detect allograft rejection. In preliminary studies, the effects of lymphocyte stimulation on serum levels of interleukin-1,[29] transferrin receptor,[30] urinary thromboxane excretion,[31] and prolactin[32] have all been proposed as useful adjuncts in establishing a diagnosis of allograft rejection. However, to date, no clinically available serologic test has been validated that can accurately detect rejection. In summary, the diagnosis of acute cardiac allograft rejection remains limited to the histologic criteria established in the early 1970s. No substitute for routine surveillance endomyocardial biopsy has emerged, resulting, unfortunately, in the necessity of repetitive biopsies in which adequate tissue samples are obtained to guide immunosuppression following cardiac transplantation.

Treatment

The number of available immunosuppressive agents was limited during the early clinical phase of human cardiac transplantation. As a result, the immunosuppressive agents used prior to transplantation, immediately after the surgery, and during long-term therapy were identical. The only therapeutic option for the treatment of established cardiac allograft rejection, therefore, was intensification of the maintenance immunosuppressive therapy, which in most instances resulted in an increase in the dose of corticosteroids. The frustrating lack of potent immunosuppressive agents is demonstrated by the immunosuppressive regimen used in the first successful human cardiac transplant recipient, which included cobalt cardiac irradiation for the first week following transplantation and actinomycin D to treat clinically evident rejection.[33] The use of a crude antilymphocyte globulin (ALG) was first reported at Stanford in 1969 by Stinson and associates.[34] A potent rabbit antithymocyte globulin (ATG) preparation was later developed at that institution and introduced into the care of cardiac transplant patients by 1973.[35]

In initial trials at Stanford, rabbit ATG was given as immunoprophylaxis against rejection during the first week following transplantation. In a similar manner, English and colleagues[36] at the Papworth Hospital incorporated equine antithymocyte globulin (ATG) into a prophylactic protocol. The polyclonal cytolytic agents also could be used as therapy for corticosteroid-resistent acute rejection. Chronic maintenance immunosuppression by 1980 remained the prednisone equivalent dose of 0.3 mg/kg and azathioprine in doses to 2 mg/kg, adjusted based on the white blood cell count.[10] The Registry of the International Society for Heart Transplantation reported a 1-year survival of approximately 60 percent and a 5-year survival of approximately 35 percent in this precyclosporine era.[37]

In 1975, a unique endecapeptide from the fungus imperfectus, Tolypocladium inflatum gams, called cyclosporine, was isolated and found to have immunosuppressive properties without affecting the white blood cell count.[38] Cyclosporine exerts its immunosuppressive effects by primarily suppressing the production of interleukin-2, which is necessary for the helper T cells to signal clonal expansion of undifferentiated cytotoxic T lymphocytes. Cyclosporine was first applied to human clinical cardiac transplantation in December 1980 at Stanford University and was widely used following approval by the Food and Drug Administration in 1983. Cyclosporine improves survival and reduces the incidence of purulent bacterial and fungal infections.[39] Although rejection was not eliminated, rejection episodes occurred less frequently and tended to be slower in onset and less severe. As a result, the overall amount of immunosuppression required was reduced and corticosteroid use was lessened. In that context, Yacoub and colleagues[40] at Harefield Hospital recognized the morbidity of corticosteroids and instituted an immunosuppressive protocol in which cyclosporine, azathioprine, and antithymocyte globulin were combined with attempts to eliminate all maintenance corticosteroids. Using this protocol, they reported an 82 percent actuarial 21-month survival rate. At the University of Pittsburgh, where prophylactic cytolytic therapy was not given, low dose prednisone and cyclosporine alone were not sufficient in preventing cardiac allograft rejection, and rejection episodes required rescue antithymocyte globulin to achieve acceptable results.[41] More recently, prednisone, azathioprine, and cyclosporine have been utilized together in so-called triple therapy, first applied at the University of Minnesota in 1981.[42] With this combination therapy, the 1-year survival rate now exceeds 85 percent.[1]

Despite these improvements in immunosuppression (Table 9–4), the major causes of death following cardiac transplantation remain rejection and infection, and, as a result, further development of potent specific immunosuppressive agents must be encouraged. Because of differences in the mode of action and the toxicity of immunosuppressive agents, the combination used for the prevention of rejection may differ in the immediate postoperative period as compared with the chronic maintenance phase. Furthermore, agents used to treat acute rejection may not be the same as those used for early prophylaxis (induction). As an example, the principal mechanism of action of cyclosporine, the attenuation of production of interleukin-2, limits the use of this agent to prevention of clonal expansion; therefore, once cytotoxic T-cell proliferation has occurred and rejection is well established, other agents may be required to reverse the process. Although investigators at the Texas Heart Institute successfully applied high-dose cyclosporine as a treatment of allograft rejection,[44] cyclosporine and azathioprine dosages usually are not altered when acute rejection is established.

Table 9–4. Development of Immunosuppressive Protocols

Year	Center	Regimen
1967	Capetown[33]	Prednisone, azathioprine, cardiac irradiation, actinomycin D
1968	Stanford[34]	Actinomycin D, prednisone, azathioprine, antilymphocyte globulin
1973	Stanford[35]	Introduction of rabbit ATG
1979	Papworth[36]	Prophylactic equine ATG
1980	Stanford[16]	Introduction of cyclosporine
1982	Harefield[40]	Trials of steroid-free protocols
1982	Pittsburgh[41]	Cyclosporine, prednisone—RATG rescue
1983	Minnesota[42]	Triple therapy—prednisone, azathioprine, cyclosporine
1985	UTAH[43]	OKT*3 monoclonal antibody for rescue and prophylaxis

In the UTAH Cardiac Transplant Program, where 153 cardiac transplant operations have been performed from March 1985 through April 1988 with an actuarial 2-year survival over 90 percent, an immunosuppressive philosophy using aggressive early immunoprophylaxis has been instituted. The approach optimally results in the prevention of rejection during the immediate postoperative recovery period (2 weeks), so that wound healing is not interrupted by the introduction of high-dose corticosteroids as a result of early allograft rejection, and the decreased early incidence of rejection may result in a state of immunologic tolerance in which maintenance corticosteroid therapy may be eliminated, with a concomitant reduction in morbidity. The first immunosuppressive protocol implemented was a modification of the Harefield protocol in which a 7-day course of equine ATG, azathioprine, and low-dose corticosteroid was employed. This protocol was quickly abandoned because of a high incidence of rejection following discontinuation of ATG. As a result, a corticosteroid oral pulse was introduced in which a daily dose of prednisone 1 mg/kg was added for 1 week beginning the day following discontinuation of cytolytic therapy. Corticosteroids were then tapered to discontinuation over 2 weeks.

The immunoprophylactic protocol underwent a second evolutionary phase when the murine monoclonal CD3 antibody (OKT*3) was developed. This murine IgG 2a specifically binds to the CD3 human lymphocyte antigen (Fig. 9–2) that is found on all human T lymphocytes and is physically linked to the T-cell receptor responsible for antigen recognition.[45] When administered intravenously, OKT*3 binds to the CD3 antigen, and the opsonized cells are cleared from the circulation by the reticuloendothelial system. The T-cell lysis results in the release of vasoactive mediators into the circulation, and a systemic reaction consisting of malaise, arthralgia, fever, and vasodilatation occurs. Following the early phase of T-lymphocyte elimination, CD2-positive T cells are seen in the circulation devoid of the CD3 antigen and presumably the T-cell receptor. The cells, therefore, are functionally normal but incapable of recognizing alloantigen, and hence cell-mediated rejection will be prevented.

OKT*3 was first applied to cardiac transplantation for the treatment of the refractory rejection.[46–49] OKT*3 therapy was found to be effective in more than 90 percent of patients whose rejection had previously been resistant to conventional immunosuppression with high dose corticosteroids and the polyclonal cyclolytic agents, ATG and Minnesota ALG. In a randomized study, we com-

MECHANISM OF ACTION OF OKT3 MONOCLONAL
ANTIBODY (OKT*3)

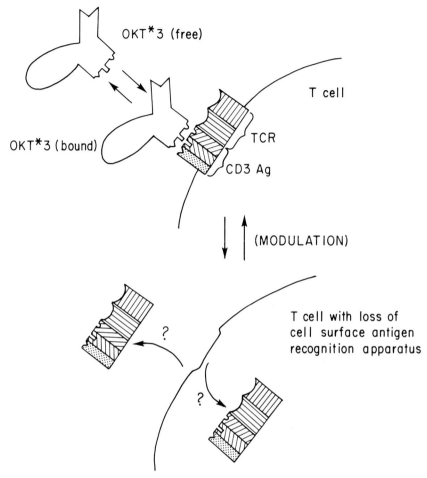

Figure 9–2. The mechanism of action of OKT*3 monoclonal antibody. OKT*3 binds to the CD3 antigen associated with the T-cell receptor on all human T lymphocytes. The bound OKT*3 stimulates phagocytosis of coated lymphocytes and modulation by shedding or internalizing the CD3-TCR complex, creating a population of T lymphocytes that are incapable of recognizing antigen. (From Bristow et al.,[45] with permission.)

pared the effects of an OKT*3-based with an ATG-based early prophylaxis protocol.[43] Patients receiving the OKT*3-based protocol had a lower incidence of rejection in the first 4 months, which was sustained beyond the first year following transplantation, and a delay in the onset of the first episode of rejection. The favorable response was not at the expense of increasing infection rate, which remained the same in both groups. When attempts were made to eliminate maintenance corticosteroids, using the criteria that patients became dependent (0.1 to 0.2 mg/kg prednisone equivalent) if they experienced three or more episodes of rejection in the first four months after transplantation, more than 80 percent of patients receiving OKT*3 were able to be successfully weaned from all cortico-

Table 9–5. Outcome of Corticosteroid-Free Maintenance*

N	Steroid 33	Steroid-Free 47	p Value
Age (years)	44.0 ± 2.7	46.9 ± 2.4	NS
Rejection incidence	4.0 ± 0.3	1.8 ± 0.2	<0.001
Infections	1.2 ± 0.2	0.7 ± 0.1	0.028
Percentage over ideal body weight	22 ± 4	12 ± 0	0.048
Cushingoid	15	4	<0.001
Diabetes mellitus	2	1	NS
Serum cholesterol (mg%)	269 ± 13	200 ± 8	<0.001

*Modified from Renlund et al,[50] with permission.

steroid therapy. Corticosteroid withdrawal resulted in less morbidity (Table 9–5) as manifested by one-half the infection incidence, less obesity and cushingoid appearance, and a significantly lower serum cholesterol level.[50]

This early prophylaxis study suffers two basic flaws in design. Patients could not be randomized with an arbitrary computer allocation, because of the intermittent lack of availability of the equine ATG (ATGAM). Patient allocation to protocol was, therefore, assigned based on drug supply. The protocols differed in the quantity of corticosteroid used in the first five weeks (less in the ATG group), timing of institution of cyclosporine (preoperative in the ATG group versus day 4 in the OKT*3 group), and duration of cytolytic therapy (8 days in the ATG group versus 14 days in the OKT*3 group). Although it seems logical that these minor protocol variations did not have a great impact on the results, this conclusion cannot be excluded. Because renal transplant studies are clear in that freedom from rejection correlates with the duration of OKT*3 administration[51] and the effect of ATG on lymphocyte suppression will not likely be sustained for 2 weeks, direct comparison of OKT*3 with ATG may not be feasible. When a 10- versus a 14-day OKT*3 based immunoprophylactic protocol were compared in cardiac transplantation, the longer duration of therapy was more successful in preventing rejection than the shorter course without an increase in the incidence of infection.[52]

Because of the antigenicity of a murine monoclonal antibody, the feasibility of retreatment for rejection rescue was considered in the decision to use an OKT*3-based early immunoprophylactic protocol. When antibodies against this murine protein were measured, 20 percent of the patients had low-titer antibody following the early prophylactic protocol. Yet when retreatment was attempted in 11 patients with rejection resistant to cytolytic agents and corticosteroids, 10 of the 11 patients responded successfully, demonstrating that immunoprophylaxis does not prevent the reuse of OKT*3 for rejection rescue.[53]

Once rejection is firmly established, the treatment should be dependent upon the histologic severity and the presence or absence of demonstrable evidence of cardiac dysfunction. Controversy exists regarding the point in the spectrum of histologic severity of rejection at which treatment should be instituted. Because approximately 50 percent of patients with lymphocytic infiltrates in the absence of myocyte necrosis will not show progressive histologic abnormalities or cardiac dysfunction, most centers do not treat rejection until myocyte necrosis is identified. Myocyte necrosis, however, is difficult to accurately appreciate histologically, and, therefore, this approach may result in the undertreatment of patients with acute rejection.

In general, the scheme for the treatment of rejection in the UTAH Cardiac Transplant Program is dependent upon the presence of hemodynamic compromise (Table 9–6). Hemodynamic compromise is said to be present when changes in systolic function are detected echocardiographically or when evidence of restricted filling is noted by unexplained elevation in jugular venous pressure, the presence of a new S3 gallop, or a pseudonormalization of the blood pressure in a previously hypertensive patient.

At our center the maintenance immunosuppressive protocol does not call for chronic corticosteroid therapy, and less morbidity is associated with a short "pulse" of oral corticosteroids in the presence of mild histologic rejection. Hence, we treat mild rejection with a 3-week oral prednisone course. If patients with mild rejection are receiving corticosteroid maintenance or if they are receiving corticosteroids as part of prophylaxis, the dose of prednisone is arrested, and biopsy is repeated at a shorter interval than scheduled. If the patient is not receiving oral corticosteroids, prednisone (50 mg twice daily for 5 days) is administered followed by tapering to discontinuation over 2 weeks. Followup biopsies are performed 1 week after institution of therapy and 1 week after the discontinuation of corticosteroids. Mild rejection rarely occurs in the presence of hemodynamic compromise and, if present, suggests either sampling error or the possibility of humoral-mediated rejection.

Moderate rejection without hemodynamic compromise is treated with pulse intravenous methylprednisolone (1 g daily for 3 days) followed by prednisone (50 mg twice daily for 2 days), followed by tapering to discontinuation with 2 weeks. Biopsies are repeated as described for mild rejection.

Moderate rejection hemodynamic compromise or severe rejection is treated by pulse methylprednisolone with a cytolytic agent, initially, ATG or Minnesota ALG (10 mg/kg IV daily for 7 to 10 days) followed by a pulse of oral prednisone (50 mg twice daily for 5 days), followed by tapering to discontinuation over two weeks. If a previous episode of moderate or severe rejection with hemodynamic compromise has been identified or the patient has previously been treated with the above regimen without resolution, retreatment OKT*3 (5 mg rapid IV push daily for 10 days) is instituted. If rejection does not respond or worsens despite this dramatic intensification of immunosuppression, consideration should be

Table 9–6. Treatment of Rejection

Mild	
Without hemodynamic compromise	Prednisone × 3 wk
With hemodynamic compromise	Methylprednisolone 1 g IV qd × 3 with prednisone × 3 wk
Moderate/Severe	
Without hemodynamic compromise	Methylprednisolone 1 g IV qd × 3 with prednisone × 3 wk
With hemodynamic compromise	Methylprednisolone 1 g IV qd × 3 with prednisone × 3 wk and cytolytic therapy (ATG, ALG, OKT*3)

given for retransplantation with mechanical support if necessary. Retransplantation should be reserved, however, for those patients with severe hemodynamic compromise requiring intravenous inotropic support.

In general, the vast majority of acute rejection episodes can be reversed and the rejection episodes that lead to death are typically unrecognized until they have progressed beyond salvage.

FUTURE PROSPECTS

Continued effort should be made to establish more specific immunosuppressive agents and protocols that prevent rejection and the attendant damage to the allograft. Such approaches may include the addition of agents that had been used previously only for cancer chemotherapy or for autoimmune disease, such as methotrexate[54] or doxorubicin,[55] or, more importantly, the development of monoclonal antibodies directed toward subpopulations of human lymphocytes or their byproducts. Preliminary studies in renal transplantation of IL-2 receptor antibodies (anti-TAC) are encouraging and strongly support continued experimentation.[56] With improved immunosuppressive techniques, early post-transplant survival may approach 100 percent. However, the effects of newer immunosuppressive agents on chronic rejection and coronary artery disease, the major cause of death beyond the early post-transplant period, have yet to be explored. It may be that immunosuppression directed toward reversing the immune response to vascular endothelial antigens may be different than that required to prevent the conventional acute cardiac allograft rejection.

REFERENCES

1. Kaye, MP: The Registry of the International Society for Heart Transplantation: Fourth official report—1987. J Heart Transplant 6:63, 1987.
2. Kirkpatrick, CH: Transplantation immunology. JAMA 251:2993, 1987.
3. Hess, M: Transplantation atherosclerosis. Cardiovasc Clin (in press).
4. Minakuchi, J, Takahashi, K, Toma, H, et al: Removal of preformed antibodies of plasmapheresis prior to kidney transplantation. Transplant Proc 18:1083, 1986.
5. Zhu, L-P, Cupps, T-R, Whalen, G, et al: Selective effects of cyclophosphamide therapy on activation, proliferation, and differentiation of human B cells. J Clin Invest 79:1082, 1987.
6. Bolman, RM III, Anderson, RW, Elick B, et al: Cardiac transplantation without a prospective crossmatch. Transplant Proc 17:209, 1985.
7. O'Connell, JB, Renlund, DG, DeWitt, CW, et al: Cardiac transplantation in sensitized recipients without a prospective crossmatch (abstrt). J Heart Transplant 7:74, 1988.
8. Stinson, EB, Dong, E, Bieber, CP, et al: Cardiac transplantation in man. I. Early rejection. JAMA 207:2233, 1969.
9. Nora, JJ, Cooley, DA, Fernbach, DJ, et al: Rejection of the transplanted human heart. Indexes of recognition and problems in prevention. N Engl J Med 280:1080, 1969.
10. Oyer, PE, Stinson, EB, Reitz, BA, et al: Cardiac transplantation: 1980. Transplant Proc 13:199, 1981.
11. Hastillo, A, Hess, ML, and Lower, RR: Cardiac transplantation: Expectation and limitation. Mod Conc Cardiovasc Dis 50:13, 1981.
12. Caves, PK, Billingham, ME, Stinson, EB, et al: Serial transvenous biopsy of the transplanted human heart. Improved management of acute rejection episodes. Lancet 1:821, 1974.
13. Sakakibara, S and Konno, S: Endomyocardial biopsy. Jpn Heart J 3:537, 1962.
14. Billingham, ME: Diagnosis of cardiac rejection by endomyocardial biopsy. Heart Transplant 1:25, 1982.
15. Spiegelhalter, DJ and Stovin, PGI: An analysis of repeated biopsies following cardiac transplantation. Stat Med 2:33, 1983.

16. Schroeder, JS and Hunt, S: Cardiac transplantation: Update 1987. JAMA 258:3142, 1987.

17. Warnecke, H, Schueler, S, Goetze, H-J, et al: Noninvasive monitoring of cardiac allograft rejection by intramyocardial electrogram recordings. Circulation 74 (Suppl III):III-72, 1986.

18. Keren, A, Gillis, AM, Freedman, RA, et al: Heart transplant rejection monitored by signal-averaged electrocardiography in patients receiving cyclosporine. Circulation 70 (Suppl I):I-124, 1984.

19. Hansen, DE, Daughters, GT II, Alderman, EL, et al: Effect of acute human cardiac allograft rejection or left ventricular systolic torsion and diastolic recoil measured by intramyocardial markers. Circulation 76:998, 1987.

20. Novitsky, D, Cooper, DKC, Boniaszczuk, J, et al: Prediction of acute cardiac rejection using radionuclide scanning to detect left ventricular volume changes. Transplant Proc 17:218, 1985.

21. Dawkins, KD, Oldershaw, PJ, Billingham, ME, et al: Noninvasive assessment of cardiac allograft rejection. Transplant Proc 17:215, 1985.

22. Valantine, HA, Fowler, MB, Hunt, SA, et al: Changes in Doppler echocardiographic indexes of left ventricular function as potential markers of acute cardiac rejection. Circulation 76 (Suppl V):V-86, 1987.

23. Eisen, HJ, Eisenerg, SB, Saffitz, JE, et al: Noninvasive detection of rejection of transplanted hearts with indium-111-labeled lymphocytes. Circulation 75:868, 1987.

24. Alivizatos, PA, Rose, ML, Aikenhead, J, et al: Migration of ^{111}In-labeled autologous leukocytes to the grafts of heart transplant patients. Transplant Proc 17:614, 1985.

25. Addinizio, LJ, Michler, RE, Marboe, C, et al: Imaging of cardiac allograft rejection in dogs using indium-111 monoclonal antimyosin. Fab J Am Coll Cardiol 9:555, 1987.

26. First, W, Yasuda, T, Segall, G, et al: Noninvasive detection of human cardiac transplant rejection with indium-111 antimyosin (Fab) imaging. Circulation 76 (Suppl V):V-81, 1987.

27. Aherne, T, Tscholakoff, D, Finkbeiner, W, et al: Magnetic resonance imaging of cardiac transplants: The evaluation of rejection of cardiac allografts with and without immunosuppression. Circulation 74:145, 1986.

28. Ertel, W, Reichenspurner, H, Hammer, C, et al: Cytoimmunologic monitoring: A method to reduce biopsy frequency after cardiac transplantation. Transplant Proc 17:204, 1985.

29. Maury, CPF and Teppo, A-M: Serum immunoreactive interleukin-1 in renal transplant recipients. Association of raised levels with graft rejection episodes. Transplantation 45:143, 1988.

30. Mohanakumar, T, Hoshinaga, K, Wood, NL, et al: Enumeration of transferrin-receptor-expressing lymphocytes as a potential marker for rejection in human cardiac transplant recipients. Transplantation 42:692, 1986.

31. Kawaguchi, A, Goldman, MH, Shapiro, R, et al: Urinary thromboxane execretion of cardiac allograft rejection in immunosuppressed rats. Transplantation 43:346, 1987.

32. Carrier, M, Emery, RW, Wild-Mobley, J, et al: Prolactin as a marker of rejection in human heart transplantation. Transplant Proc 19:3442, 1987.

33. Barnard, CN: The operation. A human cardiac transplant: An interim report of a successful operation performed at Groote Schurr Hospital, Cape Town. South Afr Med J 41:1271, 1967.

34. Stinson, EB, Dong, E Jr, Bieber, CP, et al: Cardiac transplantation in man. II. Immunosuppressive therapy. J Thorac Cardiovasc Surg 58:326, 1969.

35. Bieber, CP, Griepp, RB, Oyer, PE, et al: Use of rabbit antithymocyte globulin in cardiac transplantation. Relationship of serum clearance rates to clinical outcome. Transplantation 22:478, 1976.

36. English, TAH, Cory-Pearce, R, McGregor, C, et al: Cardiac transplantation: 3.5-year experience at Papworth Hospital. Transplant Proc 15:1238, 1983.

37. Kaye, MP: The International Heart Transplantation Registry. First Official Report—May, 1984. Heart Transplant 3:278, 1984.

38. Borel, JF: Cyclosporine: Historical perspectives. Transplant Proc 15 (Suppl 1):3, 1983.

39. Kahan, BD: Immunosuppressive therapy with cyclosporine for cardiac transplantation. Circulation 75:40, 1987.

40. Yacoub, M, Alivizatos, P, Khaghani, A, et al: The use of cyclosporine, azathioprine, and antithymocyte globulin with or without low-dose steroids for immunosuppression of cardiac transplant patients. Transplant Proc 17:221, 1985.

41. Griffith, BP, Hardesty, RL, Trento, A, et al: Cardiac transplantation. Emerging from an experiment to a service. Ann Surg 204:308, 1986.

42. Bolman, RM III, Elick, B, Olivari, MT, et al: Improved immunosuppression for heart transplantation. Heart Transplant 4:315, 1985.

43. Bristow, MR, Gilbert, EM, O'Connell, JB, et al: OKT*3 monoclonal antibody in heart transplantation. Am J Kidney Dis 11:135, 1988.

44. Radovancevic, B and Frazier, OH: Treatment of moderate heart allograft with cyclosporine. J Heart Transplant 5:307, 1986.
45. Bristow, MR, Gilbert, EM, Renlund, DG, et al: Use of OKT3 monoclonal antibody in heart transplantation: Review of the initial experience. J Heart Transplant 7:1, 1988.
46. Gilbert, EM, DeWitt, CW, Eiswirth, CC, et al: Treatment of refractory cardiac allograft rejection with OKT3 monoclonal antibody. Am J Med 82:202, 1987.
47. Costanzo-Nordin, MR, Silver, MA, O'Connell, JB, et al: Successful reversal of acute cardiac allograft rejection with OKT*3 monoclonal antibody. Circulation 76 (Suppl V):V-71, 1987.
48. Sweeney, MS, Sinnott, JT IV, Cullison, JP, et al: The use of OKT3 for stubborn heart allograft rejection: An advance in clinical immunotherapy? J Heart Transplant 6:324, 1987.
49. Klein, JB, McLeish, KR, Bunke, CM, et al: Sustained periods without rejection after treatment of cardiac allograft recipients with OKT3. Transplant Proc 20 (Suppl 1):260, 1988.
50. Renlund, DG, O'Connell, JB, Gilbert, EM, et al: Feasibility of discontinuation of corticosteroid maintenance therapy in heart transplantation. J Heart Transplant 6:71, 1987.
51. Debure, A, Chkoff, N, Chatenoud, L, et al: One-month prophylactic use of OKT3 in kidney transplant recipients. Transplantation 45:546, 1988.
52. Hegewald, MG, O'Connell, JB, Renlund, DG, et al: OKT3 monoclonal antibody given for 10 vs. 14 days as immunosuppression prophylaxis in cardiac transplantation. J Heart Transplant (in press).
53. O'Connell, JB, Renlund, DG, Gilbert, EM, et al: Treatment of refractory cardiac allograft rejection with OKT*3 monoclonal antibody in recipients with prior OKT*3 exposure (abstract). J Heart Transplant 7:74, 1988.
54. Costanzo-Nordin, MR, Grusk, BB, Silver, MA, et al: Successful reversal of recalcitrant cardiac allograft rejection with methotrexate. Circulation 78 (Suppl III): III–47, 1988.
55. Mikich, E and Ehrke, MJ: Immunomodulating effects of anticancer drugs: The example of adriamycin. Transplant Proc 16:499, 1984.
56. Strom, TB, Gaulton, GN, Kelley, VE, et al: Treatment of cardiac transplant recipients with anti-interleukin-2 receptor monoclonal antibody. In Kawai, C and Abelmann, WH (eds): Pathogenesis of Myocarditis and Cardiomyopathy. University of Tokyo Press, Tokyo, 1987.

CHAPTER 10

Infectious Complications of Transplantation

J. Stephen Dummer, M.D.

HISTORICAL BACKGROUND AND IMMUNOSUPPRESSION

Since the early 1980s there has been a rapid proliferation of centers performing heart transplantation.[1] At the same time, heart-lung transplantation has been introduced as an acceptable, though still difficult and limited, therapy for end-stage cardiopulmonary disease.[2,3] This rapid increase in transplant activity could not have been accomplished without the careful pioneering work performed over a decade at a few seminal transplant centers, particularly Stanford University.

Researchers at Stanford were also the first to comprehensively study the infectious complications of heart transplantation.[4] In 1972, Remington and associates reviewed the infectious complications in the first 40 heart recipients at that institution and found that 71 percent of the patients had developed severe infections and that 27 percent had died primarily of infection.[5] In this series the lung was the most common site of infection (60 percent of infections), and many nonbacterial pathogens were identified such as cytomegalovirus (CMV), *Aspergillus, Toxoplasma,* and *Pneumocystis.* Throughout the 1970s infections continued to be the most important complication of heart transplantation. Reviewing 13 years of experience at Stanford, Pennock and coworkers[6] noted that infections accounted for 58 percent of all deaths in heart recipients.[6] Although infectious mortality was most prominent in the early postoperative period, infections still accounted for one third to one half of deaths in patients surviving more than 2 years after the transplant procedure. This cumulative experience suggested that careful surveillance for infections and an aggressive diagnostic approach to infection should be part of the continuing management of heart transplant recipients.

As will be shown later, the types of infections that afflict heart recipients have not changed markedly in the 1980s, but recent data do suggest that infection may be somewhat less important a problem quantitatively.[7] There are undoubtedly many reasons for this development including standardized criteria for patient selection, improved diagnostic techniques, and a broader array of available antimicrobial agents. The most obvious change, in the 1980s, however, has been the introduction of cyclosporine. This 11–amino acid peptide appears to have a highly focused action on CD4 antigen-bearing T-helper cells, whereby it blocks the antigen directed release of interleukin-2, while generally sparing suppressor cell activity.[8,9] Although there is not universal agreement, many studies have shown reduced infection rates in patients receiving cycloporine compared with those receiving conventional azathioprine and prednisone immunosuppression with or without antithymocyte (ATG) globulin.[10–14] A historically controlled study at Stanford University demonstrated a fall in overall infection rates and a decline in infectious mortality (39 percent to 11 percent) in patients receiving cyclosporine.[7] These results coupled with the excellent survival rates achieved with cyclosporine-containing regimens have brought broad acceptance to cyclosporine despite serious side effects such as nephrotoxicity. It should be noted, however, that Copeland and colleagues[15] reported a 75 percent 1-year survival and a less than 10 percent infectious mortality in 32 patients receiving heart transplants with conventional azathioprine immunosuppression at the University of Arizona from 1979 to 1983, showing that good results can be achieved without the use of cyclosporine.

Immunoglobulins directed against T cells have long been used both in the prophylaxis and treatment of rejection. Numerous studies suggest that their use is associated with higher rates of clinical cytomegalovirus infection and their use may also promote Epstein-Barr virus infection and post-transplant lymphoproliferative disease.[16–19] Mason and coworkers[20] showed a 2½-fold increase in infections over a 90-day period in patients who received a course of ATG and intravenous steroids instead of oral prednisone for the treatment of rejection. Recently, a murine monoclonal antibody directed against the CD3 receptor on T cells (OKT3 antibodies) has been shown to be an effective agent to treat rejection in heart and other solid organ recipients.[21,22] Detailed studies of the infectious complications of OKT3 antibodies are not available. Recent experience from our liver transplant population suggest that this agent may be associated with higher rates of mucocutaneous herpes simplex infection, severe CMV infection, and pneumocystis pneumonia.[23,24]

The search continues for the ideal immunosuppressive agent and the ideal immunosuppressive regimen; with the increasing variety and complexity of regimens being used, it becomes more and more difficult to ferret out the contribution of each agent to overall infectious morbidity. The only firm recommendation that can be made at this time is to avoid, if possible, the use of ATG or OKT3 antibodies in the setting of ongoing systemic viral infection. One group, for example, has achieved very good results, in a small cohort of patients, with a regimen containing low doses of prednisone, cyclosporine, and azathioprine.[25] Continued critical evaluation is needed of both established immunosuppressive agents and the newer agents that will undoubtedly appear in the upcoming years in order that rational therapeutic decisions can be made.

CLINICAL INFECTIONS

TYPES AND TIMING OF INFECTIONS

Table 10–1 illustrates data on the types of pathogens encountered in severe infections in 119 heart transplant recipients receiving primarily cyclosporine and

Table 10–1. Distribution of Pathogens
in Severe Infections in Heart
Transplant Recipients

Type of Pathogen	Number of Episodes (% Total)	
Bacterial	107	(65%)
Viral	30	(18%)
Fungal	17	(10%)
Protozoal	11	(7%)
Total	165 = 1.39/patient	

prednisone immunosuppression and followed for an average of 980 days after transplantation at our center. As in other series, bacteria were numerically the most significant pathogens and included many types of organisms including some infections due to *Legionella, Listeria,* and *Nocardia* but none due to mycobacteria. The viral pathogens were all herpesviruses except for one case of progressive multifocal leukencephalopathy found at autopsy. The fungi were *Cryptococcus neoformans, Candida,* and *Aspergillus* species. The protozoal infections included nine episodes of pneumocystis infection and two of toxoplasmosis. The proportion of infections due to different pathogens was similar to a previous report from Stanford but showed a higher rate of fungal and protozoal infections than we previously reported.[11,26] Four of every 10 episodes were caused by an opportunistic pathogen, i.e., a microorganism that does not generally cause severe illness in a normal host. This fact highlights the need for sophisticated microbiologic and infectious disease input in the surveillance and management of these patients.

Figure 10–1 shows the incidence of infection due to various types of pathogens at various times after transplantation. The incidence in each interval is adjusted for the number of patients being followed, so that the height of the bars is a reflection of the true risk for each type of infection during the interval. As can be seen, the incidence of infections falls off steadily in the post-transplant period and levels off at a rate of about one severe infection for every four patient-years after 1 to 2 years. Bacterial infections were the most common late infections, but occasional serious viral, fungal, or protozoal infections were also encountered, so that surveillance for these infections can not be completely abandoned. Viral, fungal, and protozoal infections had slightly different periods of peak incidence in the early postoperative period. Severe viral infections were mostly encountered between 30 and 180 days after transplantation; severe fungal infections were most common in the first 2 months after transplantation; protozoal infections first appeared more than 30 days after transplantation and peaked between the third to sixth postoperative months. Because of the differences in the epidemiology of the different pathogens, an infection occurring 1½ months after transplantation was equally likely to be a bacterial or viral infection, whereas one occurring more than 2 years after transplantation was 10 to 20 times more likely to be a bacterial infection. Of the 119 patients described in Figure 10–1, 56, or 47 percent, died during the period of followup. Thirty (54 percent) of the 56 deaths had associated infections. It was thought that about one half of these deaths were caused primarily by infections, whereas in the other half infections complicated another

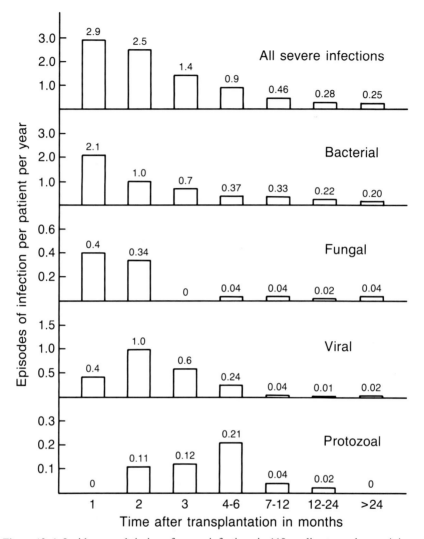

Figure 10–1. Incidence and timing of severe infections in 119 cardiac transplant recipients. The rates are corrected for the number of patients followed in each interval and the length of the interval so as to reflect the true risk for each type of infection.

terminal condition such as chronic rejection. Thus, 15 (13 percent) of the patients died primarily of infection.

COMMON SEVERE INFECTIONS

Bacterial

Table 10–2 lists the most common severe infections that occurred in the aforementioned 119 patients. The most common bacterial infection encountered

Table 10–2. Common Severe Infections
in 119 Heart Transplant Recipients

Type of Infections	Patients Infected (% Total)
Bacterial pneumonia	35 (29%)
CMV disease	21 (18%)
Bacteremia (no tissue source)	13 (11%)
Soft tissue infection	11 (9%)
Pneumocystis pneumonia	9 (8%)
Bacterial intra-abdominal	9 (8%)
Invasive *Candida*	8 (7%)
Mediastinitis	8 (7%)

in heart transplant recipients is bacterial pneumonia.[27,28] In this series, it occurred in 35 patients and accounted for 25 percent of severe infections. It occurred at all times after transplantation. Gram-negative rods were the most common group of pathogens but, notably, the pneumococcus was the single most common species encountered. Although most pneumococcal pneumonias occurred in outpatients, two cases occurred in hospitalized patients. All three legionella pneumonias occurred within 6 weeks of transplantation. The earliest bacterial pneumonia occurred 5 days after transplantation. Although transplant recipients may at times tolerate pneumonia surprisingly well, the disease can also progress rapidly and there are a broad range of diagnostic possibilities. For this reason, we hospitalize every patient with suspected pneumonia for evaluation and treatment. Empiric treatment of pneumonia in transplant recipients should be discouraged. We always evaluate a sputum gram stain as part of the initial workup. In 40 to 50 percent of cases the sputum examination, along with a history, a physical examination, and a chest radiograph, is adequate to form a presumptive diagnosis and to initiate treatment pending the results of cultures. If sputum is not obtainable or if an opportunistic pathogen is strongly suspected, we usually move quickly to invasive diagnostic procedures such as bronchoscopy with bronchoal veolar lavage. Most bacterial and many nonbacterial lung infections in transplant recipients can be diagnosed by this simple workup, but at times the diagnosis will require an open lung biopsy and we do not hesitate to perform this procedure. Examples of conditions that have been diagnosed by lung biopsy in our transplant group are viral infections such as herpes simplex or CMV pneumonia, fungal infections such as aspergillosis or cryptococcosis, and lymphoproliferative disease. In heart-lung recipients, lung biopsy may be required to establish a definite diagnosis of lung rejection and to differentiate it from infectious lung disease. Other common severe bacterial infections were mediastinitis (8 patients), intra-abdominal infections (9 patients), other soft tissue infections (11 patients), and bloodstream infections without a definite tissue source (13 patients). The bloodstream infections included six cases of line-related bacteremia. The remainder of the bacteremias were mostly due to gram-negative bacilli. In the majority of these, an abdominal or biliary source was suspected because of the clinical situation but was not proved. All but one of the soft tissue infections occurred more than 6 months after transplantation, and predisposing factors such as recent catheterization, surgery, or diabetes were present in the majority of cases. Predisposing conditions for the abdominal infections were diverticulosis (five cases), peritoneal dialysis, small bowel lymphoma, and mesenteric infarction (one case each). One patient had two recurrent intra-abdominal abscesses of obscure etiology. Bacterial mediastinitis in our population has been described previously.[29] The majority of cases were due to staphylococci, and all occurred at least 13 days after surgery. The presentations were often subtle, with low-grade fever or an elevated white count persisting as an isolated finding for a number of days. The diagnosis was usually not made until local tenderness, erythema, or drainage was evident along the sternal incision. The incidence of mediastinitis in our transplant population now appears to be declining except in patients with mechanical heart implants.[30]

Viral

Cytomegalovirus infection as defined by positive viral cultures occurs in 85 to 90 percent of our heart and heart-lung transplant population.[31] Most infections produce no definite symptoms. Symptomatic disease due to CMV occurred in 21 (18 percent) of the heart recipients described here, and 6 percent of the 119 patients had proved CMV pneumonitis. Symptomatic disease is usually manifested by fever and fatigue that may persist for 2 weeks or longer and is associated with laboratory abnormalities such as atypical lymphocytosis, neutropenia, thrombocytopenia and mild elevation of liver injury tests. About one quarter to one half of patients with CMV syndromes will also develop invasive disease due to CMV such as enteritis or pneumonitis.[31-33] Severe CMV disease occurs less frequently in patients who are seropositive for CMV before transplantation and have reactivations or reinfections. Patients who are seronegative for CMV before transplantation may acquire their infection from seropositive organ donors or blood products.[31,33,34] In addition to the direct morbidity of CMV infection, the virus is thought to produce a secondary immunosuppression that may be manifested by inversion of T-helper/T-suppressor ratios.[35,36] Clinical nonviral pulmonary infections may also be increased in patients with primary CMV infections.[37]

Seventy-five percent of significant CMV infections in this series occurred between 30 and 90 days after transplantation; a few occurred between 3 and 6 months, and two late reactivations occurred more than 1 year after transplantation in two patients who were probably additionally immunosuppressed by drug-induced leukopenia in one case and end-stage liver failure in the other. The importance of CMV infection in transplant recipients has led to experimental attempts to prevent or modify the infection by such measures as active immunization with vaccines and passive immunization with intravenous immunoglobulins.[38,39] Other measures have included immunomodulation with interferons, the use of CMV seronegative blood products, and treatment with experimental antiviral agents.[16,25,33,40-43] Enough evidence supports blood as a source of CMV infections in heart recipients to justify the use of exclusively CMV-negative blood products in patients who are seronegative for CMV before transplantation, although this may be logistically difficult or even impossible in hospitals with large transplant populations.[31] The prophylactic use of intravenous immunoglobulin or antiviral therapy with Ganciclovir are potentially useful approaches but further experimental work is needed to define their role in heart and heart-lung recipients.

Fungal

The only severe fungal infection that has occurred in 5 percent or more of the patients in this series has been invasive candidiasis. In the 119 heart recipients, there were eight cases of invasive candidiasis; these included six cases of disseminated disease, one case of esophagitis, and one case in which candida was a copathogen with staphylococci in purulent mediastinitis. All of the cases of disseminated disease occurred in patients who were residents of the intensive care unit, had other major infections, and were receiving broad-spectrum antibiotics. Four of the six cases occurred more than 2 years after transplantation in patients with severe renal, heart, or liver failure. Three of the patients were diagnosed premortem but only one of them, a patient with candidal mediastinitis, had long-term survival. Candida will continue to be a vexing problem until better diagnostic methods are developed and less toxic antifungal agents are available for prophylaxis in high-risk patients.

Protozoal

Pneumocystis carinii pneumonia occurs in 3 to 15 percent of transplant recipients who do not receive oral sulfamethoxasole-trimethoprim (SMX-TMP) prophylaxis.[7,23,27,28] Nine (8 percent) of the patients in this study had *Pneumocystis* infection. The only death occurred in a patient who was admitted to another hospital. Patients classically present with symptoms of dyspnea and dry cough that evolve over a period of a few days to a few weeks with the appearance of a diffuse infiltrate on their chest radiograph. About two thirds of patients have fever, and one patient in this series had a fever of unknown origin over a period of 2 weeks with minimal pulmonary symptoms. Another interesting occurrence in our series was the appearance in two patients of *Pneumocystis* infection within 1 to 3 weeks of the diagnosis of lymphoproliferative disease related to primary Epstein-Barr virus infection. Cytomegalovirus infection may increase the risk for *Pneumocystis* infection.[44] In a recent retrospective study of liver transplant recipients at our institution, we noted significantly higher rates of *Pneumocystis* infection in patients who had received OKT3 antibodies for the treatment of rejection.[23] There are a variety of reasonable approaches to *Pneumocystis* infection in a heart recipient population. Three possibilities are (1) prophylaxis for the entire population with SMX-TMP during the period of greatest risk, i.e., until 9 to 12 months after transplantation; (2) selective prophylaxis for patients who are thought to be at high risk because they have systemic viral infections or are heavily immunosuppressed; and (3) a high level of awareness for the infection and rapid treatment when it occurs. We have opted for the latter approach largely because increases in patients' serum creatinines with SMX-TMP therapy have created confusion with cyclosproine nephrotoxicity and because many patients have complained about gastrointestinal side effects while on SMX-TMP. Newer approaches such as the use of intermittent SMX-TMP deserve careful consideration.[45]

The diagnosis of pneumocystis infection can be made readily with methenamine silver stains of cytospin smears of fluid obtained from bronchoalveolar lavage. We generally administer 2 weeks of intravenous SMX-TMP for therapy. Although many patients will defervesce after 24 to 36 hours of therapy, a response in respiratory symptoms may not occur for 3 to 5 days. If the patient has not stabilized after 4 to 5 days of SMX-TMP, a switch to pentamadine therapy should be considered. We generally do not advise rapid reduction of immunosuppression in the first few days of treatment because of the fear that this may cause an abrupt enhancement of inflammation in the lung and lead to worsening hypoxemia. A gradual reduction in immunosuppression, however, seems reasonable. The major difficulty with high-dose intravenous SMX-TMP has been side effects of anorexia, nausea and vomiting. Inhaled pentamidine has been shown recently to be effective therapy in patients with AIDS with *Pneumocystis* infection of mild or moderate severity. This regimen deserves study in transplant recipients.[46]

OTHER SEVERE INFECTIONS

Infections due to nocardia species were documented in 13 percent of transplant recipients at Stanford receiving azathioprine but in only 3 percent of patients receiving cyclosporine.[7,47] Twenty-two cases of *Nocardia* infection in heart recipients were described and analyzed by Simpson and associates,[47] who found that the infection was confined to the lung in 81 percent of patients. Three patients disseminated the infection to the skin but there were no cases of nocardiosis of the central nervous system. The symptoms in these patients were usually mild, and in 40 percent of the patients the disease was diagnosed after a lung nodule or lung cavity was found on routine chest radiograph. The response to therapy, which usually consisted of oral sulfisoxazole, was excellent and no patient died primarily of nocardia infection. Four patients in this series developed *Nocardia* infection betwen 93 and 1251 days after transplantation. All were cured with antibiotic therapy but, unlike in the Stanford series, two patients had cerebral abscesses due to nocardia. These two patients required prolonged hospitalization at the onset of therapy and were initially treated with multiple drugs (sulfisoxazole, amikacin, and a third-generation cephalosporin).

Although CMV was the predominant viral pathogen causing severe infection in our heart recipients, we also noted four cases of severe herpes simplex infection. Two cases of herpes simplex esophagitis and one case of herpes simplex pneumonia were diagnosed in the first few weeks after transplantation and resolved with acyclovir therapy. The other patient developed multiple fatal opportunistic infections including herpes simplex esophagitis with dissemination after an open hip replacement almost 3 years after transplantation. This case highlights the need to consider severe herpes simplex infection even in the late post-transplant period. None of these patients had primary herpes simplex infection, a disease that occurs rarely in transplant recipients but is frequently associated with fulminant hepatitis and a fatal outcome.[48,49]

Twenty-two percent of the first 175 heart recipients at Stanford developed aspergillosis and it was one of the major causes of infectious mortality.[27] The incidence has fallen to 11 percent since the introduction of cyclosporine.[7] Five (4 percent) of the patients in this series developed invasive aspergillosis, including one case of isolated pulmonary aspergillosis, three cases of disseminated disease, and one unusual case of urinary tract aspergillosis. Only the patient with urinary tract aspergillosis was cured with amphotericin B therapy. Cryptococcal disease was diagnosed in four patients. It was extremely variable in its presentation, and included one case of an isolated lung nodule, one case of cryptococcal skin disease without fungal meningitis or fungemia, one case of isolated meningitis, and one case of acute pneumonia with fungemia. Although Rubin has suggested that cryptococcal disease is generally a late post-transplant infection in renal transplant recipients, two of these cases were diagnosed in the first 5 weeks after transplantation. Both of these patients suffered from extreme debilitation before transplantation, and one had received prednisone and cytotoxic drugs as treatment for myocarditis. Although all of the fungal infections in our series have been caused by a small group of fungi, other transplant groups have recorded infections with *Coccidioides immitis, Histoplasma capsulatum,* species of Mucor, and other fungi so that these may have to be considered in a diagnostic workup.[50-52]

Two patients in this series had active toxoplasmosis. The most severely affected patient had a primary infection and had involvement of the heart, pericardium, lungs, and brain at autopsy. The other patient was seropositive for *Toxoplasma* before transplantation, and a few focal areas of active toxoplasmosis were found in his heart after he died of *Pneumocystis* infection. Studies from other institutions suggest that symptomatic toxoplasmosis is usually the result of transplanting a *Toxoplasma*-seronegative patient with a heart from a seropositive donor and that most infections occur between 3 and 6 weeks after transplantation.[53] The rates of clinical toxoplasmosis were 4 percent (4/102) in one study and 3 percent (10/290) in another.[7,54] It appears that one should perform studies for antibodies to *Toxoplasma gondii* before transplantation on heart recipients and on donors and carefully monitor those seronegative patients who receive hearts from seropositive donors. Prophylactic treatment with pyrimethamine has been recommended for these "mismatched" recipients and deserves consideration.[7]

Recently we described *Mycoplasma hominis* as a cause of mediastinitis in patients, including transplant recipients, undergoing cardiac surgery.[55] The causative organism is a microaerophilic *Mycoplasma* species that can colonize the genitourinary tracts of men and women and occasionally causes postpartum infections.[56] Although there were no infections due to this agent among the 119 heart recipients described here, we have subsequently encountered six cases of *M. hominis* infection in heart and heart-lung recipients; five of these were cases of mediastinitis and one was a *Mycoplasma* bloodstream infection. In each case, a heavy growth of mycoplasma appeared on anaerobic culture plates after 2 to 4 days of incubation as very tiny, pinpoint translucent colonies. The *Mycoplasma* bloodstream infection was rapidly fatal. The cases of mediastinitis responded to treatment with clindamycin and doxycycline with clearing of the organism, but all of the patients died later of rejection or other infections.

Transplant recipients are at an increased risk of developing neoplasms of the lymphoid system.[57] Many of these lymphoproliferative lesions contain the genome of Epstein-Barr virus (EBV), and these tumors have occurred most frequently in association with serologic evidence of EBV infection.[58] Starzl and colleagues[59] have made the observation that many of these tumors regress after reduction of immunosuppression. The biology of these tumors is being investigated at a number of centers, and many factors are still unclear. Hanto and associates[60] suggest that transplant recipients with lymphoproliferative disease fall into at least two different clinical groups: (1) a younger population with symptoms suggesting infectious mononucleosis such as fever and pharyngitis who present in the early post-transplant period and usually have polyclonal tumors and (2) an older population of patients who present in the late post-transplant period with solitary tumor masses composed of a monoclonal population of lymphoid cells.[60] In our experience most, though not all, of the tumors have appeared in the first year after transplantation, and a single reliable prognostic factor has not been identified.[59] We have observed an enhanced risk for these tumors after primary EBV infection.[58,61] This is an important observation inasmuch as antibody testing before and after transplantation may identify high-risk patients. The proper treatment of these tumors is also controversial; currently we recommend that cyclosporine doses be reduced to bring blood levels to about 200 ng/ml (RIA) and that doses of other immunosuppressive medications be kept to a minimum. High-dose acyclovir has also been recommended because of its known ability to inhibit EBV replication.[62] We as well as others have noted regression of tumor during acyclovir therapy but this has generally occurred in the context of lowered immunosuppression. Some tumors that are localized may respond to irradiation or resection. Even though many of these tumors regress after reduction of immunosuppression, some do not and there is no reliable information on whether these patients might benefit from some form of chemotherapy. More research is needed into the nature of these tumors, particularly in the areas of molecular virology, immunology, and cytogenetics.

MINOR INFECTIONS

The most frequent minor infections encountered in heart transplant recipients are mucocutaneous infections caused by herpes simplex virus and herpes zoster. About one half of all transplant recipients will shed herpes simplex virus in the post-transplant period, and about one half of the virus-positive patients will develop some clinical manifestations of herpes infection, most often intraoral ulcerations.[11,64] At times these may cause severe mouth pain or be associated with esophagitis. Genital herpes also occurs, but less frequently. The usual time of onset is 7 to 21 days after transplantation. Later recurrences are usually mild unless the patient has been heavily immunosuppressed for the treatment of rejection. We generally treat oral or genital disease that is mild or moderate in intensity with oral acyclovir for about 7 days. Intravenous therapy is reserved for esophagitis and other visceral disease. Herpes zoster occurs in about 5 to 10 percent of transplant recipients during the first post-transplant year and occurs sporadically thereafter.[11] Most cases are uncomplicated and antiviral therapy is not always necessary; it should be employed if there is evidence for visceral or cutaneous dissemination. We also routinely hospitalize patients with ophthalmic zoster for evaluation and intravenous acyclovir therapy. Other patients with shingles are managed on a case-by-case basis. Unfortunately, good dosing guidelines for the use of oral acyclovir in the treatment of herpes zoster infection are not currently available. *Varicella* infection (chickenpox) developing after transplantation often has a fatal outcome, and antiviral therapy is indicated as soon as the diagnosis is made by physical examination. We monitor all heart recipients for antibodies to *Varicella zoster* before transplantation in order to determine susceptibility to chickenpox. Most adults are seropositive and these patients can be reassured that exposure to shingles or chickenpox does not represent a risk for them. The seronegative patients are candidates for treatment with *Varicella zoster* immune globulin (VZIG) within 96 hours after a household or other close exposure to shingles or chickenpox.[65]

INFECTIONS IN HEART-LUNG RECIPIENTS

Shortly after heart-lung transplantation was begun in Pittsburgh it became clear to us that infectious problems in this group were both frequent and severe. This has not been documented by published data from both our own group and the Stanford group.[66,67] Brooks from Stanford has stressed the importance of bacterial pneumonia, but also high rates of some nonbacterial infections such as

CMV and *Pneumocystis* pneumonia. We have recently updated our findings in a report on infectious complications in the first 31 operative survivors of heart-lung transplantation.[68] Although the types of pathogens encountered were quite similar to those described for 119 heart transplant recipients, the overall incidence of severe infections was more than twice that for the heart recipients, despite a much shorter mean followup (492 versus 980 days). Infections that appeared to be particularly frequent were bacterial pneumonia, CMV pneumonia, *Pneumocystis* pneumonia, and mediastinitis. Table 10–3 compares the incidence of these infections in the two populations. All the comparisons show a significantly higher frequency of infections in the heart-lung recipients.

The most striking aspect of infections in heart-lung recipients is the susceptibility of the allografted lung to infections.[67] The reasons for this susceptibility are multifactorial and probably include anatomic factors such as disruption of lymphatics and denervation of the transplanted lung, immunologic factors such as lung injury arising from local allograft reactions, and side effects of surgery such as transient injury to nerves supplying the glottis or diaphragm.[69] In some cases, infection may actually be present in the donated lung but not detected by routine donor screening.[67] In the late post-transplant period, airway injury from obliterative bronchiolitis may predispose to recurrent episodes of bacterial bronchitis and pneumonia.[68–71] The proper way to monitor and manage infectious complications in heart-lung recipients is still not clear and the development of clear guidelines will depend on further research and experience. The high rates of *Pneumocystis* infection suggest that one should employ antibiotic prophylaxis with SMX-TMP. To improve patient tolerance and compliance, we are currently using an intermittent regimen (SMX-TMP, 1 to 2 double-strength tablets for 7 days out of each month) for prophylaxis. Too few patients have been followed on this regimen to be certain how effective it will be, but no cases of *Pneumocystis* pneumonia have been encountered yet in patients on the regimen. CMV infection in heart-lung recipients remains a serious concern and we have been able to supply seronegative blood products to our CMV seronegative heart-lung recipients over the last year and a half. We also follow patients very carefully for CMV infection in the postoperative period and consider data from viral cultures and serologies when deciding on the level of immunosuppression. The clinical investigation of these patients centers on a program of serial bronchoscopies with bronchoalveolar lavages set up by our pulmonary division (Drs. Irvin Paradis and James Dauber). The two primary goals of the program are to define methods to separate pulmonary rejection from infection and to obtain samples of lympho-

Table 10–3. Severe Infections in Heart-Lung and Heart Transplant Recipients—A Comparison of Key Infections

Type of Infection	Number (%) of Patients Infected*	
	Heart-Lung (N = 31)	Heart (N = 119)
Bacterial pneumonia	26 (84%)	35 (29%)
CMV pneumonia	10 (32%)	7 (6%)
Pneumocystis pneumonia	8 (20%)	9 (8%)
Mediastinitis	7 (23%)	8 (7%)

*All comparisons are significantly different: $p < 0.01$ (χ^2)

cytes and other immune cells for *in vitro* studies. The bronchoalveolar lavages also provide samples for microbiologic stains and cultures and have been of enormous help in making precise diagnoses of infections in this group. Readers interested in a detailed description of the immunologic data collected from the bronchoalveolar lavage program may consult a recent review on the subject.[72]

INFECTIOUS DISEASE SURVEILLANCE

Both the frequency and variety of infections encountered in heart transplant recipients mandate an orderly and informed approach to the surveillance for infections. Probably the most important type of surveillance is studies that are ordered before transplantation on candidates and donors. Table 10–4 lists the studies that we currently recommend. This should be construed as a minimal list, and some centers may want to conduct more extensive studies.[43] Testing may also be determined by the geographic location. For instance, in the southwest United States, serologic and skin testing for coccidioidomycosis would be reasonable. The recipient studies are primarily helpful in assessing the risk for certain infections after transplantation and providing a baseline for later serologic studies. The donor studies are designed to test for the possibility of transmission of infections by the donated organ. A positive PPD skin test in a patient never treated for tuberculosis indicates an increased risk of developing tuberculosis by reactivation after institution of immunosuppression. Although we generally give isoniazid prophylaxis after transplantation to patients with positive PPDs, not all authorities agree that prophylaxis should be given routinely.[73] At a minimum these patients should be carefully followed for the development of tuberculosis. Stools for ova and parasites are primarily ordered to detect carriers of *Strongyloides stercoralis,* which may cause a hyperinfection syndrome and fatally disseminate in patients who are immunosuppressed.[74] The risk of carriage is highest in patients who come from tropical or subtropical areas.

After transplantation the aforementioned serologic studies are only reordered to assess clinical problems. We do generally obtain viral cultures (urine, throat wash, and buffy coat) for CMV and herpes simplex virus at intervals of every 2 to 4 weeks for the first 2 to 3 months after transplantation. In a hospital where virology services are not available, serologies for CMV should probably be

Table 10–4. Pretransplant Screening of Heart Recipients and Donors

Recipients	Donors
History and physical	CMV IgG
CMV IgG	*Toxoplasma* IgG
Toxoplasma IgG	Hepatitis B screen
EBV IgG (VCA)	HIV antibodies
Varicella zoster IgG	Clinical assessment
HIV antibodies	
Hepatitis B screen	
PPD skin test	
Stool for ova and parasites	
Urinalysis	

ordered at routine intervals instead. However, we prefer the use of viral cultures because the results are not influenced by transfusion. No routine bacterial or fungal cultures are ordered on heart recipients. Heart-lung recipients, as already mentioned, undergo routine bronchoalveolar lavage. We also order frequent (2 to 3 times per week) sputum cultures and Gram stains on heart-lung recipients while they are intubated in the intensive care unit, to provide a baseline for comparison if fevers or pulmonary infiltrates develop.

After discharge from the hospital the patient is seen at intervals for endomyocardial biopsy and clinical evaluation. Between these visits we attempt to maintain telephone contact with the patients to answer questions and to assist in managing illnesses that arise. If the patient develops a significant illness we prefer to manage them in Pittsburgh, if possible. This is particularly true for heart-lung recipients in whom our own ideas about management are still in a constant state of evolution. Although the antibody response to immunization in transplant recipients may be diminished, we recommend that patients receive pneumococcal vaccine once and influenza vaccinations yearly.[75,76] The only other prophylactic measures currently employed are oral nystatin during the initial transplant hospitalization and sulfa-trimethoprim prophylaxis for heart-lung recipients. The protocols, however, are under periodic reevaluation and may change in the future as our experience increases or new information appears in the medical literature.

DIRECTIONS FOR THE FUTURE

Transplantation is a rapidly changing specialty. Future research will likely change the ways in which we diagnose, manage, and attempt to prevent infections after transplantation. Inasmuch as transplant recipients suffer from some of these same infectious problems as patients with AIDS, it is likely that the intense research activity in AIDS will create some useful spinoff for the clinician dealing with transplant recipients. There are a number of areas in which major advances would have an immediate impact on transplantation. The most important is probably in the area of chemotherapy and prevention of CMV infection. Effective and safe agents are needed to treat CMV infection. The ideal agent would have low enough toxicity that it could be administered prophylactically. Fungal diseases, though less frequent that CMV disease, are often fatal, and noninvasive diagnostic tests and less toxic therapeutic agents are needed. Many of the pathogens that threaten transplant recipients are newly acquired during or after transplantation, and effective ways to immunize patients, either actively or passively, against these pathogens would be a major advance. Given the current pace of change in biomedical science, it is likely tht some advances will be made in these areas in the next decade. At the same time, new immunosuppressive drugs and emerging technologies such as the mechanical heart bridge may create new infectious complications that will require novel solutions. All of these changes will introduce progressively greater complexity into transplantation that will accentuate the need for an integrated team approach.

REFERENCES

1. Solis, E and Kaye, MP: The registry of the international society for heart transplantation: Third official report—June 1986. J Heart Transplant 5:2, 1986.

2. Reitz, BA, Wallwork, JL, Hunt, SA, et al: Heart-lung transplantation. N Engl J Med 306:557, 1982.

3. Jamieson, SW, Reitz, BA, Oyer, PE, et al: Combined heart and lung transportation. Lancet 1:1130, 1983.

4. Stinson, EB, Bieber, CP, Griepp, RB, et al: Infectious complications after cardiac transplantation in man. Ann Intern Med 74:22, 1971.

5. Remington, JS, Gaines, JD, Griepp, RB et al: Further experience with infection after cardiac transplantation. Transplant Proc 3:699, 1972.

6. Pennock, JL, Oyer, PE, Reitz, BA, et al: Cardiac transplantation in perspective for the future. J Thorac Cardiovasc Surg 83:168, 1982.

7. Hofflin, JM, Potasman, I, Baldwin, JC, et al: Infectious complications in heart transplant recipients receiving cyclosporine and corticosteroids. Ann Intern Med 106:209, 1987.

8. Hess, AD and Tutschka, PJ: Effect of cyclosporin A on human lymphocyte responses *in vitro.* I. CsA allows for the expression of alloantigen-activated suppressor cells while preferentially inhibiting the induction of cytolytic effector lymphocytes in MLR. J Immunol 124:2601, 1980.

9. Bunjes, D, Hardt, C, Rollinghoff, M, et al: Cyclosporin A mediates immunosuppression of primary cytotoxic T cell responses by impairing the release of interleukin 1 and interleukin 2. Eur J Immunol 11:657, 1981.

10. Dummer, JS, Hardy A, Poorsattar, A, et al: Early infections in kidney, heart, and liver transplant recipients on cycloporine. Transplantation 36:259, 1983.

11. Ho, M, Wajszczuk, CP, Hardy, A, et al: Infections in kidney, heart, and liver transplant recipients on cyclosporine. Transplant Proc 15:2768, 1983.

12. Ferguson, RM, Rynasiewicz, JJ, Sutherland, DER, et al: Cyclosporin A in renal transplantation: A prospective randomized trial. Surgery 92:175, 1982.

13. Barnhart, GR, Hastillo, A, Goldman, MH, et al: A prospective randomized trial of pretransfusion/ azathioprine/prednisone versus cyclosporine/prednisone immunosuppression in cardiac transplant recipients: Preliminary results. Circulation 72(Suppl II):227, 1985.

14. The Canadian Multicentre Transplant Study Group: A randomized clinical trial of cyclosporine in cadaveric renal transplantation. N Engl J Med 314:1219, 1986.

15. Copeland, JG, Mammana, RB, Fuller, JK, et al: Heart Transplantation: Four years' experience with conventional immunosuppression. JAMA 251:1563, 1984.

16. Cheeseman, SH, Rubin, RH, Stewart, JA et al: Controlled clinical trial of prophylactic human-leukocyte interferon in renal transplantation: Effects on cytomegalovirus and herpes simplex virus infections. N Engl J Med 300:1345, 1979.

17. Pass, RF, Whitley, RJ, Diethelm, AG, et al: Cytomegalovirus infection in patients with renal transplants: Potentiation by antithymocyte globulin and an incompatible graft. J Infect Dis 142:9, 1980.

18. Rubin, RH, Tolkoff-Rubin, NE, Oliver, D, et al: Multicenter seroepidemiologic study of the impact of cytomegalovirus infection on renal transplantation. Transplantation 40:243, 1985.

19. Bieber, CP, Herberling, RL, Jamieson, SW, et al: Lymphoma in cardiac transplant recipients associated with cyclosporin A, prednisone and anti-thymocyte globulin (ATG). In Purtilo, DT (ed): Immune Deficiency and Cancer. Plenum Press, New York, 1984.

20. Mason, JW, Stinson, EB, Hunt, SA, et al: Infections after cardiac transplantation: Relation to rejection therapy. Ann Intern Med 85:69, 1976.

21. Cosimi, AB, Colvin, RB, Burton, RC, et al: Use of monoclonal antibodies to T-cell subsets for immunologic monitoring and treatment in recipients of renal allografts. N Engl J Med 305:308, 1981.

22. Gilbert, EM, Eiswirth, CC, Renlund, DG, et al: Use of ORTHOCLONE OKT3 monoclonal antibody in cardiac transplantation: Early experience with rejection prophylaxis and treatment of refractory rejection. Transplant 19:45, 1987.

23. Kusne, S, Dummer, JS, Singh, N, et al: Infections after liver transplantation: An analysis of 101 consecutive cases. Medicine 67:132, 1988.

24. Singh, N, Dummer, JS, Kusne, S, et al: Infections with cytomegalovirus and other herpesviruses in 121 liver transplant recipients: Transmission by donated organ and the effect of OKT3 antibodies. J Infect Dis 158:124, 1988.

25. Andreone, PA, Olivari, MT, Elick, B, et al: Reduction of infectious complications following heart transplantation with triple-drug immunotherapy. J Heart Transplant 5:13, 1986.

26. Baumgartner, WA, Reitz, BA, Oyer, PE, et al: Cardiac homotransplantation. Curr Probl Surg 16:1, 1979.

27. Copeland, JG and Stinson, EB: Human heart transplantation. Curr Probl Cardiol 3:4, 1980.
28. Dummer, JS, Bahnson, HT, Griffith, BP, et al: Infections in patients on cyclosporine and prednisone following cardiac transplantation. Transplant 15:2779, 1983.
29. Trento, A, Dummer, JS, Hardesty, RL, et al: Mediastinitis following heart transplantation: Incidence, treatment and results. Heart Transplant 3:336, 1984.
30. Griffith, BP, Kormos, RL, Hardesty, RL, et al: The artificial heart: Infection-related morbidity and its effect on transplantation. Ann Thorac Surg 45: 409, 1988.
31. Dummer, JS, White, LT, Ho, M, et al: Morbidity of cytomegalovirus infection in recipients of heart or heart-lung transplants who received cyclosporine. J Infect Dis 152:1182, 1985.
32. Peterson, PK, Balfour, HH Jr, Marker, SC, et al: Cytomegalovirus disease in renal allograft recipients: A prospective study of the clinical features, risk factors and impact on renal transplantation. Medicine 59:283, 1980.
33. Pollard, RB, Arvin, AM, Gamberg, P, et al: Specific cell-mediated immunity and infections with herpes viruses in cardiac transplant recipients. Am J Med 73:679, 1982.
34. Chou, S: Cytomegalovirus infection and reinfection transmitted by heart transplantation. J Infect Dis 155:1054, 1987.
35. Schooley, RT, Hirsch, MS, Colvin, RB, et al: Association of herpes virus infections with T-lymphocyte-subset alterations, glomerulopathy, and opportunistic infections after renal transplantation. N Engl J Med 308:307, 1983.
36. Dummer, JS, Ho, M, Rabin, B, et al: The effect of cytomegalovirus and Epstein-Barr virus infection on T-lymphocyte subsets in cardiac transplant patients on cyclosporine. Transplantation 38:433, 1984.
37. Rand, KH, Pollard, RB, and Merigan, TC: Increased pulmonary superinfections in cardiac-transplant patients undergoing primary cytomegalovirus infection. N Engl J Med 298:951, 1978.
38. Plotkin, SA, Friedman, HM, Fleisher, GR, et al: Towne-vaccine-induced prevention of cytomegalovirus disease after renal transplants. Lancet 1:528, 1984.
39. Snydman, DR, Werner, BG, Heinze-Lacey, B, et al: Use of cytomegalovirus immune globulin to prevent cytomegalovirus disease in renal-transplant recipients. N Engl J Med 317:1049, 1987.
40. Collaborative DHPG Treatment Group: Treatment of serious cytomegalovirus infections with 9-(1,3 dihydroxy-2-propoxymethyl) guanine in patients with AIDS and other immunodeficiencies. N Engl J Med 314:801, 1096.
41. Erice, A, Jordan, MC, Chace, BA, et al: Ganciclovir treatment of cytomegalovirus disease in transplant recipients and other immunocompromised hosts. JAMA 257:3082, 1987.
42. Shepp, DH, Dandliker, PS, Miranda, P, et al: Activity of 9-[2-hydroxy-1-(hydroxymethyl)ethoxymethyl] guanine in the treatment of cytomegalovirus pneumonia. Ann Intern Med 103:368, 1985.
43. Snyder, MB, Markowitz, N, Saravolatz, LD, et al: Infection surveillance in cardiac transplantation. Am J Infect Cont 16:54, 1988.
44. Hardy, AM, Wajszczuk, CP, Suffredini, AF, et al: *Pneumocystis carinii* pneumonia in renal-transplant recipients treated with cyclosporine and steroids. J Infect Dis 149:143, 1984.
45. Hughes, WT, Rivera, GK, Schell, MJ, et al: Successful intermittent chemoprophylaxis for *Pneumocystic carinii* pneumonitis. N Engl J Med 316:1627, 1987.
46. Conte, JE, Hollander, H, and Golden, JA: Inhaled or reduced-dose intravenous pentamidine for *Pneumocystis carinii* pneumonia. Ann Intern Med 107:495, 1987.
47. Simpson, GL, Stinson, EB, Egger, MJ, et al: Nocardial infections in the immunocompromised host: A detailed study in a defined population. Rev Infect Dis 3:492, 1981.
48. Elliott, WC, Houghton, DC, Bryant, RE, et al: Herpes simplex type 1 hepatitis in renal transplantation. Arch Intern Med 140:1656, 1980.
49. Taylor, RJ, Saul, SH, Dowling, JN, et al: Primary disseminated herpes simplex infection with fulminant hepatitis following renal transplantation. Arch Intern Med 141:1519, 1981.
50. Baumgartner, WA: Infection in cardiac transplantation. Heart Transplant 3:75, 1983.
51. Cohen, IM, Galgiani, JN, Potter, D, et al: Coccidioidomycosis in renal replacement therapy. Arch Intern Med 142:489, 1982.
52. Davies, SF, Sarosi, GA, Peterson, PK, et al: Disseminated histoplasmosis in renal transplant recipients. Am J Surg 137:686, 1979.
53. Luft, BJ, Noat, Y, Araujo, FG, et al: Primary and reactivated toxoplasma infection in patients with cardiac transplants. Ann Intern Med 99:27, 1983.
54. Wreghitt, TG, Hakim, M, Cory-Pearce, R, et al: The impact of donor-transmitted CMV and *Toxoplasma gondii* disease in cardiac transplantation. Transplant Proceed 18:1375, 1986.

55. Steffensen, DO, Dummer, JS, Granick, MS, et al: Sternotomy infections with *Mycoplasma hominis*. Ann Intern Med 106:204, 1987.
56. Cassell, GH and Coe, BC: Mycoplasma as agents of human disease. N Engl J Med 304:80, 1981.
57. Penn, I: Malignancies associated with immunosuppressive or cytotoxic therapy. Surgery 83:492, 1981.
58. Ho, M, Miller, G, Atchison, RW, et al: Epstein-Barr virus infections and DNA hybridization studies in posttransplantation lymphoma and lymphoproliferative lesions: The role of primary infection. J Infect Dis 152:876, 1985.
59. Starzl, TE, Porter, KA, Iwatsuki, S, et al: Reversibility of lymphomas and lymphoproliferative lesions developing under cyclosporin-steroid therapy. Lancet 1:583, 1984.
60. Hanto, DW, Gajl-Peczalska, KJ, Frizzera, G, et al: Epstein-Barr virus (EBV) induced polyclonal and monoclonal B-cell lymphoproliferative disease occurring after renal transplantation. Ann Surg 198:356, 1983.
61. Ho, M, Jaffee, R, Miller, G, et al: The frequency of EBV infection and associated lymphoproliferative syndrome after transplantation and its manifestations in children. Transplantation 45: 719, 1988.
62. Colby, BM, Shaw, JE, Datta, AK, et al: Replication of Epstein-Barr virus DNA in lymphoblastoid cells treated for extended periods with acyclovir. Am J Med 73(Suppl 1A):77, 1982.
63. Thiru, S, Calne, RY, and Nagington, J: Lymphoma in renal allograft patients treated with cyclosprin-A as one of the immunosuppressive agents. Transplant Proc 13:359, 1981.
64. Rand, KH, Rasmussen, LE, Pollard, RB, et al: Cellular immunity and herpesvirus infections in cardiac-transplant patients. N Engl J Med 296:1372, 1976.
65. Weller, TH: Varicalla and herpes zoster: Changing concepts of the natural history, control and importance of a not-so-benign virus. N Engl J Med 309:1362, 1983.
66. Brooks, RG, Hofflin, JM, Jamieson, SW, et al: Infectious complications in heart-lung transplant recipients. Am J Med 79:412, 1985.
67. Dummer, JS, Montero, CG, Griffith, BP, et al: Infections in heart-lung transplant recipients. Transplantation 41:725, 1986.
68. Dummer, JS: Infectious complication of heart-lung transplantation. In Cooper, DKC (ed): Heart and Lung Replacement. Medical and Technical Press, (in press).
69. Thompson, ME, Dummer, JS, Paradis, I, et al: Heart-lung transplantation—the courage to succeed. In Yu, P (ed): Progress in Cardiology. Vol 16. Lea and Febiger, Philadelphia, 1987.
70. Burke, CM, Theodore, J, Dawkins, KD, et al: Post-transplant obliterative bronchiolitis and other late lung sequelae in human heart-lung transplantation. Chest 86:824, 1984.
71. Yousem, SA, Burke, CM, and Billingham, ME: Pathologic pulmonary alterations in long term human heart-lung transplantation. Human Pathol 16:911, 1985.
72. Dauber, JH and Zeevi, A: Lung transplantation: Lessons learned about local immune function and pulmonary defense mechanisms. In Daniele, RP (ed): Pulmonary Immunology. McGraw Hill, New York, 1988.
73. Rubin, RH and Young, LS: Clinical Approach to Infection in the Compromised Host. Plenum Press, New York, 1981.
74. Scowden, EB, Schaffner, W, and Stone, WJ: Overwhelming strongyloidiasis. Medicine 57:527, 1978.
75. Huang, KL, Armstrong, JA, and Ho, M: Antibody response after influenza immunization in renal transplant patients receiving cyclosporin A or azathioprine. Infect Immunol 40:421, 1983.
76. Linneman, CC Jr, First, MR, and Schiffman, G: Response to pneumococcal vaccine in renal transplant and hemodialysis patients. Arch Intern Med 141:1637, 1981.

CHAPTER 11

Hypertension Following Orthotopic Cardiac Transplantation*

Alvin P. Shapiro, M.D.
Gale H. Rutan, M.D., M.P.H.
Mark E. Thompson, M.D.
R. L. Nigalye, M.B., B.S.

Since the achievement of successful orthotopic cardiac transplantation, it has become apparent that hypertension arising *de novo* is an inevitable complication in many patients. In fact, in our first reports of this event in 1983 from our series at the University of Pittsburgh, it was apparent that the majority of our patients receiving cyclosporine became hypertensive.[1,2] This development was not related to pre-existing hypertension but instead it appeared and progressed during the postoperative course, with a mean onset in this initial series of 50 days post-transplant (ranging from 1 week to 6 months after surgery). Although the extent to which the hypertension contributes to *mortality* in these patients is unclear, it makes a significant contribution to *morbidity* and it is a source of continuous concern to the surgeons and cardiologists who care for these patients because it represents an additional threat to the integrity of the transplanted heart.

Our interest in this unique form of hypertension has been directed primarily at two aspects of the problem—namely, its *etiology* and its *treatment*. It has been difficult to do carefullly controlled studies of these considerations because of the large variety of complications and the complex problems that these individuals experience, and the need for these ailments, particularly rejection and infection, to command priorities in their management. Consequently, most of the data that we have gathered to understand the hypertension have been descriptive and often retrospective. In this chapter, we review our experiences from 1980 to 1986 and attempt to summarize our viewpoints about the current status of the problem of hypertension.

*Supported in part by NHLBI Grant #HL-07011.

ETIOLOGIC MECHANISMS

Volume

During the immediate postoperative phase, these patients tend to be over-expanded, and a major component of their hypertension is probably the same type of extracellular and intravascular volume expansion that is encountered in patients with hypertension secondary to renal parenchymal disease, or postoperatively after a variety of surgical procedures. Our evidence for this association is related to the initial need for diuretics and the blood pressure response, albeit modest in some patients, after the use of diuretics in management. Increased intravascular and extracellular volume in these patients may be secondary to sodium and water retention from the renal dysfunction that they exhibit so frequently postoperatively, which is aggravated by cyclosporine.[3,4]

Peripheral Resistance

Most patients who undergo cardiac transplantation have been in low output heart failure for a significant period of time. Under these circumstances, the systemic vascular resistance is increased,[5] and it is of interest that it does not return to normal in the presence of the "new heart." In fact, increased peripheral resistance persists as long as 1 year after the transplant.[6] After transplant, however, the "new heart" has replaced the depressed cardiac output of the recipient's "old heart" with a normal cardiac output. Accordingly, we have a situation with a normal cardiac output and a persistently increased systemic vascular resistance, which by definition of the two major factors that control blood pressure (i.e., $CO \times PR = BP$), will inevitably produce a hypertensive individual.

Cardiac Denervation and Heart Rate

The transplanted heart is a denervated organ; it is not subject to vagal slowing or to heart rate increase via sympathetic nervous system stimulation. Circulating catecholamines may modulate the rate but the baroreceptor control, which operates through cardioacceleratory and cardiac-inhibitory reflexes to the heart, is absent. One of the striking things we noted early in our study of these patients is that when we monitored their 24-hour ambulatory blood pressures, they failed to show the 10 to 15 percent fall in blood pressure during recumbency/sleep at night that we find in most normotensive and hypertensive individuals.[1,7] Along with the failure of the blood pressure to fall at night, there was also an accompanying diminution in the nocturnal decline in heart rate. The other situation in which failure of decline in blood pressure with sleep had been noted prior to our observations, was in patients with neurogenic orthostatic hypotension;[8,9] we have shown it also in diabetics, usually type I, with autonomic neuropathy.[10]

The phenomenon of loss of nocturnal decline in blood pressure and heart rate is quite striking, and we have reported it in a series of 69 transplanted patients.[10] Furthermore, we have demonstrated its presence as long as 1 year after the surgery, apparently because the human heart does not appear to reinnervate even after it has been *in situ* for at least this period of time. The first manifestation of elevated blood pressure may occur during the nocturnal recumbent hours in patients who are normotensive during the day; this phenomenon has been the cause of early morning headaches in some of our patients.

The reason for this failure of blood pressure to decline when recumbent/

asleep has not been demonstrated conclusively in these patients with denervated, transplanted hearts but the mechanism can be hypothesized from known hemo-dynamic data. When recumbency is assumed at night, central pooling of blood volume tends to increase stroke volume and cardiac output. In the normal indi-vidual, this tendency is blunted by a drop in heart rate of sufficient degree so that the increased central blood volume does not cause a rise in cardiac output and blood pressure, but instead a blood pressure decline ensues; this decline is prob-ably further encouraged by an increased vasodilatation, which results from a drop in systemic vascular resistance. Both of these phenomena—fall in heart rate and decrease in systemic vascular resistance—probably occur only to a minimal extent in the transplanted subject during recumbency/sleep, thus resulting in the failure of the blood pressure to decline, and sometimes even a blood pressure rise.

Catecholamines

In our original survey of these patients in the early phases of their hyperten-sion, measurements of urinary excretion of norepinephrine, epinephrine, and dopamine were all within normal limits. We have not studied them during the later course of the hypertension.[1,2]

Corticosteroids

Transplanted patients all receive steroids in addition to their other immu-nosuppressive agents. Steroids by their effect on arteriolar sensitivity and with some preparations by producing sodium retention, may be a contributing factor to the hypertension, but their exact impact is not known.

The Renin-Angiotensin System

Plasma renin activity (PRA) was studied from the start of our experience with these patients. Serial determinations were obtained both in the immediate postoperative period as well as regularly during the course of their followup. In our initial report in these patients, we noted that PRA levels were usually within normal limits or somewhat low.[1,2] This finding was in keeping with our hypothesis that in the early stages of the hypertension in these subjects, volume overexpan-sion was present owing to a fall in sodium excretion and/or administration of excess fluids. Thus, we did not think that the renin-angiotensin system played a significant role in the hypertension at that point.

However, during the course of followup in these patients, a rise in PRA to significantly elevated levels was noted in association with a rise in serum creati-nine and a persistent, and sometimes further, elevation in blood pressure. This development is believed related to continued cyclosporine administration, as will be discussed further on. This late rise in PRA has also influenced our approach to pharmacologic therapy in these patients, as we will also discuss later.

Cyclosporine

The administration of cyclosporine is an established cause of slowly progres-sive renal impairment. In studies at our institution, only 55 percent of cardiac transplant patients retain normal renal function 6 months after transplant, and at 1 year only 17 percent. This percentage falls further over time, and no patients who have survived as long as 3 years exhibit normal renal function.[3,4] The kidney disease in these patients has the characteristics expected from the tubular atrophy and interstitial fibrosis that have been observed on biopsy, but there also seems to be a significant vascular component. Cyclosporine has a direct renal vasoconstrictor effect, and scarring of arterioles leading to narrowing or occlusion of these vessels has been noted.[11,12] The relationship of slowly progressive renal dysfunction to cyclosporine observed in the later period of followup in these individuals has been treated by reduction of cyclosporine dosage and by the introduction of azathioprine in their management, which has resulted in some lowering of blood pressure, although not to normotensive levels, and at least stabilization of the rising creatinine.[4,13]

Thus, there are both acute and chronic components to the nephrotoxicity and its accompanying hypertension in the transplant patient. Initially, at the time of the cardiac transplantation, renal dysfunction related to the ischemia of the kidney during surgery and aggravated by large doses of cyclosporine, is characterized by volume overexpansion and increased sodium avidity, which are associated with hypertension but from which most patients recover. Whereas as many as 60 percent of patients receiving cyclosporine may show evidence of this renal functional impairment in the immediate postoperative period, this incidence has been reduced by lowering the dose of cyclosporine during the acute ischemic phase.[3,4,13]

Chronic hypertension appears to be associated with increasing vascular damage to the kidney and a slow rise in both creatinine levels and PRA. These changes occur to a significantly lesser extent in patients receiving azathioprine. Inasmuch as we do not have a comparable series of patients who were treated exclusively with azathioprine at our institution we compared a series of our patients with a series who underwent heart transplantation during a comparable period of time at the Medical College of Virginia (MCV). One year postoperatively, the series operated upon at the MCV had a significantly lower blood pressure (average of 124/84 mmHg; mean blood pressure of 98 mmHg) as compared with the group at our institution (average 154/95 mmHg; mean blood pressure of 116 mmHg). At that time, the average creatinine in the group at our hospital was 2.2 mg/dl versus 1.1 mg/dl in the MCV group. Eighteen patients had been followed for 1 year at our hospital as compared with 12 patients from MCV. The group of 18 long-term survivors at our hospital came from a total of 33 operated on through the period from 1981 to 1982, during the early part of our experience. Twenty-seven of them had survived 1 month or more; of these, 25 had developed hypertension. The 18 patients were those of the 25 on whom we had 1-year followup data. The 12 patients from MCV were part of a larger group of 24 who were operated on during the same time period and also had survived for up to 1 year.[14]

We then turned our attention to the effects of the long-term administration of cyclosporine on both creatinine and PRA levels.[15] By 1986 there were 144 patients in whom we had been able to follow PRA regularly along with creatinine and blood pressure. The median creatinine level for these 144 transplant patients was 1.5 mg/dl. The patients with creatinine values less than the median had significantly lower diastolic and systolic blood pressures than those patients with creatinine above 1.5 mg/dl. This difference, although small (145/97 mmHg in the higher creatinine group versus 141/92 mmHg in the lower creatinine group), was nevertheless statistically significant ($p = 0.05/0.01$). Moreover, the supine PRA was 17.1 ng/ml in the higher group and 10.6 ng/ml in the lower group ($p = 0.05$) (normal 1.5 to 5 ng/ml/3 hours incubation). It was also apparent that the average PRA levels in the transplant patients were now elevated in contrast to the levels in the early group of patients reported previously. Furthermore, the level of serum creatinine and the level of PRA were significantly correlated ($r = 0.4$; $p < 0.001$) in recipients with creatinine levels above 1.5 mg/dl and not in those whose creatinine level was less than 1.5 mg/dl.[15]

We then examined the data in patients whose PRAs were measured on at least two occasions over a period from 6 to 30 months between their initial PRA and a followup outpatient PRA. Thus, these individuals had survived at least more than 6 months and up to a maximum of 30 months. A total of 42 of the 144 patients fit these criteria and in this sample, PRA rose from 8.9 ng/ml to 19.6 ng/ml over the time period, with creatinine also increasing significantly from a mean of 1.1 mg/dl to 2.1 mg/dl.[15]

Our interpretation of these data is that although PRA at most may play only a minor role in the hypertension of the patients during the early period after transplant, with cyclosporine contributing only to sodium retention and volume overexpansion, as the administration of cyclosporine continues, the significant renal dysfunction that develops is associated with a gradually rising PRA and continued hypertension. The sequence of events suggests to us that renal arteriolar damage ensues with elaboration of increasing renin activity, and hence angiotensin II, which begins to make a major contribution to the hypertension; the hypertension then in turn may feed back to further injure kidney function. Cyclosporine therefore emerges as a major contributor to the persistent hypertension of the transplanted patient, adding to the other aforementioned etiologies, and in particular contributing to the sustained increase in systemic vascular resistance. Such a sequence and this hypothesis are consistent with the multifactorial etiology of all types of hypertension.[16]

THERAPY OF HYPERTENSION

Our initial approach to therapy of hypertension in cardiac transplant patients was somewhat empiric but stepwise, and basically aimed at the various etiologic factors that have been described earlier. Thus, we have handled the problem with the following treatments.

Diuretics

Diuretics were the cornerstone of initial management based upon our impression that volume overexpansion and sodium retention were present. Thiazide diuretics were used if the creatinine was 1.5 mg/dl or less; above this level, loop diuretics were employed.

Vasodilators

If the diuretic alone failed to control blood pressure, which was often the situation, a vasodilator, usually *hydralazine,* was added. An occasional patient was advanced to *minoxidil* as the vasodilator drug, but this was unusual because of concern that the degree of vasodilation induced by minoxidil might lead to cardiac dilatation and hypertrophy, an outcome to be avoided in these transplanted hearts. It was of interest that the use of these vasodilators seemed to produce minimal tachycardia—an event predicted by the fact that the denervated heart would not respond to vasodilatation with increased heart rate, as is usually the case when these drugs are given.

Other occasionally prescribed vasodilators were *prazosin* and *nifedipine.* These drugs were particularly helpful for their short-term effect on those patients in whom the major manifestation of the hypertension was the night-time rise in blood pressure.

Beta Blockers

As might be predicted, beta blockers failed to produce much of a fall in heart rate in these patients with denervated hearts and absent connections between cardiac accelerating neurogenic stimuli and the beta receptors. Most of these hearts have rates of 90 beats per minute or above, which are relatively unaffected by the usual neurogenic stimuli that slow or increase heart rate. To the extent that these patients do have circulating norepinephrine, beta blockade may cause some slowing but primarily the heart continues to act as a vagally denervated organ with a relatively fixed rate above 90 per minute. It should be emphasized that these are empiric observations and as with the failure to increase heart rate after vasodilators are given, these comments are based primarily on clinical retrospective observations.

Sympatholytics

Sympatholytic drugs (e.g., *guanethidine*) and centrally acting alpha agonists (e.g., *clonidine* and *alpha methyldopa*) were used sparingly. The latter drug was occasionally useful in acute situations but not as continued therapy.

Frequency of the Use of the Above Drugs and Comments on the Efficacy

At various times during the course of our followup, diuretics were used in up to 98 percent of the patients. Hydralazine was used in up to 50 percent of the patients, and minoxidil in up to 10 percent. Beta blockers were administered in 10 percent of the patients at the time of the first PRA and 21 percent at the time of the second PRA, and prazosin was given to 5 percent and 17 percent, respectively. As indicated, sympatholytics and calcium channel blockers were used sparingly—5 percent received clonidine and 2 percent nifedipine.[15]

In spite of our continuing attention to the problem of hypertension, control was only modest. We were able to reduce blood pressure but it tended to be resistant. Only occasionally was normotension achieved in patients who were not rejecting or were not otherwise compromising their cardiac output.

ACE Inhibitors

Initially we were concerned about using angiotensin converting enzyme (ACE) inhibitors because the first clinically available ACE inhibitor, *captopril,* had been reported to produce neutropenia and thus we thought that it was inappropriate to use this agent in already immunocompromised patients. However, with the advent of *enalapril,* which does not have the sulfhydryl radical allegedly responsible for many of captopril's untoward effects, we felt more comfortable about using this drug in the treatment of resistant hypertension. It was again not possible for us to examine the effectiveness of enalapril in a controlled fashion, but we have now retrospectively examined the data on the relationship of renal function, blood pressure and PRA in the 29 subjects in whom this drug was initiated. These patients were already receiving a variety of antihypertensive medications, as described previously, which were maintained at a stable dose at the time of the initiation of the enalapril. The last blood pressure recorded just prior to the initiation of enalapril was compared with the blood pressure obtained after a stable dose of the latter drug was established. Levels of serum potassium and creatinine measured before and after introduction of enalapril also were compared. Most patients were started on a 5 mg dose of enalapril, which was increased by 5 mg increments usually to no more than 20 mg.

The results of this retrospective analysis, reported for the first time in this chapter, indicated that the initial PRA in these 29 subjects averaged 15.0 ng/ml/ 3 hours incubation. Figure 11–1 indicates the results. Blood pressure dropped from 152/103 mmHg to 147/96 mmHg; the diastolic drop was statistically significant (p = 0.04). Creatinine also showed a significant decline from 2.0 mg/dl before talking enalapril to 1.8 mg/dl while taking enalapril (p = 0.02). As might be anticipated, potassium showed a rise from 4.15 to 4.51 (p<0.001). The rise in potassium, in fact, was the limiting factor to the use of the drug or to further increases in its dosage.

These data, although retrospective, gleaned from only single determinations of blood pressure, creatinine, and potassium, both before and after initiation of enalapril, and indicating changes that were only modest in degree, are nevertheless important clinically because the changes occur in the predicted directions. As stated earlier, the rise in PRA and the accompanying rise in blood pressure and creatinine with progressive use of cyclsosporine, implicates PRA as a major factor in both the hypertension and the ensuing events in the kidney. If this is a valid hypothesis, an ACE inhibitor should be quite specific in lowering blood pressure and perhaps creatinine as well. A rise in potassium is predictable because of the antialdosterone effect on ACE inhibition and clearly represents the limiting factor to the use of enalapril or other ACE inhibitors. Nevertheless, these observations

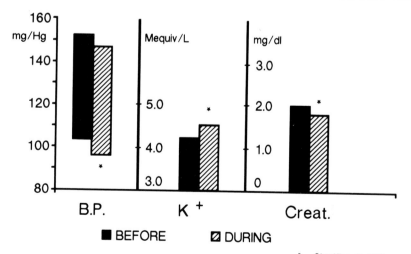

Figure 11–1. Changes in blood pressure, serum potassium, and creatinine after treatment of transplant patients with enalapril.

add another class of drugs to the therapeutic armamentarium for these transplant patients, particularly in the later phase when their hypertension appears to be motivated by a significant renin-angiotensin component.

SUMMARY AND DISCUSSION

It seems established that hypertension, to some degree, is a frequent consequence of cardiac transplantation. The hypertension occurs de novo and is not related to whether hypertension was present in association with the heart disease that led to the need for transplantation. The etiology of this hypertension is multifactorial and varies depending on the time that has ensued after transplantation. Acutely, it is primarily a problem related to intravascular volume expansion and persistently increased systemic vascular resistance. Although it may be modest in severity, it seems to be particularly resistant to therapy with most antihypertensive drugs. Moreover, the total "hyperbaric impact" of the hypertension is rendered greater because the blood pressure and heart rate in these patients with denervated hearts fails to show the usual 10 to 15 percent fall when recumbent/asleep at night, which occurs in normotensive individuals and in most with hypertension of other etiologies.

The major factor in the persistence of the hypertension through the later stages post-transplantation appears to be the cyclosporine that is used as an immunosuppressive. Although cyclosporine has been the major contributor to reduced rejection in these individuals, and to their increasingly prolonged survival, it inevitably produces slowly progressive impairment of renal function. The damage to the kidney is reflected both in tubular as well as glomerular and vascular damage, with a steady fall in glomerular filtration and a rise in creatinine. From our studies it appears that the renal alterations are associated with a gradual rise in plasma renin activity and angiotensin II, which perhaps further damages the kidney and causes persistence of the increased systemic vascular resistance. The use of lower doses of cyclosporine during the ischemic phase in the kidney that immediately follows surgery and of reduced doses over time, often with azathioprine added, seems to minimize the renal damage, or at least to stabilize it and to slow progression of the renal dysfunction and hypertension.

Treatment of the hypertension with conventional drugs has definite but limited value. Diuretics and vasodilators have been the mainstay of our approach during the early phases of the hypertension but our recent data indicate that ACE inhibitors may become relatively specific in management during the later phases of the post-transplantation period as PRA levels rise in response to vascular damage by cyclosporine.

ACE inhibitors have inherent dangers that require careful monitoring.[17] Captopril, which contains a sulfhydryl group in its molecular structure, is prone to produce skin rashes, either of an urticarial type or a skin lesion that is due to a vasculitis, and also has occasionally been implicated as a cause of proteinuria and neutropenia. The latter is an outcome to be avoided in these patients who are immunosuppressed. Enalapril, which does not have the sulfhydryl group, can produce urticaria, and cough is a common complaint. Blocking the production of angiotensin II also inhibits aldosterone secretion, with resultant rise in serum potassium, which is of particular concern in patients who have progressive renal damage and a rising creatinine level. Hyperkalemia is the limiting factor both to the use of the ACE inhibitor in general and to the dosage given. In addition to its peripheral effects on systemic vasoconstriction, angiotensin II also has the intrarenal effect of constricting the postglomerular (efferent) arteriole. The fall in glomerular filtration rate (GFR) produced by ACE inhibition can lead to increasing renal failure, with a rise in creatinine in those individuals in whom the GFR is already depressed. Theoretically, this might occur in some of the heart transplant patients who have suffered the most severe renal damage.

Until a "better" immunosuppressive than cyclosporine is developed, its use will continue in the cardiac transplant patient. However, in addition to avoiding rejection, a major goal in these patients is protection of myocardial function by decreasing unnecessary cardiac stress as much as possible. Because of its effects on the left ventricle and its tendency to accelerate atherosclerosis and perhaps increase coronary artery disease in the transplanted heart, hypertension is a disorder to be avoided and/or treated as soon as it is evident. It therefore behooves transplant surgeons and cardiologists who follow these patients to be aware of the almost universal expression of hypertension in these patients and the need for aggressive and properly designed antihypertensive therapy.

REFERENCES

1. Thompson, ME, Shapiro, AP, Johnsen, AM, et al: New hypertension following cardiac transplantation. Proceedings, Abstract #3, 1983. (Presented at 37th Annual Session of the Council of High Blood Pressure Research, American Heart Association, Cleveland, September 1983.)
2. Thompson, ME, Shapiro, AP, Johnsen, AM, et al: New onset of hypertension following cardiac transplantation: A preliminary report and analysis. Transplant Proc 15 (Suppl 1):2573, 1983.
3. Greenberg, A, Egel, JW, Thompson, ME, et al: Early and late forms of cyclosporine nephrotoxicity: Studies in cardiac transplant recipients. Am J Kidney Dis 9:12, 1987.
4. Greenberg, A and Thompson, ME: Cyclosporine-related hypertension and renal failure after cardiac allografting. Proceedings of Venetian Conference on Cardiac Transplantation, March, 1987, U.T.E.T. (in press).
5. Zelis, R and Flaim, SF: The circulations in congestive heart failure. Mod Concepts Cardiovasc Dis 51:79, 1982.
6. Greenberg, ML, Uretsky, BF, Reddy, PS, et al: Long-term hemodynamic follow-up of cardiac transplant patients treated with cyclosporine and prednisone. Circulation 71:487, 1985.
7. Reeves, RA, Johnsen, AM, Shapiro, AP, et al: Ambulatory blood pressure monitoring: Methods to assess severity of hypertension, variability and sleep changes. In Weber, MA and Drayer, JIM (eds): Ambulatory Blood Pressure Monitoring. New York, Springer-Verlag, 1984, pp 27–34.
8. Bristow, JD, Honour, AJ, Pickering, TG, et al: Cardiovascular and respiratory changes during sleep in normal and hypertensive subjects. Cardiovasc Res 3:476, 1969.
9. Mann, S, Altman, DG, Raftery, EB, et al: Inverted daily blood pressure pattern in autonomic impairment. In Proceedings of the 9th Annual Meeting of the International Society of Hypertension, Mexico City, February, 1982, No 267.
10. Reeves, RA, Shapiro, AP, Thompson, ME, et al: Loss of nocturnal decline in blood pressure after cardiac transplantation. Hypertension 73:410, 1986.
11. Baxter, CR, Duggin, GG, Willis, NS, et al: Cyclosporine-A induced increases in renin storage and release. Res Comm Chem Pathol Pharmacol 37:305, 1982.
12. Murray, BM, Paller, MS, and Ferris, TF: Effect of cyclosporine administration on renal hemodynamics in conscious rats. Kid Int 28:767, 1985.
13. Griffith, BP, Hardesty, RL, Lee, A, et al: The response of cyclosporine toxicity to azathioprine and reduced cyclosporine dose. Heart Transplant 4:148, 1985.
14. Thompson, ME, Shapiro, AP, Johnsen, AM, et al: The contrasting effects of cyclosporine-A and azathioprine on arterial blood pressure and renal function following cardiac transplantation. Int J Cardiol 11:219, 1986.
15. Rutan, GH, Shapiro, AP, Thompson, ME, et al: Hypertension, creatinine and plasma renin activity in heart transplant recipients. (Submitted for publication.)

16. Shapiro, AP: Essential hypertension—why idiopathic? Am J Med 54:1, 1973.
17. Gavras, H and Gavras, I: Angiotensin converting enzyme inhibitors: Properties and side effects.Hypertension 11(Suppl):37, 1988.
18. Hollenberg, NK: Renal perfusion and function; the implications of converting enzyme inhibition. Am J Med 84(Suppl 4A):9, 1988.

CHAPTER 12

Renal Failure in Cardiac Transplantation

Arthur Greenberg, M.D.

Renal dysfunction complicated the first use of cyclosporine.[1] Initially, only the acute form of nephrotoxicity was appreciated but chronic cyclosporine nephrotoxicity is now well recognized. Inasmuch as it is difficult to study nephrotoxicity in renal or liver transplant patients because of the occurrence in these populations of numerous potential causes of renal failure, bone marrow[2] and especially cardiac[3,4] transplants have provided an opportunity to study cyclosporine nephrotoxicity with fewer confounding variables. The drug's potential to cause nephrotoxicity also has been evident with its use as an immunosuppressant in a number of nontransplant disorders. These include myasthenia gravis,[5] autoimmune uveitis and other ocular disorders,[6] rheumatoid arthritis,[7] incipient diabetes,[8] multiple sclerosis,[9] and systemic lupus erythematosus.[10] While focusing on cyclosporine nephropathy in cardiac transplant patients, this chapter also draws from the considerable experience in other settings.

COURSE AND INCIDENCE

The acute form of cyclosporine nephrotoxicity occurs within the first few days of transplantation. Its course in an early series of patients undergoing cardiac transplantation at our institution is shown in Figure 12–1. Typically, BUN rises much more than serum creatinine, but both peak at approximately 4 to 5 days after surgery. In this group of 43 patients, 25 (58 percent) developed moderate azotemia, with serum creatinine levels between 2 and 8 mg/dl, and an additional 5 (12 percent) developed more severe renal dysfunction. Four of these latter patients required dialysis. Renal failure of this severity was encountered only with the use of cyclosporine; in a comparison group of azathioprine-treated patients from Richmond, no patient developed severe renal dysfunction and only 14 of 41 (34 percent) developed even moderate azotemia. With an inactive sediment, oliguria, and low urine sodium, this form of renal dysfunction resembles prerenal azotemia, despite the improved cardiac output noted in such patients after trans-

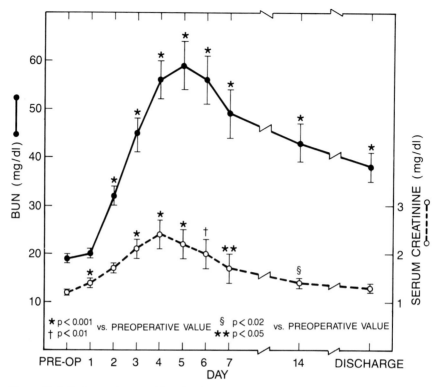

Figure 12–1. Perioperative renal function in 43 patients undergoing cardiac transplantation during the period March 1981 through June 1983 and receiving cyclosporine. The dose varied but, by current standards, was high in all cases. (From Greenberg et al.,[4] with permission.)

plantation. Hyper-reninism has been noted in some patients.[11] Coexisting volume depletion may worsen the azotemia. Renal function rapidly improves after reduction in dosage of cyclosporine. By the time of hospital discharge, serum creatinine levels had fallen in our group from their peak of 2.4 ± 0.3 mg/dl to 1.2 ± 0.6 mg/dl.[4]

Acute nephrotoxicity is clearly dose-related. The high incidence rate and marked severity described here occurred with use of as much as 17.5 mg/kg cyclosporine preoperatively. Current practice (see further on) recognizes the propensity for serious nephrotoxicity, and the incidence is much lower with currently used dosing regimens.

This form of rapid-onset acute renal failure, which resolves as doses are reduced, is common to all clinical situations in which cyclosporine is used, and frequent dosage manipulation in relation to serum creatinine is performed at all transplant centers. There is no clearcut division between the self-limited acute form of cyclosporine toxicity and the much more serious chronic toxicity. The chronic form is characterized principally by a slow rise in creatinine. It may begin with the initiation of cyclosporine treatment or may not become apparent until several weeks or months of therapy.[4] It may follow acute nephrotoxicity but need not do so, as it occurs in virtually all cardiac transplant patients given a sufficient dose of cyclosporine for a sufficient length of time whether or not acute nephrotoxicity was present. In our experience, the cumulative probability of developing renal dysfunction, defined as a serum creatinine above 1.7 mg/dl, increased linearly from 1 to 15 months after transplant with 45 percent, 83 percent, 96 percent, and 100 percent of patients receiving cyclosporine developing renal dysfunction at 1, 2, 3, and 4 years after transplantation, respectively. At Stanford, there was virtually no overlap in inulin clearance at 1 year after transplant among patients treated with cyclosporine and control subjects treated with azathioprine. Inulin clearance averaged 51 ± 4 ml/min in the cyclosporine group and 93 ± 3 ml/min in the patients receiving azathioprine.[3]

Only the Pittsburgh, Richmond, Stanford, and Arizona[3,4,12,13] groups have provided comparisons of azthioprine- and cyclosporine-treated patients, whereas reports of significant chronic nephrotoxicity come from numerous centers.[14-18]

CLINICAL AND PATHOLOGIC FEATURES OF CYCLOSPORINE NEPHROTOXICITY

The histopathologic findings in cyclosporine nephrotoxicity are mainly confined to the interstitium and vasculature. The principal effects are tubular atrophy, proximal tubular vacuolization, interstitial fibrosis, and arterial luminal thickening.[3,4,19,20] The latter changes are indistinguishable from hypertensive changes but may occur in nonhypertensive subjects. The biopsy of a typical case is shown in Figure 12–2. Glomerular findings are minimal, with sclerosis without

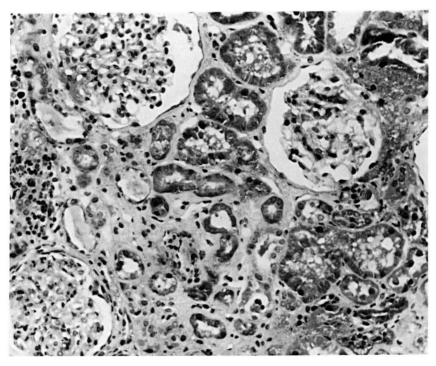

Figure 12–2. Renal biopsy obtained 19 months after cardiac transplantation. The patient received cyclosporine for 18 months with a rise in serum creatinine to 4.0 mg/dl, at which point his cyclosporine was stopped and azathioprine substituted. This biopsy was obtained 1 month later, when the serum creatinine was 2.1 mg/dl. Findings included extensive interstitial fibrosis and tubular atrophy with periglomerular sclerosis but no primary glomerular disease. (Trichrome, magnification ×325.)

inflammatory changes the main abnormality. The glomerular thrombosis observed in bone marrow or renal transplant patients[21-23] has been reported in only one cardiac allograft recipient.[24] Ultrastructurally, wrinkling of glomerular basement membranes (an ischemic change) is observed. Mitochondrial changes have also been described[25] but their specificity has been questioned.[26] The interstitial fibrosis may occur in bands corresponding to the vascular distribution. In autoimmune uveitis patients, the severity of fibrosis correlated with the duration of time the serum creatinine was elevated but not with cumulative dose of cyclosporine or severity or duration of hypertension.[20]

As with most forms of nonproliferative renal disease, proteinuria in this disorder is minimal. In five patients studied a mean of 31 ± 3 months after transplantation, creatinine clearance averaged 30 ± 3 ml/min and 24-hour protein excretion 381 ± 185 mg. The urine sediment typically shows only a few hyaline casts.

Hyperkalemia disporportionate to any decline in glomerular filtration rate has been noted in cardiac transplant patients[4] and in nontransplant cyclosporine recipients[6,7] but has been best documented in renal transplantation in which azathioprine control subjects are more readily available.[27] The hyperkalemia may be caused by hyporeninemic hypoaldosteronism inasmuch as suppression of renin and aldosterone release[28] and diminished responsiveness to aldosterone with hyperchloremic acidosis despite normal ability to lower urine pH[29] have been documented. In renal transplant recipients, the basis for renin suppression may be chronic volume expansion.[30] Use of beta blockers, which are known to suppress renin release, may exacerbate the hyperkalemia.[29] Data from heart transplant patients are conflicting. Acute infusion of cyclosporine stimulates renin production, which may contribute to acute cyclosporine toxicity.[11] In one report, chronically treated patients showed low plasma renin activity with a probable block in intrarenal conversion of inactive prorenin to active renin since levels of the former were high when compared with azathioprine control subjects.[24] An earlier study, however, showed no depression of renin in chronic patients.[31]

Independent of the need to use antiuricosuric diuretics to treat hypertension, hyperuricemia and an increased incidence of gout have also been described in renal transplant patients.[32,33] In the most systematic study of tubular function in chronic nephrotoxicity (undertaken in patients with ocular inflammatory disorders), Fanconi's syndrome defects such as bicarbonate or phosphate wasting, hyperuricosuria, hypokalemia, glucosuria, or aminoaciduria were absent. Instead, cyclosporine caused an increase in serum potassium and urate, magnesium wasting with a modest fall in serum magnesium, and lysozymuria.[34] Maximal diluting ability may also be impaired.[3]

PATHOPHYSIOLOGY OF CYCLOSPORINE NEPHROTOXICITY

The mechanism of cyclosporine nephrotoxicity has been extensively reviewed but there remains considerable controversy whether direct turbular toxicity or hemodynamic effects cause the damage.[35-37] Cyclosporine deposits in kidneys with nephrotoxicity,[38] and high-dose administration in animals causes proximal tubular histologic alterations.[39,40] However, the latter may only be secondary to renal perfusion changes. Furthermore, interstitial fibrosis has not been demonstrated in animal models. Both acute infusion and chronic administration of cyclosporine increase renal vascular resistance and decrease renal plasma flow and glomerular filtration rate.[41,42] Alpha-adrenergic blockade and renal denervation also protect against the decline in renal perfusion.[41] The latter may be especially pertinent in cardiac transplants since, in contrast to renal transplants, the kidney is not denervated. Although acute infusion increases renin production, pretreatment with captopril does not abolish the fall in renal plasma flow, suggesting that renin and angiotensin do not mediate the renal vasoconstriction. Prostaglandin synthesis rises after cyclosporine and the prostaglandin synthetase inhibitor meclofenamate worsens the vasoconstrictive effect of cyclosporine, suggesting a role for prostaglandins in compensatory vasodilation. The overall role of prostaglandins, however, is controversial.[43] Prostacyclin synthesis is depressed by cyclosporine,[44] and thromboxane synthesis stimulated.[45] Use of a fish oil vehicle for cyclosporine that decreases thromboxane synthesis is associated with diminished nephrotoxicity in animals.[46]

Although no unifying hypothesis has been proved, it seems plausible that independent of any direct tubular toxicity, cyclosporine-induced vasoconstriction may produce both an acute and reversible decline in renal blood flow and glomerular filtration rate as well as chronic ischemia that leads to irreversible renal fibrosis. Prostaglandins, angiotensin, adrenergic tone, and catecholamines may modulate the severity of the vasoconstriction and toxicity. This model fits well with the clinical observations that chronic toxicity is partly but not completely reversible with dosage reduction (see further on) and that a profound rise in creatinine may follow the use of prostaglandin synthesis inhibitors for treatment of pain or gout in transplant patients.

PHARMACOLOGIC CONSIDERATIONS

Cyclosporine is a fungal-derived cyclic endecapeptide with molecular weight 1203 Daltons. Its pharmacokinetics have been extensively reviewed.[47] The drug is lipophilic, highly bound to erythrocytes and plasma proteins, and extensively metabolized in the liver. Radioimmunoassay (RIA) using a commercial kit is comparatively simple and widely available but the antiserum reacts with a number of metabolites devoid of immunosuppressive activity. The relative distribution between metabolites and native drug may be affected by hepatic disease and the coadministration of a variety of drugs. Cyclosporine alone may be measured by high-performance liquid chromatography (HPLC) but the procedure is more cumbersome. The relative proportion of unbound cyclosporine in serum is dependent upon hematocrit. Red cell binding is temperature dependent; serum or plasma levels may vary significantly depending upon how the separation from red cells is accomplished in the laboratory.

It is not surprising therefore that there is no agreement on how cyclosporine levels should be measured, with various institutions using HPLC or RIA of either serum or whole blood.[48,49] The lack of consensus and the increasing recognition that the needed therapeutic level falls with time make it impossible to make a definite statement about a single therapeutic level for the drug. At our institution, whole blood RIA is most widely used. Acute toxicity is unusual at trough levels below 600 ng/ml and is common at levels above 1000 ng/ml. High levels are generally required in the immediate postoperative period, with lower levels desirable later. Serum RIA levels of 100 to 250 ng/ml or whole blood HPLC levels of 100 to 300 ng/ml are general therapeutic ranges.[47,48]

Table 12–1. Drugs that Alter Cyclosporine Metabolism

Drug	Mechanism	Comment
	Drugs Raising Cyclosporine Levels	
Erythromycin		
Ketoconazole	Interfere with metabolism	Reduce dose
Diltiazem		
	Drugs Lowering Cyclosporine Levels	
Rifampin		
Phenytoin	Induce cyclosporine metabolizing enzymes	Increase dose
Phenobarbital		

A number of drugs interfere with cyclosporine metabolism or independently affect serum creatinine and thus must be taken into account when cyclosporine is used.[47,48] Cyclosporine metabolism depends on cytochrome P-450 activity. Inhibitors of this enzyme system may increase cyclosporine levels thereby predisposing to nephrotoxicity, whereas inducers may result in reductions in cyclosporine levels and lead to rejection episodes. Some drugs interfere with creatinine secretion and consequently raise serum creatinine levels. This is not a nephrotoxic effect, but it does complicate management of patients since dosage is usually adjusted in accordance with serum creatinine level. This condition may be suspected if serum creatinine rises after a drug is started but BUN remains constant. Some drugs that are nephrotoxins in their own right, including amphotericin and the aminoglycosides, may have an additive effect with cyclosporine although this is difficult to demonstrate rigorously.[50] A drug interaction bearing special mention is that of methylprednisolone. Given in high dose boluses for rejection crises, it increases RIA but decreases HPLC cyclosporine levels, presumably by affecting relative distribution of native drug metabolites that are measured by RIA but not HPLC.[51] The principal cyclosporine drug interactions are summarized in Tables 12–1 and 12–2.

AVOIDANCE OF NEPHROTOXICITY

The doses of cyclosporine first used in the immediate postoperative period were, in retrospect, clearly too high.[4,11,15,52] A number of groups successfully used lower doses with less nephrotoxicity and without unacceptable rejection rates. At Alabama, five of nine patients identified as at high risk for acute renal failure and given 12 to 17 mg/kg cyclosporine preoperatively developed acute renal failure. None of seven similarly identified patients receiving 0.1 to 1 mg/kg cyclosporine developed acute renal failure. To prevent rejection, rabbit antithymocyte globulin (R-ATG) was administered until cyclosporine levels became therapeutic.[52] In Berlin, perioperative serum creatinine values rose sharply in patients receiving 18 mg/kg loading doses to achieve immediate cyclosporine levels of 800 to 1000 ng/ml by whole blood RIA. Addition of perioperative R-ATG with low dose cyclosporine targeted at levels of 400 to 600 ng/ml and not begun until postoperative day four was associated with better renal function but unacceptable rejection rates. Institution of cyclosporine at 12 hours after surgery with use of R-ATG until cyclosporine levels reached 350 to 500 ng/ml produced adequate immunosuppression without nephrotoxicity.[11] The immunosuppressive protocol currently in use at our institution calls for prednisone and azathioprine preopera-

Table 12–2. Cyclosporine Drug Interactions

Drug	Comment
Trimethoprim-sulfa	Interferes with creatinine secretion; confounds nephrotoxicity monitoring; suspect if creatinine rise not paralleled by BUN rise
Cimetidine	Same as above; may also interfere with cyclosporine metabolism; avoid.
Methylprednisolone (bolus)	Alters distribution between parent cyclosporine- and RIA-reactive metabolites, raises RIA but lowers HPLC; follow cautiously
Nonsteroidal anti-inflammatory drugs	Reduce renal function as in other patients with pre-existing renal disease but effect exaggerated; avoid

tively but no cyclosporine until a good urine flow is established 24 to 36 hours after surgery. Then, 2.5 mg/kg cyclosporine is begun and rapidly increased to achieve a level of 700 ng/ml by whole blood RIA. Renal failure is less frequent, less severe, and of shorter duration than it was when prednisone and 10 to 17.5 mg/kg loading doses of cyclosporine were used with 1000 to 1200 ng/ml target cyclosporine levels.

In our early experience, no patient retained normal renal function beyond 4 years after transplantation. Mean serum creatinine at 3 years was 2.5 ± 0.5 mg/dl,[4] a value similar to the 2.2 ± 1 mg/dl noted in Paris.[15] Although we could not confirm it,[4] some have suggested that early nephrotoxicity may condemn patients to late nephrotoxicity. In one study, patients receiving a higher initial loading dose of cyclosporine had serum creatinines of 2.6 ± 0.6 mg/dl at 6 months, a value significantly higher than the 1.6 ± 0.3 mg/dl found in patients who received lower doses in the early perioperative period. Both groups were receiving similar doses of cyclosporine at 6 months.[53] In an uncontrolled study using low-dose perioperative cyclosporine with equine antithymocyte globulin to prevent initial rejection, serum creatinine levels at one year were the same, 1.6 mg/dl, as preoperatively.[54] Interpretation of this result requires some caution because of the high preoperative level.

Quite apart from any effect of high perioperative doses to foreordain late nephrotoxicity, it is clear in cardiac transplant and in other patients receiving cyclosporine that reduction of dosage late in the course of nephrotoxicity, results in an improvement in renal function.[4,9,15,18,20,55,56] In Alabama, conversion from cyclosporine to azathioprine a mean of 11.5 months after transplantation was accompanied by a fall in creatinine from 2.6 ± 0.2 mg/dl to 1.8 ± 0.1 mg/dl.[18] In 20 patients at our institution whose cyclosporine dosage was dropped from a mean of 6.4 mg/kg at 1 year after transplant to 2 mg/kg as azathioprine was added at a mean dose of 2.3 mg/kg, creatinine fell from a mean of 3.7 mg/dl to 2.2 mg/dl, and the fall persisted. Cyclosporine levels fell from the original target of 1000 ng/ml to approximately 300 to 400 ng/ml.[55]

Unquestionably, long-term nephrotoxicity may be severe. Two patients in our program have required chronic hemodialysis—the first, 1 year and the second, 7 years after transplantation. At Stanford, end-stage renal disease developed in six patients.[24]

With the recognition that cyclosporine toxicity could be alleviated by dosage reduction, reduction of cyclosporine dosing in response to development of chronic nephrotoxicity is now a standard feature of management. This has made it quite difficult to determine whether cyclosporine nephrotoxicity is progressive over long periods of followup.[57]

Most of our long-term nephrotoxicity patients have undergone some reduction in dosing, and the progression rate for serum creatinine is modest, with values of 2.3 ± 0.2 mg/dl at 1 year after surgery, 2.2 ± 0.3 mg/dl at 2 years, and 2.5 mg/dl at 3 years.[4] The results of the few long-term studies are all similar.[9,15,24] Nine patients transplanted at our program in 1981 and 1982 have now survived at least 5 years. Their mean serum creatinine an average of 37.2 months after transplantation was 2.2 ± 0.1 mg/dl. At most recent followup a mean of 70 ± 2 months after transplantation, serum creatinine averaged 2.6 ± 0.3 mg/dl, a modest change that did not reach statistical significance. Of the nine patients in this group, seven had azathioprine added to prednisone and cyclosporine as the dose of the latter was reduced. Our current regimen calls for such "triple therapy" from the start, with much lower initial cyclosporine dosing than was used in this early group of patients.

Although this relatively slow progression provides some reassurance that cyclosporine may be used long-term without prohibitive nephrotoxicity, caution is still in order. These results all depend on serum creatinine as a marker for glomerular filtration rate, a notoriously bad practice. Serum creatinine levels also vary with muscle mass, which decreases with aging. More importantly, creatinine is not an ideal filtration marker because it is secreted by the renal tubules. At normal glomerular filtration rate, the contribution of secretion to creatinine excretion is minimal. However, as glomerular filtration rate falls, the relative contribution of secretion becomes much more significant and may be as much as 20 percent. The normal range for serum creatinine is quite broad. Because of all of these factors, it has been demonstrated that in cardiac transplantation, glomerular filtration rate may fall by 50 percent before serum creatinine rises above normal.[58] In three patients with autoimmune uveitis receiving cyclosporine with serum creatinines of 1.3, 1.9, and 2.4 mg/dl, the measured inulin clearances were 42, 29, and 19 ml/min, respectively.[20]

The presence of fibrosis on kidney biopsy is the best indicator of irreversible damage. It has been shown to correlate poorly with serum creatinine or inulin clearance but reasonably well with the length of time the serum creatinine has been supranormal. Severe fibrosis with a marked fall in inulin clearance may occur with the modest rises in serum creatinine generally considered acceptable in cardiac transplantation.[20]

CONCLUSION

Although considerable progress has been made in using this powerful new immunosuppressive agent to achieve better survival in cardiac transplantation, nephrotoxicity may still prove to be limiting. Thus far, no congeners of cyclosporine with less nephrotoxicity are forthcoming.

REFERENCES

1. Calne, RY, White, DJG, Thiru, S, et al: Cyclosporin A in patients receiving renal allografts from cadaver donors. Lancet 2:1323, 1978.

2. Kennedy, MS, Yee, GC, McGuire, TR, et al: Correlation of serum cyclosporine concentration with renal dysfunction in marrow transplant recipients. Transplantation 40:249, 1985.

3. Myers, BD, Ross, J, Newton, L, et al: Cyclosporine-associated chronic nephropathy. N Engl J Med 311:699, 1984.

4. Greenberg, A, Egel, JW, Thompson, ME, et al: Early and late forms of cyclosporine nephrotoxicity: Studies in cardiac transplant recipients. Am J Kid Dis 19:12, 1987.

5. Tindall, RSA, Rollins, JA, Phillips, JT, et al: Preliminary results of a double-blind, randomized, placebo-controlled trial of cyclosporine in myasthenia gravis. N Engl J Med 316:719, 1987.

6. Palestine, AG, Nussenblatt, RB, and Chan, CC: Side effects of systemic cyclosporine in patients not undergoing transplantation. Am J Med 77:652, 1984.

7. Berg, KJ, Forre, O, Bjerkhoek, F, et al: Side effects of cyclosporin A treatment in patients with rheumatoid arhtritis. Kidney Int 29:1180, 1986.

8. Stiller, CR, Dupre, Gent, M, et al: Effects of cyclosporine immunosuppression in insulin-dependent diabetes mellitus of recent onset. Science 223:1362, 1984.

9. von Graffenried, B and Harrison, WB: Renal function in patients with autoimmune diseases treated with cyclosporine. Transplantation Proc 27 (Suppl 1):215, 1985.

10. Feutren, G, Querin, S, Noel, LH, et al: Effects of cyclosporine in severe systemic lupus erythematosus. J Pediatr 111:1063, 1987.

11. Schuler, S, Thomas, D and Hetzer, R: Cyclosporine A-related nephrotoxicity after cardiac transplantation: The role of plasma renin activity. Transplant Proc 19:3998, 1987.

12. Emery, RW, Cork, R, Christensen, R, et al: Cardiac transplant patient at one year. Cyclosporine vs. conventional immunosuppression. Chest 89:29, 1986.

13. Barnhart, GR, Hastillo, A, Goldman, MH, et al: A prospective randomized trial of pretransfusion/azathioprine/prednisone versus cyclosporine/prednisone immunosuppression in cardiac transplant recipients: Preliminary results. Circulation 72 (Suppl 2):227, 1985.

14. McKenzie, N, Keown, P, Stiller, C, et al: Effects of cyclosporine on renal function following orthotopic heart transplantation. Heart Transplant 4:400, 1985.

15. Rottenbourg, J, Mattei, MF, Cabrol, A, et al: Renal function and blood pressure in heart transplant recipients treated with cyclosporine. Heart Transplant 4:404, 1985.

16. Goldstein, J, Thoua, Y, Wellens, F, et al: Cyclosporine nephropathy after heart and heart-lung transplantation. Proc Eur Dialysis Transplant Assoc 21:973, 1984.

17. Loertscher, R: Cyclosporine-associated nephrotoxicity is not intractable. Transplant Proc 19:3486, 1987.

18. McGiffin, DC, Kriklin, JK, McVay, RF, et al: Conversion from cyclosporine to azathioprine following heart transplantation. J Heart Transplant 5:99, 1986.

19. Chomette, G, Auriol, M, Beaufils, H, et al: Morphology of cyclosporine nephrotoxicity in human heart transplant recipients. J Heart Transplant 5:273, 1986.

20. Palestine, AG, Austin, HA, Balow, JE, et al: Renal histopathologic alterations in patients treated with cyclosporine for uveitis. N Engl J Med 314:1293, 1986.

21. Shulman, H, Striker, G, Deeg, HJ, et al: Nephrotoxicity of cyclosporin A after allogeneic marrow transplantation. N Engl J Med 305:1392, 1981.

22. Atkinson, K, Biggs, JC, Hayes, J, et al: Cyclosporin A associated nephrotoxicity in the first 100 days after allogeneic bone marrow transplantation: Three distinct syndromes. Br J Haematol 54:59, 1983.

23. Van Buren, D, Van Buren, CT, Flechner, SM, et al: De novo hemolytic uremic syndrome in renal transplant recipients immunosuppressed with cyclosporine. Surgery 98:54, 1985.

24. Myers, BD, Sibley, R, Newton, L, et al: The long-term course of cyclosporine-associated chronic nephropathy. Kidney Int 33:590, 1988.

25. Mihatsch, MJ, Olivieri, W, Marbet, U, et al: Giant mitochondria in renal tubular cells and cyclosporin A. Lancet 1:1162, 1981.

26. Verani, R: Giant mitochondria in renal tubular cells and cyclosporin. Lancet 2:285, 1983.

27. Foley, RJ, Hamner, RW, and Weinman, EJ: Serum potassium concentrations in cyclosporine- and azathioprine-treted renal transplant patients. Nephron 40:280, 1985.

28. Bantle, JP, Nath, KA, Sutherland, DER, et al: Effects of cyclosporine on the renin-angiotensin-aldosterone system and potassium excretion in renal transplant recipients. Arch Intern Med 145:505, 1985.

29. Adu, D, Turney, J, Michael, J, et al: Hyperkalaemia in cyclosporin-treated renal allograft recipients. Lancet 2:370, 1983.

30. Bantle, JP, Boudreau, RJ, and Ferris, TF: Suppression of plasma renin activity by cyclosporine. Am J Med 83:59, 1987.

31. Thompson, ME, Shapiro, AP, Johnsen, A-M, et al: The contrasting effects of cyclosporin-A and azathioprine on arterial blood pressure and renal function following cardiac transplantation. Int J Cardiol 11:219, 1986.

32. Chapman, JR, Griffiths, D, Harding, NGL, et al: Reversibility of cyclosporin nephrotoxicity after three months' treatment. Lancet 1:128, 1985.

33. West, C, Carpenter, BJ, and Hakala, TR: The incidence of gout in renal transplant recipients. Am J Kid Dis 10:369, 1987.

34. Palestine, AG, Austin, HA, and Nussenblatt, RB: Renal tubular function in cyclosporine-treated patients. Am J Med 81:419, 1986.

35. Bennett, WM: Basic mechanisms and pathophysiology of cyclosporine nephrotoxicity. Transplant Proc 17 (Suppl 1):297, 1985.

36. Kahan, BD: Cyclosporine nephrotoxicity: Pathogenesis, prophylaxis, therapy, and prognosis. Am J Kid Dis 8:323, 1986.

37. Bennett, WM and Pulliam, JP: Cyclosporine nephrotoxicity. Ann Intern Med 99:851, 1983.

38. Kolbeck, PC, Wolfe, JA, Burchett, J, et al: Immunopathologic patterns of cyclosporine deposition associated with nephrotoxicity in renal allograft biopsies. Transplantation 43:218, 1987.

39. Whiting, PH, Thomson, AW, Blair, JT, et al: Experimental cyclosporin A nephrotoxicity. Brt J Exp Pathol 63:88, 1982.

40. Farthing, MJG and Clark, ML: Nature of the toxicity of cyclosporin A in the rat. Biochem Pharmacol 30:3311, 1981.

41. Murray, BM, Paller, MS, and Ferris, TF: Effect of cyclosporine administration on renal hemodynamics in conscious rats. Kidney 28:767, 1985.

42. Jackson, NM, Hsu,C-H, Visscher, GE, et al: Alterations in renal structure and function in a rat model of cyclosporine nephrotoxicity. J Pharmacol Exp Therap 242:749, 1987.

43. Barros, EJG, Boim MA, Ajzen, H, et al: Glomerular hemodynamics and hormonal participation on cyclosporine nephrotoxicity. Kidney Int 32:19, 1987.

44. Neild, GH, Rocchi, G, Imberti, L, et al: Effect of cyclosporin A on prostacyclin synthesis by vascular tissue. Thromb REs 32:373, 1983.

45. Kawaguchi, A, Goldman, MH, Shapiro, R, et al: Increase in urinary thromboxane B_2 in rats caused by cyclosporine. Transplantation 40:214, 1985.

46. Elzinga, L, Kelley, VE, Houghton, DC, et al: Modification of experimental nephrotoxicity with fish oil as the vehicle for cyclosporine. 43:271, 1987.

47. Ptachcinski, RJ, Venkataramanan, R, and Burckart, GJ: Clin Pharmacokinetics 11:107, 1986.

48. Kahan, BD: Immunosuppressive therapy with cyclosporine for cardiac transplantation. Circulation 75:40, 1987.

49. Faynor, SM, Moyer, TP, Sterioff, S, et al: Therapeutic drug monitoring of cyclosporine. Mayo Clin Proc 59:571, 1984.

50. Wood, AJ and Lemaire, M: Pharmacologic aspects of cyclosporine therapy: Pharmacokinetics. Transplant Proc 17 (Suppl 1):27, 1985.

51. Klintmalm, G and Saw, J: High dose methylprednisolone increases plasma cyclosporin levels in renal transplant recipients. Lancet 1:731, 1984.

52. McGiffin, DC, Kirklin, JK, and Naftel, DC: Acute renal failure after heart transplantation and cyclosporine therapy. Heart Transplant 4:396, 1985.

53. Bolmam, RM, Elick, B, Olivari, MT, et al: Improved immunosuppression for heart transplantation. Heart Transplant 4:315, 1985.

54. Sprat, P, Esmore, D, Baron, D, et al: Effects of low-dose cyclosporine A on toxicity and rejection in cardiac transplantation. Transplant Proc 19:2847, 1987.

55. Griffith, BP, Hardesty, RL, Lee, A, et al: Management of cyclosporine toxicity by reduced dosage and azathioprine. Heart Transplant 4:410, 1985.

56. Stiller, CR, Keown, PA, Heinrichs, D, et al: The effect of cyclosporine on renal function in newly diagnosed diabetics. Transplant Proc 17 (Suppl 1):202, 1985.

57. Porter, GA, and Bennett, WM: Chronic cyclosporine-associated nephrotoxicity. Transplant Proc 18 (Suppl 1):204, 1986.

58. Tomlanovich, S, Golbetz, H, Perlroth, M, et al: Limitations of creatinine in quantifying the severity of cyclosporine-induced chronic nephropathy. Am J Kid Dis 8:332, 1986.

CHAPTER 13

Accelerated Coronary Atherosclerosis in Cardiac Transplantation*

David M. Eich, M.D.
Danna E. Johnson, M.D.
Andrea Hastillo, M.D.
James A. Thompson, M.D.
Glenn R. Barnhart, M.D.
Daijin Ko, Ph.D.
Richard R. Lower, M.D.
Michael L. Hess, M.D.

HISTORIC PERSPECTIVE

In 1969, Thomson reported the pathologic findings in the first long-term cardiac transplant patient who survived 19 months. In his report, he commented on the irony of the death of Dr. Phillip Blaiberg who had succumbed to the "same disease" that had caused the dysfunction of his original heart.[1] Indeed, a number of early transplant patients were subsequently noted to develop an aggressive form of coronary artery disease (CAD), which prompted Kosek and associates in 1971 to suggest that this group of patients could represent a model population for studying coronary artery disease.[2] These early reports substantiated pathological findings in the canine cardiac allograft model in which severe coronary occulsive disease was also noted.[3] The unsettling reoccurrence of this aggressive CAD in patients with successful cardiac allografts coupled with grim short-term survival statistics led many institutions to abandon the procedure. Advances in immunosuppressive protocols and organ procurement, as well as an increased awareness of the problems inherent in long-term immunosuppression, resulted in marked improvements in survival. As a consequence of improved survival and the initiation of third-party reimbursement in the early 1980s, there was an expo-

---

*Supported in part by RR00065 to the Clinical Research Center of the Medical College of Virginia.

nential increase in the number of cardiac transplant procedures. By 1987, approximately 1500 cardiac transplant procedures had been performed worldwide, with a greater than 80 percent 1-year survival.[4] As improvements were made in the diagnosis and therapy for rejection and infection, CAD became the leading cause of death among those who survive at least 1 year after cardiac transplantation.

A number of centers have acquired sufficient data to ascertain the incidence of accelerated CAD. The Stanford group in 1982 reported that coronary atherosclerosis was the cause of death in 11 percent of their long-term survivors.[5] At the Medical College of Virginia approximately 20 percent of deaths in heart transplant patients have been caused by significant coronary disease. At present, the incidence of allograft CAD, as determined by angiographic and autopsy studies, appears to be between 1 and 4 percent at 1 year, and 40 to 50 percent at 5 years following transplantation.[5,6] Autopsy studies have documented that virtually all long-term survivors have some degree of significant coronary artery pathology.[7-10] Both the severity of luminal narrowing and the frequency of complications, such as arterial thrombosis and myocardial infarction, seem to increase in parallel with graft survival.[9] It is believed therefore that all allograft recipients will develop CAD, but the question becomes what are the factors that predispose these patients to this aggressive form of coronary artery disease.

PATHOLOGY

In human transplant patients, two forms of CAD exist. One form of CAD affects primarily the large epicardial arteries, and a second diffusely involves the coronary arterial system.[9-10] Evidence of proximal artery disease has been demonstrated as early as 2 to 3 weeks after transplantation as concentric fibrous thickening of the intima[7-10] (Fig. 13–1). Progressive intimal thickening can occur over

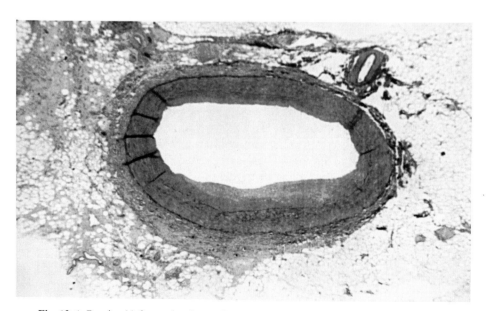

Fig. 13–1. Proximal left anterior descending (LAD) artery from a transplant recipient who died 3 months postoperatively of an infection. Mild fibrous thickening of the large vessel is present, whereas a small branch is normal. (Elastic von Gieson, magnification ×5.)

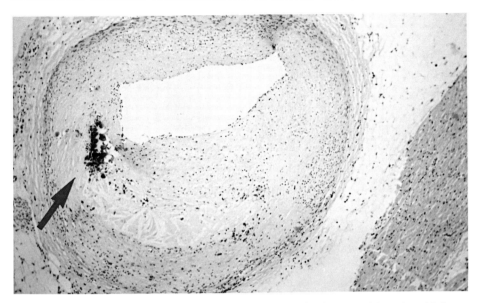

Fig. 13–2. An eccentric atheromatous lesion with focal calcification *(arrow)* from the mid circumflex artery of a long-term survivor of cardiac transplantation. (Hematoxylin and eosin, magnification ×13.)

time. At 1 year following transplantation, lipid deposits in the form of fat-filled intimal cells are observed. These lesions eventually accumulate extracellular lipid, calcify, and develop eccentric plaques. Thus, these proximal, often focal lesions in long-term survivors closely resemble those of natural atherosclerosis (Fig. 13–2). The diffuse form of CAD, on the other hand, may begin as a severe widespread necrotizing vasculitis of the coronary arteries[7–10] (Fig. 13–3). This destructive arteritis heals by scarring of the media and proliferative changes of the intima, leading to obliterative lesions of both the epicardial and intramyocardial arteries (Fig. 13–4). Coronary angiography reveals pruning of the distal arborization patterns in such cases[11] (see Fig. 13–11). Although secondary thrombosis and myocardial infarction may occur in patients with either proximal or diffuse disease, these complications develop more frequently in patients who develop diffuse CAD.

ETIOLOGY

From the debate over the pathogenesis of atherosclerosis in the general population, two principal theories have evolved: one that evokes hyperlipidemia and plaque formation as the primary mechanism and another that implicates cellular injury. A number of risk factors have been shown to have an association with the development of spontaneously occurring atherosclerotic cardiovascular disease. These include male sex, hypertension, hyperlipidemia, tobacco abuse, and diabetes mellitus. The majority of patients referred for cardiac transplantation are skewed toward an increase in risk factors, partly as a consequence of the prevalence of male patients with ischemic heart disease. However, the exact role of these risk factors in cardiac allograft CAD has been little studied and is poorly

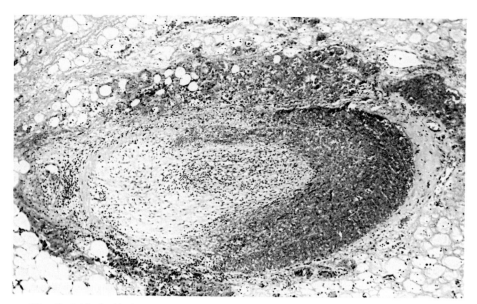

Fig. 13–3. Marked intimal thickening, patchy inflammation and necrosis, with intramural hemorrhage are found in this small epicardial artery. The patient died 13 months after transplantation as a result of an acute myocardial infarction. At autopsy, widespread, severe coronary arteritis and multiple myocardial infarcts were discovered. (Hematoxylin and eosin, magnification ×33.)

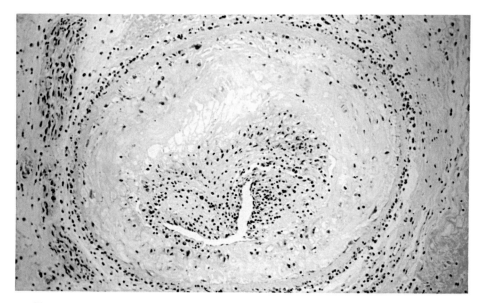

Fig. 13–4. A small epicardial artery with severe luminal encroachment caused by an atheromatous plaque. The features of a healing arteritis are also present. These features include thinning and complete fibrous replacement of the media with scattered residual lymphocytes and plasma cells. (Hematoxylin and eosin, magnification ×40.)

understood. The assimilation of data has been difficult because of the small sample sizes of the varied protocols.

It is widely believed that allograft rejection and subsequent endothelial injury play a key role in transplant CAD. The most attractive hypothesis implicates chronic rejection in conjunction with associated risk factors, such as hyperlipidemia[2,12,13] (Fig. 13–5). It has been suggested that viral infection also may have some role in the endothelial injury of these immunocompromised hosts.[14] The presumed role of immune-mediated injury to the donor endothelium and the association with allograft CAD is supported by the injury model of atherosclerosis. In accordance with the injury theory of naturally occurring atherosclerosis, loss of the endothelial cell layer of transplant coronary arteries could result in adhesion of platelets and monocytes, release of stimulatory factors such as platelet-derived growth factor, and intimal smooth muscle cell proliferation with collagen deposition.[15] Histologic evidence of endothelial cell damage and/or denudation has been frequently observed in the acutely rejecting cardiac allograft.[3,7] Endothelial injury can result from either cell-mediated or humoral mechanisms.[15,16] Palmer and coworkers used immunofluorescent techniques to discover immunoglobins in the disrupted endothelium of a patient with widespread large and small vessel coronary artery disease.[17] At the Medical College of Virginia, Hess and associates found circulating cytotoxic antibodies against vascular endothelium in some long-term survivors of acclerated CAD.[13]

The intensity of the immune response that any given transplant recipient mounts in an attempt to reject the transplanted organ is known to be highly variable. There can be a wide degree of variance on a case by case basis in the amount of ongoing rejection. Some patients, surprisingly, require no additive immunosuppressive efforts to control rejection, whereas others require repeated courses of high-dose steroids, antithymocyte globulin, and/or OKT3. Although our present immunosuppressive regimens have allowed us to preempt life-threatening rejection, we are still unable to preclude immunologic injury to the donor coronaries. Thus, some vascular injury must be accepted, given the present limitations of our immunosuppressive protocols. The University of Pittsburgh group recently has reported the suspected relationship between bouts of rejection necessitating treatment and the genesis of clinically significant CAD.[18] These findings have not been substantiated by others.[19]

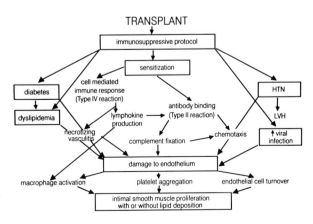

Fig. 13–5. Factors predisposing the cardiac transplant recipient to CAD.

The selection of patients for transplantation from the pool of individuals with end-stage cardiomyopathy creates a rather narrow patient profile. The treatment of the individuals after transplantation with a set regimen of drugs further intensifies this homogeneity. In this regard, the vast majority of patients transplanted at the Medical College of Virginia are male (86 percent). Another idiosyncrasy unique to the transplant population is that they are nearly uniformly hypertensive as a result of cyclosporine immunosuppression. Tobacco abuse is a risk factor that clearly has been associated with atherosclerosis in the general population. Although strongly discouraged, some patients continue to smoke after transplantation. The majority of patients, however, are nonsmokers and thus the experience has been largely anecdotal. No statistically significant association has been drawn between tobacco abuse and allograft CAD to date.

The presence of diabetes has been a relative contraindication to transplantation in the past. Occasionally, patients on prednisone protocols become hyperglycemic. Katz and Barhnart reported a 10 percent incidence of steroid-induced diabetes in patients treated with cyclosporine and prednisone.[20] Despite the well-known association of atherosclerotic vascular disease in the general diabetic population, we have been unable to demonstrate an association with accelerated CAD.[21] Again, the problem of few patients exists. It has been noted, however, that those few patients with poor glucose control have significant hyperlipidemia.[22]

Hyperlipidemia is another factor that has clearly been associated with atherosclerosis in the general population. The incidence of hyperlipidemia is quite high among the transplant population as a result of patient selection and the medications employed in immunosuppression. The appearance of hyperlipidemia can be dramatic, although it is rare for the pretransplant patient to manifest high serum cholesterol values owing to the presence of class IV congestive failure and concomitant cardiac cachexia. After surgery, these patients manifest a significant weight gain and often develop hyperlipidemia. These observations have been made at our institution regardless of the predisposing cardiomyopathy. Sixty-six percent of our patients on the cyclosporine/prednisone protocol were hyperlipidemic (mean total cholesterol 266 mg/dl) 1 year following transplantation.[22]

In 1984, Hess and colleagues reported an association between hypercholesterolemia, humoral injury to the endothelium, and accelerated CAD.[13] Further anecdotal experience supported these observations. A review of serum lipid profiles of patients on conventional, azathioprine/prednisone, and cyclosporine/prednisone immunosuppression conducted at the Medical College of Virginia in 1986 revealed some interesting observations between those patients with CAD at two years following surgery and those without CAD at 5 years after surgery (Figs. 13–6 through 13–9). These data suggest a clear trend toward "inferior" lipid profiles in those patients who develop CAD. Most recently, the Medical College of Virginia reported that high-risk total cholesterol levels when indexed for age at 6 months after transplantation are predictive of clinically significant CAD by the third year.[20] Given the ongoing endothelial injury associated with donor rejection, and the extraordinary prevalence of risk factors in the cardiac transplant population, the incidence of cardiac allograft CAD is easily understood. Clearly, there is a spectrum of presentations, which at the Medical College of Virginia has been from 1 year to 15 years following transplantation. This time-course would suggest a possible long-term interaction between the cellular injury of rejection and associated risk factors.

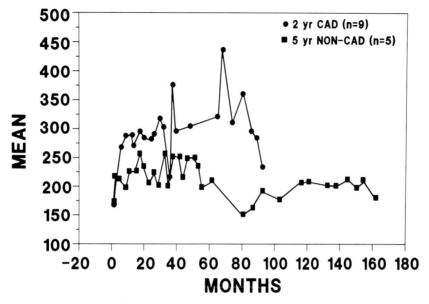

Fig. 13–6. Serum total cholesterol values.

CLINICAL PRESENTATION AND MANAGEMENT

The insidious presentation of allograft coronary artery disease complicates the diagnosis and management of this frustrating problem. Sympathetic denervation precludes the perception of typical anginal pain and thus eliminates the usual warning symptoms of infarction. Patients most often present with a progressive decline in ejection fraction heralded by nonspecific complaints such as

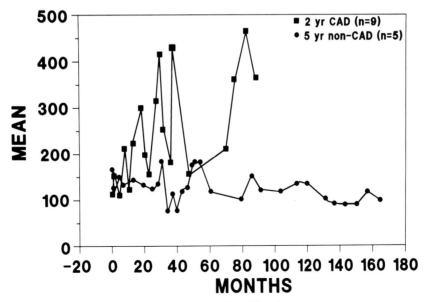

Fig. 13–7. Serum triglyceride values.

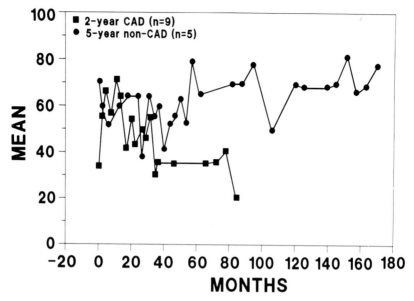

Fig. 13–8. Serum HDL values.

upper respiratory symptoms, persistent cough, or increasing fatigue. The deterioration of graft function is most often associated with multiple small myocardial infarcts, but may be related to acute coronary occlusion with a much more precipitous decline.

A variety of protocols have been adopted by different institutions for the detection of graft CAD. These protocols include some combination of studies used in a complementary fashion annually or semiannually. Exercise thallium

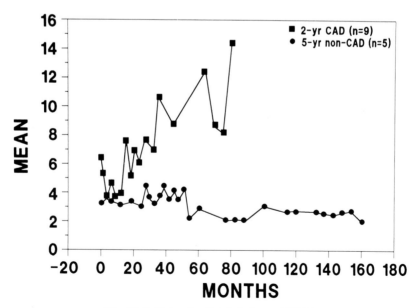

Fig. 13–9. Risk ratios (total cholesterol/HDL).

studies are utilized for detection of exercise-induced ischemia.[23] Nuclear ventriculography and echocardiography are employed to evaluate systolic function and regional wall motion abnormalities. Cardiac cathetarization provides direct visualization of the epicardial vessels.

Serum lipid profiles are followed prospectively as a means of shaping one's index of suspicion, as well as monitoring risk modification. Total serum cholesterol values of less than 200 mg/dl with an HDL of 45 mg/dl or greater, an LDL of less than 150 mg/dl, and risk ratios less than 4 are considered to be ideal. Although endomyocardial biopsy has been reported to demonstrate CAD, it has rarely proven to be of benefit in making the direct diagnosis of CAD.[17] Thus the use of this procedure in post-transplant followup should be restricted to that of assessing the degree of ongoing rejection and endothelial injury. Holter monitoring was reported by Romhilt and coworkers to provide some insight into the diagnosis of allograft CAD. Those patients on azathioprine and prednisone who were noted to have complex ventricular ectopy were observed to have a higher incidence of CAD.[24] These data have not been verified with the currently used cyclosporine protocols, and the true value of Holter monitoring in the surveillance for clinically significant CAD is uncertain.

When noninvasive evidence supports the diagnosis of CAD, angiography is performed. As one might expect given the range of pathologic presentations, the angiogram may reveal either large or small vessel disease (Figs. 13–10, 13–11).

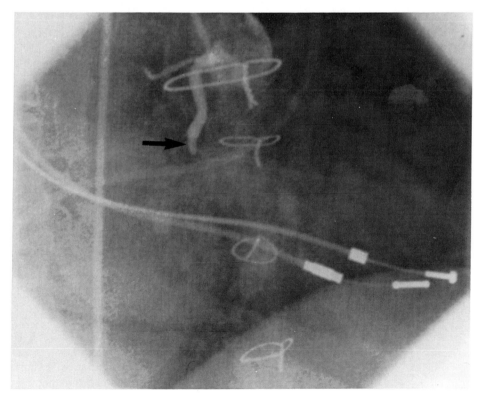

Fig. 13–10. Right coronary injection demonstrating complete occlusion of the right coronary artery *(arrow)* in this patient 10 years after transplantation.

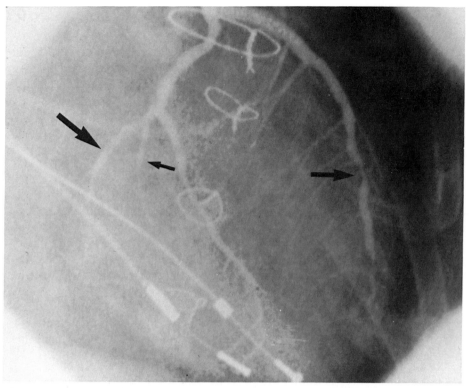

Fig. 13–11. Left coronary injection demonstrates discrete focal lesions in the LAD (*large arrow, right*) as well as pruning of the A-V groove circumflex (large arrow, left) marginal branch *(small arrow)*.

However, angiography may be difficult to evaluate in that the epicardial arteries may appear normal despite the presence of significant diffuse coronary disease in either the epicardial vessels or the intramyocardial branches.[25] Given this diverse angiographic presentation, and occasionally misleading data, many have sought to increase the sensitivity and specificity of the angiogram. Presently, coronary flow reserve studies are being performed by some investigators. Coronary flow reserve is diminished by both epicardial and intramyocardial stenosis. However, abnormal coronary flow reserve patterns are also noted in patients with left ventricular hypertrophy, and with endothelial injury.[26] Therefore, if an individual presents with noninvasive studies suggestive of CAD, without diagnostic angiographic evidence, then a negative flow reserve study would virtually exclude possible coronary pathology. However, a diminished flow reserve would raise the differential diagnosis of CAD, endothelial injury with ongoing rejection, or left ventricular hypertrophy.

TREATMENT

The only treatments for cardiac allograft CAD are retransplantation or balloon dilation of discrete lesions. Neither approach is completely satisfactory. Therefore, the best approach appears to be risk modification and prevention. Given the range of time that it takes for the transplant population to develop

CAD, it follows that there may be some modifiable factors that would alter an individual's predisposition.

Clearly, every effort must be made to minimize rejection. Although the process cannot be completely ameliorated, careful donor and recipient cross-matching and aggressive management of rejection episodes hopefully can minimize endothelial injury.

Unfortunately, our greatest tools in managing the postoperative transplant patient become our greatest liability. As stated previously, those risk factors known to predispose patients to coronary artery disease are exacerbated by our immunosuppressive protocols. Prednisone and cyclosporine have long been noted to have significant side effect profiles. In 1986, the Medical College of Virginia Transplant Program began treating patients with maintenance azathioprine/cyclosporine immunosuppression. Prednisone is added to the regimen only if rejection episodes are particularly recalcitrant. Long-term followup reveals a small increase in the mean number of episodes of rejection, but a significant drop in total cholesterol and HDL, and a significant decrease in the incidence of diabetes.[19,21] It remains to be seen whether the elimination of prednisone will have an impact upon the development of graft CAD.

Certainly, dietary moderation of cholesterol consumption is encouraged. Diets with less than 300 mg cholesterol daily and less than 30 percent total calories in fat are recommended. Progressive ambulation and daily exercise are also encouraged. These measures have had little effect on weight gain, increases in serum lipid levels, and hypertension in the patient after transplantation.

Pharmacologic interventions in the control of acclerated CAD have been disappointing. Initial reports suggested that platelet inhibitors and warfarin might reduce the incidence of allograft coronary disease, but more recent data failed to support these conclusions.[27] Theoretically, calcium channel blockers should be of some benefit. There have been recent reports in the literature of regression of atherosclerotic lesions using calcium channel blockers.[28,29] Handley and Van-Vasen found a 44 percent decrease in atherosclerotic lesions induced in the rabbit carotid using a new calcium antagonist.[30] These agents also have been shown to be effective in the treatment of hypertension and thus may serve a dual purpose in the transplant population.

Hypertension is a particularly vexing problem. The appearance of hypertension has proven to be inevitable in transplant recipients as a result of cyclosporine immunosuppression. Aggressive treatment of hypertension in these patients often culminates in triple drug regimens. Traditional first-line agents such as diuretics and beta-blockers are rarely effective and often further aggravate dyslipidemia. Angiotensin-converting enzyme inhibitors may be effectively employed, but with care to avoid further exacerbation of cyclosporine-induced renal insufficiency.

The development of the HMG CoA reductase inhibitor lovastatin was initially felt to hold great promise for the treatment of hyperlipidemia after transplantation. Reports of rhabdomyolysis in patients treated with lovastatin while on cyclosporine proved to be very disappointing.[31] Subsequently, anecdotal experience has suggested that very low doses of lovastatin may be used safely and effectively, although the clinical data are insufficient to advocate its use.

Angiographically demonstrated critical epicardial stenosis have been documented clearly as part of the diverse coronary pathology associated with accelerated CAD. These specific lesions have been successfully approached using percutaneous transluminal coronary angioplasty.[32,33] Although typically one is most apt to find distal vessel disease, the presence of a threatening epicardial stenosis deemed physiologically significant by thallium warrants aggressive intervention.

Frequently, progressive atherosclerosis results in decreasing left ventricular function, which culminates in recurrent class IV failure. For these patients, the only treatment alternative becomes retransplantation. Although technically feasible, the long-term success of a second transplantation has not been as favorable.[34] One must, therefore, consider all of the ramifications prior to making this difficult decision.

SUMMARY

The implications of this new aggressive form of coronary disease for the transplant population are obvious. It appears that for the majority of transplant patients we have simply bought some time. We have given them a temporary respite from congestive failure and cardiomyopathy while they surmount the daily challenges imposed by immunosuppression. Clearly, this issue now looms as a major stumbling block toward improving long-term survival. It is no longer enough to simply perform the procedure and submit the patient to the rigors of transplantation, only to obtain 50 percent 5-year survival. We must pay particular attention to the patient postoperatively and make those modifications necessary to improve the individual's risk profile. Moreover, we must continue to concentrate our research efforts on interventions in accelerated coronary disease.

REFERENCES

1. Thomson, JG: Production of severe atheroma in a transplanted human heart. Lancet 2:1088, 1969.
2. Kosek, JC, Bieber, C, and Lower, RR: Heart graft arteriosclerosis. Transplant Proc 3:512, 1971.
3. Lower, RR and Cleveland, RJ: The current status of heart transplantation. Proceedings of the First International Conference of the Transplant Society, 1967, p 657.
4. Solis, EK and Kaye, MP: The Registry of the International Society for Heart Transplantation: Third Official Report-June 1986. Heart Transplant 5:2, 1986.
5. Pennock, JL, Oyer, PE, et al: Cardiac transplantation in perspective for the future. J Thorac Cardiovasc Surg 83:168, 1982.
6. Barnhart, GR, Pascoe, EA, et al: Accelerated coronary atherosclerosis in cardiac transplant recipients. Transplant Review 1:31, 1988.
7. Bieber, CP, Stinson, EB, Shumway, NE, et al: Cardiac transplantation in man. VII. Cardiac allograft pathology. Circulation 41:753, 1970.
8. Uys, CJ and Rose, AG. Pathologic findings in long-term cardiac transplants. Arch Pathol Lab Med 108:112, 1984.
9. Johnson, DE, Gao, SZ, Schroeder, JS, et al: The spectrum of coronary artery pathology in human cardiac allografts. Heart Transplantation (in press).
10. Billingham, ME: Cardiac transplant atherosclerosis. Transplant Proc 19 (Suppl 5):19, 1987.
11. Gao, SZ, Alderman, E, Schroeder, J, et al: Accelerated coronary vascular disease in the heart transplant patient: Coronary arteriographic findings. J Am Coll Cardiol 12:334, 1988.
12. Alonso, DR, Starek, PK, and Minick, CR: Studies on the pathogenesis of atheroarteriosclerosis induced in rabbit cardiac allografts by the synergy of graft rejection and hypercholesterolemia. Am J Pathol 87:415, 1977.
13. Hess, ML, Hastillo, A, Mohanakumar, DVM, et al: Accelerated atherosclerosis in cardiac transplantation: Role of cytotoxic B-cell antibodies and hyperlipidemia. Circulation 68 (Suppl II):II-94, 1983.
14. Virella, G and Lopes-Virella, MF: Infections and atherosclerosis. Transplant Proc XIX (Suppl 5):26, 1987.

15. Ross, R: The pathogenesis of atherosclerosis: An update. N Engl J Med 314:488, 1986.
16. Cramer, DV: Cardiac transplantation: Immune mechanisms and alloantigens involved in graft rejection. CRC, Crit Rev Immunol 7:1, 1987.
17. Palmer, DC, Tsai, CC, Roodman, ST, et al: Heart graft arteriosclerosis. An ominous finding on endomyocardial biopsy. Transplantation 39:395, 1985.
18. Uretsky, BF, Murali, S, Reddy, PS, et al: Development of coronary artery disease in cardiac transplant recipieints receiving immunosuppressive therapy with cyclosporine and prednisone. Circulation 76:827, 1987.
19. Gao, SZ, Schroeder, JS, et al: Clinical and laboratory correlates of accelerated coronary artery disease in the cardiac transplant patient. Circulation 76 (Suppl 5):56, 1987.
20. Katz, MR and Barhnart, GR: Are steroids essential for successful maintenance of immunosuppression in heart transplantation? Heart Transplant 6:293, 1987.
21. Thompson, JA and Eich, DM: Hypercholesterolemia: An early maker of accelerated coronary artery disease in the cardiac allograft. Circulation 76:167, 1987.
22. Taylor, DO, Thompson, JA, et al: Hyperlipidemia following clinical cardiac transplantation. Heart Transplantation (in press).
23. McKillop, JH and Goris, ML: Thallium 201 myocardial imaging in patients with previous cardiac transplantation. Clin Radiol 32:447, 1981.
24. Romhilt, DW, Doyle, M, et al: Prevalence and significance of arrhythmias in long-term survivors of cardiac transplantation. Circulation 66 (Suppl 1):219, 1982.
25. Mason, JW and Strafling, A: Small vessel disease of the heart resulting in myocardial necrosis and death despite angiographically normal coronary arteries. Am J Cardiol 44:171, 1979.
26. Hodgson, JM, Cohen, MD, et al: Reductions of ventricular function correlate with impairment of coronary flow reserve but not with endomyocardial biopsy following cardiac transplantation. J Am Coll Cardiol 9:116A, 1987.
27. Nitkin, RS, Hunt, SA, and Schroeder JS: Accelerated atherosclerosis in a cardiac transplant patient. J Am Coll Cardiol 6:243, 1985.
28. Henry, PD: Atherosclerosis, calcium and calcium antagonists. Circulation 72:456, 1985.
29. Weinstein, DB: Anti-atherogenic properties of calcium antagonists. Am J Cardiol 59:163B, 1987.
30. Handley, PA and VanVasen, RO: Suppression of rat carotid lesion development by the calcium channel blocker, PN 200-110. Am J Path 124:88, 1986.
31. Norman, DJ, Illingworth, DR, et al: Letter to the Editor: Myolysis and acute renal failure in a heart transplant recipient receiving lovastatin. N Engl J Med 318:46, 1988.
32. Hastillo, A, Cowley, MJ, Vetrovec, GW, et al: Serial coronary angioplasty for atherosclerosis following heart transplantation. Heart Transplant 4:192, 1985.
33. Ventrovec, GW and Cowley, MJ: Application of percutaneous transluminal angioplasty in cardiac transplantation. Circulation (in press).
34. Gao, SZ, Schroeder, JS, et al: Retransplantation for severe accelerted coronary vascular disease in heart transplants. J Am Coll Cardiol 9:294, 1987.

CHAPTER 14

Management and Long-Term Followup of Outpatient Care in the Cardiac Transplant Recipient

James A. Thompson, M.D.
Sheelah Rider-Katz, R.N.
Michael L. Hess, M.D.
Alain Heroux, M.D.
Andrea Hastillo, M.D.
Richard R. Lower, M.D.

Successful long-term management of the cardiac transplant patient requires the concerted efforts of the patient, the cardiac transplant team, and the primary care physician. The increase in transplant procedures performed over the last several years coupled with improved survival has led to a large outpatient population. Inasmuch as this population will continue to increase over the next several years, it is of the utmost importance that the communication between primary care physicians and the cardiac transplant team be optimized in order to offer our patients the long-term care that they deserve. This chapter reviews in general terms the various aspects of the management of the cardiac transplant recipient once he or she has left the hospital following the initial transplant procedure.

GENERAL ASPECTS

First 3 Months After Discharge

After discharge from the initial hospitalization, our patients remain in the community for several weeks while we adjust drug dosages and monitor for evidence of rejection (with surveillance biopsies) or of infection. We generally see patients in the outpatient clinic two to three times per week for the first couple of weeks and cut back to once a week thereafter. By the time the patients are discharged to homes outside of the general area, they are being seen at 2- to 3-week intervals depending on their biopsy schedule. The average patient is discharged to his or her home community between 8 and 12 weeks after the transplant but this decision obviously depends on their clinical stability and the distance they live from Richmond.

Clinic visits generally involve routine laboratory studies plus measurement of weight, and other routine vital signs. At each clinic visit the medications are reviewed thoroughly to be absolutely certain that the patients are taking their medications properly. The clinical examination of the post-transplant patient is aimed primarily at detecting any evidence of rejection, of infection, or of side effects from the immunosuppressive protocol. Unfortunately, with the use of cyclosporine, there are almost no physical findings that help diagnose rejection. We do, however, encounter cardiomegaly, gallops, and ECG changes when patients have severe rejection. This is quite uncommon and in our experience over the past 4 years this has occurred only twice in two patients who did not comply to the prescribed drug regimen.

Routine examination of the heart and lungs are performed as well as assessment of right-sided pressure as noted by neck vein distention and pedal edema. After discharge to their home community, we continue to see the patients for biopsies and periodic checkups. The patient is seeing their primary care physician in the intervals as often as is necessary based on their clinical status.

Biopsies

After discharge from the hospital, cardiac biopsies are performed weekly for the first 2 weeks and then every other week until they return home. This schedule is soon reduced to 3 to 6 weeks depending on the previous biopsy findings. Should a patient need treatment for a rejection, the biopsy then is performed 7 to 10 days after treatment for the rejection and subsequently every other week for two more biopsies. The subsequent biopsy schedule is tailored depending on the biopsy readings. The average number of biopsies during the first year after transplant is 16, and biopsies are then done three to six times during the second year depending on the number of rejection episodes in the initial postoperative period and whether the immunosuppressive therapy needs to be tapered.

We currently perform biopsies in our outpatient surgical department with results available the same day or the next afternoon. Because of the increasing number of patients who are maintained at a distance from Richmond, those requiring frequent biopsies sometimes have their biopsies performed by a cardiologist or cardiothoracic surgeon in their area by one who is experienced with the procedure. The tissue then is sent to our pathologists for review. Unfortunately, at this time the endomyocardial biopsy is the only reliable way to detect rejection in the cyclosporine-treated patient.[1]

Laboratory Data

Initially after discharge, we monitor laboratory panels three times per week for the first several weeks and then taper to once a week if possible. We currently recommend continuing once a week laboratory work until approximately 3 months. If by this time the patient is clinically stable, we decrease the frequency of laboratory work to once or twice per month. For long-term survivors who have demonstrated clinical stability for long periods of time, laboratory work may be decreased to once every 2 to 3 months. Routine laboratory work should include the following:

1. *Complete blood count with differential and platelet count.* We are concerned primarily about following the white blood cell (WBC) count because all patients are on azathioprine. We do not use prednisone in the majority of our patients and have found that we need to lower the WBC into the 4000 to 4500 range to achieve good immunosuppression without prednisone. We also monitor the hemoglobin and platelet counts for evidence of excessive immunosuppression or other ongoing illnesses such as cytomegalovirus infection.[2]

2. *Chemistry panel.* This panel includes electrolytes, glucose, blood urea nitrogen (BUN), creatinine, calcium, phosphate, total protein, albumin, uric acid, cholesterol, SGOT, SGPT, total bilirubin, and alkaline phosphatase. We continue to follow this panel for evidence of hepatic or renal dysfunction during the postoperative period, as a sign of cyclosporine toxicity.[3]

3. *Cyclosporine trough levels.* We believe that levels are necessary but do not adjust medicine changes because of levels alone. We believe that the patient's clinical course must be taken into account, and, therefore, we do not aim for certain levels. All patients are different. The frequency of cyclosporine trough levels is dictated by how frequently the dose adjustments are needed. At the time of discharge to their home communities, the patients receive instructions on how to have blood samples sent to our laboratory for this measurement. We strongly recommend that patients continue to send samples to our laboratory because of marked laboratory variability with different assays.

4. *Electrocardiogram.* We perform routine electrocardiograms one to two times a month in the immediate postoperative outpatient clinic and once every 2 to 3 months during the first year after transplantation and thereafter yearly unless a patient complains of ill health. A decrease in electrocardiographic voltage is no longer considered a reliable sign of early rejection in the cyclosporine era. Nowadays the most common cause of decreased voltage is a pericardial effusion.[4] However, in some patients who are not on cyclosporine because of early protocols or who have been weaned from cyclosporine because of toxicity, we follow voltage changes closely as a method to monitor for rejection.

5. *Chest roentgenogram.* The patients receive periodic chest roentgenograms as surveillance for infection, pericardial effusion, and other postoperative complications such as a tumor. We obtain a chest roentgenogram at discharge, then at 1 and 3 months, and then at 6 months and 1 year. Thereafter we obtain chest roentgenograms every year. Additionally, chest roentgenograms are obtained whenever the patient has an undiagnosed fever or an undiagnosed illness. We recommend chest roentgenograms for every patient who has a fever, and for any patient with chest symptoms, however insignificant they may seem.

6. *Lipids.* Elevated cholesterol levels are ubiquitous in the transplant patient. Because of the suggestion that elevated cholesterol levels are in some part related to the development of coronary atherosclerosis, we now

monitor cholesterol quite frequently.[5] We obtain fasting lipid profiles at 3 and 6 months and then at least yearly thereafter. It is important to obtain the entire lipid profile inasmuch as many of our patients have very low high-density lipoprotein (HDL) values and thus high cholesterol/HDL ratios.

Immunosuppressive Protocol

Currently we are employing an immunosuppressive protocol that consists of cyclosporine and azathioprine.[6] This protocol is in contrast to most major programs that use a triple-drug regimen of prednisone, cyclosporine, and azathioprine for long-term maintenance.[7] In addition, we use rabbit antithymocyte globulin (RATG) for refractory rejections. We reserve the use of OKT3 for patients that are not responsive to RATG inasmuch as we have had several serious infections after the use of OKT3. Approximately 4 years ago we decided that cyclosporine and azathioprine could offer adequate protection without the addition of corticosteroids and thus spare the patient the long-term side effects of corticosteroids. The long-term side effects including diabetes, cataracts, and bone compression fractures were becoming quite prevalent in most of our long-term transplant patients after 4 to 14 years. This led to a poor lifestyle owing to the morbidity and pain of the side effects. Since then we have enrolled over 130 patients into this protocol and have added prednisone only for repeated rejections or if cyclosporine or azathioprine had to be severely reduced or stopped due to side effects. Currently over 80 percent of our patients who were enrolled in this protocol are not taking prednisone. When a patient is started on prednisone we attempt to wean the drug to the lowest possible dose and we have discontinued prednisone in some patients. Since we have started this program, the cardiac transplant team retains permanent responsibility for adjustment of the patient's immunosuppressive regimen.

3 Months After Discharge

At 3 months after discharge, most patients are ready to go back to their homes and are quite stable medically. Baseline studies at this juncture include physical examination, ECG, chest roentgenogram, CBC, chemistry panel, lipid profile, cardiac ultrasound, MUGA scan, and a 24-hour urine for creatinine clearance.

The patient is then sent back to their referring physician who will follow the patient clinically. Needed biopsies are performed monthly or every other month as stated earlier. All laboratory work performed by other physicians is sent to Medical College of Virginia (MCV), where the immunosuppression maintenance protocols are regulated. The patients will usually call these results into a phone line dedicated for this purpose. All laboratory examinations are perused the next day by the nurse coordinators and once per week by the physician in charge. If medications need to be changed, the patients are contacted.

Yearly Visits

All patients now have yearly examinations, which include a history and physical examination, ECG, lipid profile, exercise tolerance test, creatinine clearance, MUGA scan, cardiac ultrasound, CBC and chemistry panel, chest roentgenogram, cardiac biopsy, and cardiac catheterization.

We have begun only recently to do yearly cardiac catheterizations. Formerly, we had a protocol that employed stress or dipyridamole thallium tests, which we found to be adequate for assessment of coronary artery disease. We felt that we did not miss significant life-threatening coronary artery disease, but we did miss early disease. Therefore, we have embarked on yearly cardiac catheterization with quantitative coronary angiography. We continue to do yearly checkups during the life of the patient.

SPECIAL LONG-TERM PROBLEMS

Hypertension

In our experience, more than 80 percent of patients maintained with cyclosporine develop significant arterial hypertension.[8] The mechanism is not clearly understood, but the most current data suggest a renal mechanism as the most likely cause for both the decrease in glomerular filtration rate and the hypertension. It has been our experience that the calcium channel blockers are the most effective agents, and we maintain most patients requiring treatment on these agents. We favor diltiazem because of relatively fewer side effects encountered with this agent.

We add an angiotensin-converting enzyme inhibitor as our second drug of choice. Subsequently we will add hydralazine if the hypertension remains refractory. We have not encountered a change in blood pressure by weaning cyclosporine. We do not use beta blockers because these drugs decrease the exercise tolerance of our patients.

We believe that aggressive blood pressure management is needed, and all of our patients measure their own blood pressures. It is noteworthy that cyclosporine causes an altered diurnal pattern to blood pressure, with the highest pressures observed in the morning, and this means the regimen must be tailored to each patient.[9] This can be achieved only if the patients take their own blood pressures.

Diuretics

Patients frequently are discharged from the hospital after their initial transplant on low doses of diuretics because of pedal edema associated with mild right ventricular dysfunction that is commonly encountered after transplantation. As the right ventricle hypertrophies and the pulmonary vascular resistance improves, the edema resolves. Most patients are then tapered off diuretics. We have not found that diuretics improve hypertension unless associated with edema. We do not routinely supplement diuretics with potassium because cyclosporine can cause hyperkalemia and potassium conservation by its direct effect on the kidneys. Likewise, we do not recommend potassium sparing diuretics.

Anemia

Anemia is quite common in the transplant population and therefore we start most patients on iron supplementation for several weeks to months. We also add folate to the regimen for patients with moderate anemia. We try not to transfuse patients after transplant unless absolutely necessary.

Antibiotics

Because of their immunosuppressed state, transplant patients are more susceptible to infections involving a vast array of organisms and organ system involvement. We ask our patients and primary care physicians to check with us prior to starting any antibiotic so that we may check for possible drug interactions with their immunosuppressive regimen. The most common antibiotics that cause problems are erythromycin, which can cause dramatic changes in cyclosporine levels, and trimethoprim-sulfa, which can cause renal failure and marked neutropenia. Recently we have had problems with a new antibiotic, cipofloxicin, which causes profound renal dysfunction. Generally, penicillins and cephalosporins have been well tolerated by this population.

Antiseizure Medication

Some patients who had a focus for seizures before transplantation, because of embolic stroke or trauma, may have recurrent seizures after transplantation because cyclosporine seems to lower seizure threshold. In addition, seizures occasionally are encountered in patients without a focus and we believe this is due to early toxicity of cyclosporine. We try to taper all patients off antiseizure medications because phenytoin and phenobarbital cause dramatic falls in cyclosporine levels because of increased P-450 activity in the liver, thus requiring very large doses of cyclosporine and making it difficult to maintain therapeutic levels. Tegretol can cause a marked neutropenia.

Allopurinol

Many patients have a history of gout before transplantation or they develop the problem after transplantation owing to hyperuricemia from cyclosporine therapy. We do not recommend giving patients allopurinol while they are receiving azathioprine because the combination can cause dramatic neutropenia. We treat gout with low-dose colchicine and may treat individual episodes with short courses of corticosteroids.

Pericardial Effusions

We encounter significant pericardial effusions in approximately 1 in 10 to 20 transplantations. this complication has been encountered only since the use of cyclosporine. We have seen tamponade on several occasions and we now routinely tap large effusions prior to the onset of symptoms. This is usually done in the intensive care unit (ICU) or cardiac catheterization laboratory. Only two patients have had to have more than one pericardiocentesis. The etiology of this fluid is unknown at present.

Renal Dysfunction

We have been using cyclosporine since 1983, with renal dysfunction as the most bothersome side effect. We try to wean cyclosporine to the lowest level possible. Currently, we try to use only azathioprine and cyclosporine for long-term maintenance therapy. Should the serum creatinine continue to rise or the glomerular filtration rate fall below 40 ml/min, we then add prednisone and taper cyclosporine. Initially, we stopped the cyclosporine, but now we wean the patient from the cyclosporine until the renal function begins to improve, without totally stopping the drug.

Lipid Abnormalities

We firmly believe that hypercholesterolemia in part worsens the acceleration of coronary artery disease in the post-transplant patient.[10] Therefore, we insist on lowering the cholesterol in hypercholesterolemic patients. Some patients may have low total cholesterol but extremely low HDL levels, resulting in a high-risk ratio. Unfortunately, the treatment at present is less than satisfactory. All patients are started on a low-cholesterol, low–saturated fat diet. All too often this diet is of marginal benefit. We have a study protocol using lovastatin, but we do not recommend its use until we have further data inasmuch as patients have been known to develop lethal rhabdomyolysis from the use of this agent. Most binding agents lower cyclosporine levels or cause elevated liver enzyme abnormalities, and therefore the patient needs to be followed closely. We have encouraged the use of oat bran as a natural means of lowering cholesterol. All patients who have low HDLs are encouraged to start an exercise program, and several patients have been started on a long-acting niacin preparation but we have no data as to the safety of this therapy.

Accelerated Coronary Artery Disease

Development of accelerated coronary artery disease (CAD) in the cardiac allograft is one of the major causes of late graft failure in the heart transplant recipients. We believe that by 5 years after surgery 50 percent of patients will develop some aspect of the disease. We have had several patients develop the disease in less than 2 years, and this malignant form of the disease rapidly leads to death in weeks to months if the patient does not undergo retransplantation. Alternatively, we have had patients develop the disease later, usually after 5 years, and this form of CAD seems to be less rapid in its progression and in several patients amenable to percutaneous transluminal coronary angioplasty (PTCA).[11] Treatment or prevention of coronary artery disease is most difficult because of its diffuse distribution and our lack of understanding of its pathogenesis.

SUMMARY

Successful long-term management of the cardiac transplant patient requires the concerted effort of the patient, the cardiac transplant team, and the primary care physician. The long-term management of these patients will continue to evolve as new immunosuppressive agents are used and new methods of surveillance for rejection are found. The long-term management is indeed one of the most exciting parts of the care of the transplant patient, especially when all those involved can watch the patient enter into a normal lifestyle.

REFERENCES

1. Billingham, ME and Mason, JW: Role of endomyocardial biopsy in the management of acute rejection in cardiac allograft recipients. In Fenoglio, JJ: Endomyocardial Biopsy: Techniques and applications. CRC Press, Boca Raton, FL, 1983, 58.
2. Icenogle, TB, Petersen, E, Ray, G, et al: DHPG effectively treats CMV infection in heart and heart-lung transplant patients: A preliminary report. Heart Transplant 6:199, 1987.
3. Calne, RY, Rolles, K, White, DJG, et al: Cyclosporine-A initially as the only immunosuppressant in 34 recipients of cadaveric organs: 32 kidneys, 2 pancreases and 2 livers. Lancet 2:1033, 1979.
4. Hastillo, A, Thompson, JA, Lower, RR, et al: Cyclosporine-induced pericardial effusion in patients who have undergone cardiac transplantation. Am J Cardiol 59:1120, 1987.
5. Gao, SZ, Schroeder, JS, Alderman, EL, et al: Clinical and laboratory correlations of accelerated coronary vascular disease in the cardiac transplant patient. Circulation 76:V-56, 1986.
6. Katz, MR, Barnhart, GR, Szentpetery, S, et al: Are steroids essential for successful maintenance of immunosuppression in heart transplantation? J Heart Transplant 6:293, 1987.

7. Copeland, JG, Emery, RW, Levinson, MM, et al: Cyclosporine: An immunosuppressive panacea? J Thorac Cardiovasc Surg 91:26, 1986.

8. Myer, BD, Ross, J, Newton, L, et al: Cyclosporine associated with chronic nephropathy. N Engl J Med 311:699, 1984.

9. Reeves, RA, Shapiro, AP, Thomppson, ME, et al: Loss of nocturnal decline in blood pressure after cardiac transplantation. Circulation 73:401, 1986.

10. Laden, AMK: Experimental atherosclerosis in rat and rabbit cardiac allografts. Arch Pathol 93:240, 1972.

11. Vetrovec, GW, Cowley, MJ, Newton, M, et al: Applications of percutaneous transluminal coronary angioplasty in cardiac transplantation. Circulation 78:III-83, 1988.

PART 4

Special Populations

CHAPTER 15

Pediatric Cardiac Transplantation

F. Jay Fricker, M.D.
Alfredo Trento, M.D.
Bartley P. Griffith, M.D.

Cardiac transplantation has only recently become an accepted modality for treatment of end-stage myocardial dysfunction and palliated congenital heart disease in children. In fact, before Pennington's multicenter review in 1985[1] and reports from Pittsburgh[2] and Stanford[3] in 1987, only one report of successful transplantation in children had been published.[4] Interest in transplantation in children has been fostered by success in adult programs, effective immune suppression protocols, and improved quality of life in surviving patients.

Historically, credit for the first pediatric heart transplant is given to Kantrowitz,[5] who, in 1967, transplanted a heart from an anencephalic infant to a 3-week-old infant with tricuspid atresia. In 1968 Cooley[6] transplanted the heart and lungs from an anencephalic infant to a baby with an atrioventricular septal defect. Stanford can be credited with the first successful pediatric heart transplants.[4] In 1981 they reported their experience with cardiac transplantation in seven adolescents, one of whom had survived more than 5 years following transplantation. Extending cardiac transplantation to younger patients was a natural result of this success in adolescents. The International Heart Transplant Registry[7] and the Pediatric Heart Transplant Survey of 1978–1987[8] have gathered information from over 30 transplant centers in the United States and abroad performing heart transplantation in children. There are now over 300 children, ranging from neonates to 18 years of age, listed on those registries who have had heart, heart-lung, or heart-liver transplants.

The technical accomplishment and early success of pediatric cardiac transplantation has been established. Reports of late deaths from coronary artery disease and complications of cyclosporine-based immune suppression has tempered some of the initial enthusiasm. It is important now to reflect on the successes and failures of pediatric cardiac transplantation of the past 5 years and to direct research efforts toward solving the problems that limit long-term graft survival.

SELECTION OF THE PEDIATRIC HEART TRANSPLANT RECIPIENT

LESSONS LEARNED

Extending cardiac transplantation to young children requires scrutiny of the natural history of cardiomyopathy and palliated congenital heart disease and assessment of the benefits of transplantation in children with those diseases. Timing of transplantation surgery can be a difficult decision, and the importance of the families' expectations of length of survival cannot be overemphasized. Transplantation resulting in death should be viewed by the family as having given their child a chance for extended life, not having caused premature death.

Dilated cardiomyopathy and palliated congenital heart disease with irreversible myocardial dysfunction are the major indications for heart transplantation in children.[1-3,8] At the Children's Hospital of Pittsburgh 27 orthotopic heart transplants have been done in children between 2 weeks and 16 years of age (Fig. 15–1). Sixteen (59 percent) were performed in patients with dilated cardiomyopathy (DCM) or myocarditis and 11 (41 percent) in children with congenital heart disease. The Pediatric Heart Transplant Survey[8] reported 40 percent of patients receiving orthotopic heart transplants for congenital heart disease.[8] Children with palliated congenital heart disease represent a particular challenge to the transplant surgeon because he or she must deal with unusual relationships and connections, altered pulmonary artery anatomy from systemic-to-pulmonary-artery shunts, and patients who have had previous thoracotomy or sternotomy. These problems are responsible for a high early mortality in our institution. Perioperative mortality in a patient with cardiomyopathy is 15 percent campared with a staggering 55 percent in children with congenital heart disease. Two factors stand out as problems: technical difficulties created by previous palliative surgery, and proper estimation of pulmonary vascular resistance in the recipient.

Technical Considerations: Transplantation in Children With Congenital Heart Disease

The technique of implantation in the presence of normal atrial and great vessel arrangement has not presented a problem, even in small children. The operation requires biatrial connection and end-to-end anastomosis between donor and recipient aortas and pulmonary arteries.

Implantation in the presence of congenital heart disease creates additional

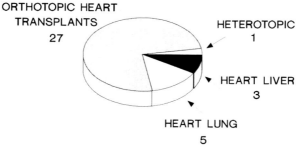

Figure 15–1. Total heart transplantation experience in children at the University of Pittsburgh, 1982 to 1988.

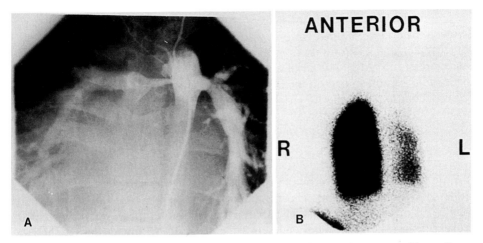

Figure 15–2. *A,* Pre-transplant cineangiogram in a patient with complex congenital heart disease and pulmonic stenosis. Palliation had been accomplished with a Potts shunt (left pulmonary artery to descending aorta) but left him with severe branch pulmonary artery stenosis. *B,* Post-transplant lung perfusion scan in this patient demonstrated marked decrease in left lung blood flow.

problems that prolong the operative procedure and graft ischemic time. A large atrial septal defect is a frequent finding, and requires a prosthetic patch or use of atrial wall tissue from the donor heart for repair. A more serious problem is distortion of the pulmonary artery anatomy from a previous systemic-to-pulmonary-artery shunt or pulmonary artery band. Figure 15–2*A* is a preoperative cineangiogram obtained in a patient with severe left branch pulmonary artery stenosis from a previous Potts anastomosis. Despite attempts to reconstruct the left pulmonary artery at transplantation, adequate left pulmonary blood flow could not be established (Fig. 15–2*B,* postoperative lung perfusion scan). This problem was the major contributing cause of early mortality in this patient. A second patient who had previously undergone a first-stage Norwood procedure and right and left modified Blalock-Taussig shunts died when bilateral pulmonary artery reconstruction was attempted. Risk is also increased by a previous sternotomy that results in dense scarring around mediastinal structures and makes surgical dissection tedious and dangerous. Thus, technical problems should be given strong consideration when selecting a patient for transplantation surgery.

Pulmonary Vascular Resistance

The major cause of early graft loss is failure of the donor right ventricle. The unpredictable response of the allograft right ventricle to elevated pulmonary vascular resistance (PVR) was recognized early in Stanford's experience with heart transplantation.[9] The major causes of elevated PVR include chronic left ventricular dysfunction with secondary pulmonary venous hypertension that is not immediately reversible with transplantation, multiple pulmonary emboli emanating from mural thrombus formation on the right ventricular endocardium, and increased muscularization and abnormal extension of muscle into pulmonary arterioles in patients with congenital heart disease.[10] Sudden exposure of the donor right ventricle to inordinantly elevated PVR will cause it to dilate or to fail.[11]

The upper limit of PVR for successful orthotopic heart transplantation is not known. Criteria developed from the adult transplant experience suggest that a PVR greater than 6 Wood units or a transpulmonary gradient (pulmonary artery mean pressure [PAM]–left atrial mean pressure [LAM] greater than 15 mmHg is a contraindication to orthotopic heart transplantation.[9,12,13] These criteria are not valid in children, and the use of pulmonary vascular resistance index below

$$\left(PVRI = \frac{TPG}{CI} \right)$$

is more appropriate. The problem of elevated PVR was reviewed by Addonizio and associates,[12] who found no perioperative mortality when PVRI was less than 6 units. In our experience, PVRI between 4 and 6 units increased perioperative morbidity and the subsequent course was determined by how prompt a decrease in PVR occurred with improved left ventricular function of the new allograft. On the other hand, orthotopic heart transplantation has been successful in children with PVR index between 6 and 12 units, particularly when it could be demonstrated that they had pharmacologic reactive pulmonary vasculature (using amrinone, nitroprusside, or prostaglandin).[1,14] If PVR is increased, an oversized heart with increased right ventricular mass may be better able to function with elevated right ventricular afterload.[15] We are unaware of any clinical or laboratory support for this argument.

Other contraindications to transplantation have become relative. Significant hepatic and renal dysfunction are invariably reversible with transplantation. The presence of pulmonary infarction once was thought to be a contraindication to heart transplant because of the risk of lung abscess with immune suppression.[16] However, we have successfully transplanted three children with lung infarction, albeit with increased morbidity. One patient did develop a lung abscess following transplantation, which required segmental lung resection.

In children with malignant disease and diabetes, decisions must be individualized. Several children with Adriamycin cardiotoxicity have now been transplanted with good early survival.[8]

It should be unusual to exclude a pediatric patient from transplantation for social reasons, but a reasonably intelligent and supportive family is necessary to manage the child after surgery. In our institution, several single-parent families have survived the stress of chronic illness, hospitalization, and unexpected problems after transplantation.

IMMUNE SUPPRESSION AND MONITORING OF REJECTION

Immune suppression therapy regimens in children have evolved with increasing adult experience.[17-19] In our early experience, cyclosporine and prednisone were used routinely and antithymocyte globulin (ATG)* was added as rescue therapy for acute rejection. In late 1986 we began to use ATG prophylactically

---

*ATG-RATG-Rabbit Antithymocyte Globulin; obtained initally from Dr. Charles Bieber at Stanford University; currently made in the laboratories of the University of Pittsburgh.

for the first 3 to 5 days following transplantation. The optimal immune suppressive regimen for children is not known. Triple-drug therapy using cyclosporine, prednisone, and azathioprine has gained popularity recently in the hope that it will minimize late toxicity from cyclosporine and prednisone.[20,21]

We also have added azathioprine to cyclosporine and prednisone for chronic immunosuppression. Currently, we attempt initially to maintain whole blood radioimmunoassay (RIA) cyclosporine levels between 700 and 1000 ng/ml. The dose necessary to achieve such blood levels varies from 4 to 20 mg/kg/day. After 6 months the cyclosporine dose is decreased to attain blood levels of 500 ng/ml by RIA and 100 to 250 ng/ml by high-performance liquid chromatography (HPLC). Prednisone dose varies between 0.1 and 0.3 mg/kg/day. Children appear to be unusually sensitive to bone marrow suppression from azathioprine, and some do not tolerate this drug or are receiving very small daily or every other day doses.

The endomyocardial biopsy (EMB) remains the only reliable monitoring method for rejection. We have encountered no major major technical difficulties in doing EMB, even in small children. Instruments have been scaled down from the original 8.5 F Caves-Schultz reusable biotome. Currently 6 or 7 F cordis and 6.3 F Caves-Schultz biotomes are used from either a right internal jugular or femoral vein approach. The use of a Mullins long sheath facilitates the procedure when done from the leg. In our institution, EMB is usually done as an outpatient procedure.

Echocardiographic measurements of wall thickness and isovolumetric relaxation time (IRT) have been reported to be good predictors of myocyte necrosis.[22,23] This has not been our experience, but echocardiography is useful to estimate the initial ischemic insult and to monitor the new graft's recovery (Fig. 15–3). Serial studies after transplantation are used to assess the effects of chronic rejection, hypertension, and coronary artery disease.

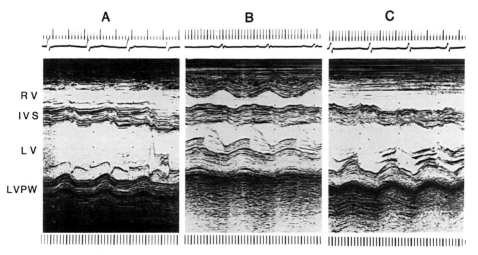

Figure 15–3. Serial M-mode echocardiograms done 1 day (*A*), 1 week (*B*), and 1 month (*C*) after orthotopic heart transplant. Notice early systolic dysfunction, paradoxical septal motion, and myocardial wall thickening (*A* and *B*). All resolved except paradoxical septal motion by 1 month after transplantation (*C*).

Radionuclide scans for left ventricular ejection fraction (LVEF) are performed at the time of each endomyocardial biopsy. A decrease in LVEF of 5 percent has been a good predictor of active or imminent rejection.[24]

Recently we have looked at the prediction of rejection by growth of activated lymphocytes from endomyocardial biopsies.[25] Endomyocardial biopsy samples are infiltrated with activated lymphocytes which can be expanded in the presence of interleukin 2. The frequency of positive cell cultures generally increase with histologic grade of rejection. Recently we have had positive cell cultures associated with histology grade of 0–1 +. Currently we are studying the predictive value of positive cell culture for subsequent allograft rejection.

ALLOGRAFT REJECTION

The Stanford group reported actuarial free-from-rejection rates (percent free from rejection) in children of less than 20 percent at 1 year after transplant.[3] In our experience, all children undergoing transplantation have had histologically proven rejection that requires treatment within the first year. The experience in adults is quite different, with actuarial free-from-rejection rates of more than 50 percent when ATG is used prophylactically along with triple-drug immune suppression.[26] Some institutions have reported low actuarial rejection rates in children with similar immune suppression protocols.[20] Reasons for this difference are unclear but may be related to institutional variability in interpretation of the EMB. Most histologic rejection is focal, and treated rejection episodes are at least Billingham grade 3 (focal perivascular interstitial lymphocytic infiltration with myocyte necrosis). Endocardial quilty effect, and subendocardial and perivascular lymphocytic infiltration are not treated with augmented immune suppression.

Clinical or histologic rejection events are treated with intravenous Solu-Medrol 500 to 750 mg/m^2 daily for 3 days. If there is persistent or progressive change on followup endomyocardial biopsy, polyclonal antibody, ATG, or monoclonal antibody (OKT3) is used. Generally, maintenance oral prednisone and cyclosporine doses are increased after a rejection episode.

COMPLICATIONS OF IMMUNE SUPPRESSION

Infection

Infection continues to be a problem in pediatric patients undergoing transplantation. Approximately 75 percent of our patients have developed infection between the time of transplantation and discharge from the hospital. Fifty percent of these infections were bacterial, 39 percent viral, 7 percent fungal, and 4 percent protozoal.[27] This distribution is similar to that reported in adults.[28,29] In our series, there were two deaths from *Pseudomonas aeruginosa* infection of the lung and mediastinum, both after exploration for bleeding. Another child died from severe cytomegalovirus pneumonia 1 month after heart-lung transplantation.

The presence of a pulmonary infarct was at one time considered a contraindication to heart transplantation, but recently some patients have survived appropriate medical and surgical treatment.[16,30] Serious morbidity occurred from a lung abscess in one patient, which required segmental lung resection. Two others survived with no unusual morbidity.

One of our patients developed *Pneumocystis carinii* pneumonia following augmentation of immune suppression for acute rejection. We do not use Bactrim routinely for prophylaxis against *Pneumocystis carinii* infection except after courses of ATG or OKT3 as rescue therapy for rejection.

Serious late infections have been unusual in our experience. Several minor infections (urinary tract, otitis media, sinusitis) have occurred with usual pathogenic organisms and have resolved without sequelae. Recently one patient presented 1 year after transplantation with reactivated Ebstein-Barr virus (EBV) infection causing hepatitis and meningoencephalitis. This infection was uncontrollable despite discontinuation of cyclosporine immunosuppression. The patient died with multiple organ involvement with lymphoproliferative disease, including the heart allograft.

In summary, the most frequent site of infection in our pediatric patients has been in the lungs. Early pneumonias have been caused by gram-negative agents and late ones by viral agents cytomegalovirus, respiratory syncytial virus, or EBV.

Hypertension

Systemic hypertension is by far the most common hemodynamic abnormality noted following transplantation and is related, at least in part, to cyclosporine therapy.[31] Essentially all recipients have required antihypertensive therapy, and nearly all patients who have survived longer than 1 year currently require chronic antihypertensive regimens. The exact mechanism of hypertension is unclear but is thought to be related to cyclosporine-induced renal vasoconstriction. The hypertension is characterized by a lack of diurnal decrease in blood pressure. Hypertension has been difficult to treat, and therapeutic regimens usually begin with diuretics and angiotensin blocking agents. Long-acting calcium channel blocking drugs such as verapamil and sustained-release combination beta and alpha adrenergic blocking agents have also been helpful.

Renal Function

Careful monitoring of renal function is necessary becuase of the known nephrotoxic effects of cyclosporine.[32] We monitor whole blood cyclosporine levels both by radioimmunoassay (RIA) and high-performance liquid chromatography methods at frequent intervals. Cyclosporine dosages are variable and adjusted to maintain high performance liquid chromatography cyclosporine levels between 150 and 250 ng/ml, depending on the time elapsed since transplantation. We have used serum creatinine as an estimate of glomerular filtration in these children because of the difficulty in obtaining complete accurately timed urine collections for creatinine clearance (Fig. 15–4).[33] Serum creatinine generally returns to normal in the first month following transplantation, as myocardial function improves. Creatinine usually rises in patients who survive longer than one year after transplantation, doubling in most patients. Over subsequent years serum creatinine has remained stable, except in our longest surviving transplant recipient. In this adolescent, serum creatinine reached a peak of just over 2 mg% and necessitated a substantial reduction in cyclosporine dose as well as the addition of azathioprine to the immunosuppression regimen. Recent evidence suggests that serum creatinine and creatinine clearance do not accurately reflect cyclosporine nephrotoxicity.[34] The abnormalities in serum creatinine that we have encountered are significant and we are concerned that long-term use of cyclosporine may cause progressive renal dysfunction in children.

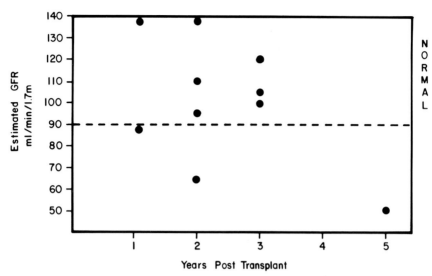

Figure 15–4. Estimated glomerular filtration rate (GFR)[33] in 10 children who have survived more than 1 year after heart transplantation.

Growth

We have assessed growth and weight gain in children surviving longer than 1 year following transplantation and have shown that linear growth has been maintained in 8 of 10 of these patients. In contrast, the majority of patients have shown a marked increase in weight, with only four patients remaining on the same weight percentile (Fig. 15–5). At their latest followup visit six patients have crossed weight percentiles and one patient is morbidly obese.

Lymphoproliferative Disease

Lymphoma in cyclosporine-treated transplant recipients is now well established in children.[35] Two of our children have had major EBV infections. One

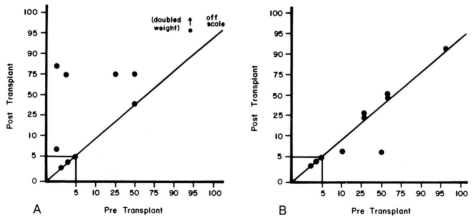

Figure 15–5. Pre- and post-transplant growth percentiles in 10 patients surviving more than 1 year after heart transplant. *A*, weight; *B*, linear growth.

heart-lung transplant recipient had biopsy-proven EBV lymphoproliferative disease of the lung. Another adolescent heart transplant recipient presented with hepatitis, meningoencephalitis, and renal failure 1 year after transplant and died with multiple organ lymphoproliferative disease. The only treatment currently available is reduction or discontinuation of immunosuppression.[35] Prevalence and future risk of lymphoproliferative disease in children on current immunosuppressive protocols is not yet known.

SURVIVAL

Since 1974 the International Heart Transplant Registry has listed more than 300 neonates, children, and adolescents who have undergone heart, heart-lung, or heart-liver transplantation.[7] Currently the Pediatric Heart Transplant Survey 1978–1987[8] is compiling a detailed profile on the majority of those patients, including information on survival, cause of death, incidence and frequency of rejection, complications of immunosuppression, and current status.

Since the beginning of the heart transplant program at the University of Pittsburgh in 1980, 1- to 5-year survival of children is comparable to that in adults (Fig. 15-6). Actuarial 1-year survival has continued to improve in most institutions and currently is 85 percent at the University of Pittsburgh. The difference between children and adult survival is exagerated if we look at the period 1982 to 1988, which is the time frame for pediatric heart transplantation at Children's Hospital. Current adult actuarial 5-year survival approaches 60 percent. In children, perioperative mortality is high at 35%. Late deaths in children are from chronic rejection, coronary artery disease, and lymphoproliferative syndromes.

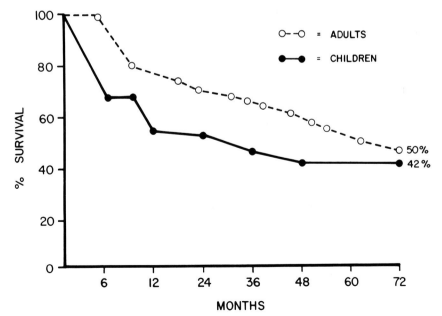

Figure 15–6. Cumulative survival in adults and children receiving heart transplants at the University of Pittsburgh Children's Hospital from February 1980 to June 1988.

The longest surviving pediatric patient in our institution is now 6 years after transplantation, and 11 children currently are alive 1 or more years following transplantation.

The issue of long-term survival in children is an important one. Everyone would agree that extending the life of a 45-year-old adult by 5 years is worthwhile. Most adults can remain productive and a part of their family. The same argument cannot be made as strongly for a young child. Depending on one's perspective, extending the life of a child through the uncertainties of cardiac transplantation may not be worthwhile. This is a most difficult decision for parents and we believe that the physician must support the decision either for or against transplantation, regardless of his or her personal view.

CORONARY ARTERY DISEASE

LIMITING FACTOR IN LONG-TERM SURVIVAL

Despite improvement in early survival after cardiac transplantation in children, accelerated coronary artery disease reamins a major obstacle to long-term graft survival. Prevalence of atherosclerosis in adult cardiac transplant recipients is estimated to be 20 percent at 1 year and 50 percent at 3 years after transplantation.[36-38] Pennington[8] did not find coronary atherosclerosis to be a major problem in children, reflecting the short followup interval of most children receiving cardiac transplants. Coronary atherosclerosis has been a major factor in four of five late deaths in our series, and our longest surviving recipeint has significant coronary artery disease 6 years after transplantation. Two children who died at 8 months and 11 months after transplantation had had multiple treated rejection episodes. At autopsy both had severe diffuse coronary artery disease and ischemic cardiomyopathy (Fig. 15–7). Two other patients died at 2 and 3 years after transplantation. One had known progressive coronary artery disease and was awaiting retransplantation. The other had mild to moderate large vessel coronary artery disease and died suddenly. He had several coronary risk factors including hyperlipidemia, hypertension, morbid obesity, and recurrent rejection episodes during the first year after transplantation.

Although pathogenesis of transplant atherosclerosis has not been determined, overwhelming evidence points to an immunologic basis.[36,37] Uretsky and associates[37] related the development of coronary artery disease to the occurrence of two or more major rejection episodes. Importance of risk factors such as age, hypertension, lipids, and obesity have yet to be determined in children.

QUALITY OF LIFE

The quality of a child's life following cardiac transplantation is an important consideration. Transplantation is a major surgical and emotional assault on a child. The child must spend several weeks in the hospital, endure frequent intrusive procedures, and emotionally incorporate another person's heart. A preliminary study measured how well the children are able to adjust to this procedure.[39] The 10 children in the study ranged in age from 6 to 15 years. The study surveyed the areas of emotional adjustment, peer relationships, school achievement, self-care, exercise tolerance, and family relationships. The tools used in the study

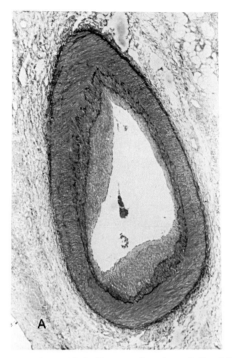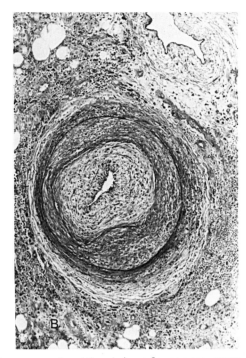

Figure 15–7. Cross-section through the right coronary artery (*A*) and circumflex coronary artery (*B*) of two patients who died of acute and chronic rejection within 1 year of transplantation.

included standardized psychologic tests, projective drawings, exercise testing, and parent interviews to determine the child's daily activities before and after transplantation. In each area measured, there was adequate functioning; in many areas functioning dramatically improved after transplantation. Therefore, for the 10 children studied, there is evidence that the quality of life did improve.

NEONATAL HEART TRANSPLANTATION

Leonard Bailey made neonatal heart transplantation a reality when he replaced the heart of an infant born with aortic atresia with a baboon's heart.[40] Subsequently he has used human allografts in 13 other infants.[41,42] Eleven of the infants are currently alive, three surviving for more than 1 year.

Neonatal transplantation presents several special problems with aortic atresia. Transplantation is a more demanding operation because of the need for aortic arch reconstruction.[41] Variable pulmonary vascular resistance in the recipient and uncertain response of the donor right ventricle to increased afterload make the postoperative period especially difficult. Scarcity of appropriate donors and the necessity of on-site procurement has added to the complexity of transplanting this group of patients.

Currently these problems are being addressed on several fronts. Expanding the donor pool by using anencephalic infants has been proposed. Modification of current brain-death criteria would be necessary because these infants have brain-stem function.[43,44] Another approach is to identify infants with aortic atresia by fetal ultrasound and plan delivery in conjunction with search for an appropriate donor. This area is still quite controversial because of the availability of alternative palliative surgery.

FUTURE OF PEDIATRIC HEART TRANSPLANTATION

Cardiac transplantation is a viable therapeutic alternative in children with terminal congenital and acquired heart disease. Appropriate selection of the pediatric transplant recipient is still difficult. The pediatric patient with palliated congenital heart disease remains a technical challenge to the transplant surgeon. Failure to identify patients with sufficiently elevated pulmonary vascular resistance to be a prohibitive risk for orthotopic heart transplant has resulted in substantial perioperative mortality. Long-term problems that affect survival remain unsolved. Hypertension, renal dysfunction, and lymphoproliferative disease related to cyclosporine immunosuppression can be addressed only by developing new immunosuppression regimens. Finally, until the problem of graft atherosclerosis is solved, cardiac transplantation in children can never be considered more than a palliative procedure.

REFERENCES

1. Pennington, DG, Sarafrin, J, and Swartz, M: Heart transplantation in children. Heart Transplant 4:441, 1985.
2. Fricker, FJ, Griffith, BP, Hardesty, RL, et al: Experience with heart transplantation in children. Pediatrics 79:138, 1987.
3. Starnes, VA, Stinson, EB, Oyer, PE, et al: Cardiac transplantation in children and adolescents. Circulation 76 (Suppl V):V43, 1987.
4. Baum, D, Stinson, EB, and Shumway, NE: The place for heart transplantation in children. Pediatric Cardiology 4:741, 1981.
5. Kantrowitz, A, Haller, SD, Joos, H, et al: Transplantation of the heart in an infant and an adult. Am J cardiol 22:782, 1968.
6. Cooley, DA, Bloodwell, RD, Hallman, GL, et al: Organ transplantation for advanced cardiopulmonary disease. Ann Thorac Surg 8:30, 1969.
7. Kaye, M: The International Heart Transplant Registry: Fifth Official Report 1988. J Heart Transplant 7:249, 1988.
8. Pennington, DG: Pediatric Heart Transplant Survey 1978–1987. Personal communication, 1988.
9. Griepp, RB, Stinson, EB, Dong, E, et al: Determinants of operative risk in human heart transplantation. Am J Surg 129, 1971.
10. Rabinovitch, M, Haworth, SG, Castaneda, AR, et al: Lung biopsy in congenital heart disease: A morphometric approach to pulmonary vascular disease. Circulation 58:1107, 1978.
11. Taquini, AC, Fermoso, JD, and Aramendia, P: Behavior of the right ventricle following acute constriction of the pulmonary artery. Circ Res 8:315, 1960.
12. Addonizio, LJ, Gersony, WM, Robbins, RC, et al: Elevated pulmonary vascular resistance and cardiac transplantation. Circulation 76 (Suppl V):V-52, 1987.
13. Kormos, RL, Griffith, BP, and Hardesty, RL: Utility of preoperative right heart catheterization data as a predictor of survival after heart transplantation. J Heart Transplant 5:391, 1986.
14. Addonizio, LJ Gersony, WM, and Rose, EA: Cardiac transplantation in children with high pulmonary vascular resistance. Am Heart J 112:647, 1986.
15. Griffith, BP and Hardesty, RL: Personal communication, 1982.
16. Young, JN Yazbeck, J, Espositio, G, et al: The influence of acute preoperative pulmonary infarction on the results of heart transplantation. J Heart Transplant 5:20, 1986.
17. Hardesty, RL, Griffith, BP, Debski, RF, et al: Experience with cyclosporine in cardiac transplantation. Transplant Proc 15:2553, 1983.
18. Griffith, BP, Hardesty, RL, and Bahnson, HT: Powerful but limited immunosuppression for car-

diac transplantation with cyclosporine and low dose steroid. J Thorac Cardiovasc Surg 87:35, 1984.

19. Griffith, BP, Hardesty, RL, Trento, A, et al: Five years of heart transplantation in Pittsburgh. Heart Transplant 4:489, 1985.

20. Ring, WS, Braulin, EA, Olivari, MT et al: Triple drug immune suppression after cardiac transplantation in children. J Heart Transplant 7:77, 1987.

21. Kormos, RL, Trento, A, Hardesty, RL, et al: Avoidance of perioperative renal toxicity by a modified immunosuppression protocol. Transplant Proc 19:2525, 1987.

22. Dawkins, KD, Oldershaw, PJ, Billingham, ME, et al: Changes in diastolic function as a noninvasive marker of cardiac allograft rejection. Heart Transplant 3:286, 1984.

23. Valantine, HA, Fowler, MB, Hunt, SA, et al: Changes in Doppler echocardiographic indexes of left ventricular function as potential markers of acute cardiac rejection. Circulation 76 (Suppl V):V-86, 1987.

24. Follansbee, WP, Kiernan, JM, and Curtiss, EI: Acute rejection in the cardiac allograft is associated with measurable decreases in left ventricular ejection fraction. Circulation 74 (Suppl II):160, 1986.

25. Duquesnoy, R, Weber, T, Zeevi, A, et al: Propagation of lymphocytes from endomyocardial biopsies: Prognostic value for patients at risk of transplant rejection. J Heart Transplant 7:79, 1988.

26. Griffith, BP and Hardesty, RH: Personal communication, 1988.

27. Green, M, Wald, ER, Fricker, FJ, et al: Infections in pediatric orthotopic heart transplant recipients. Pediatr Infect Dis J (in press).

28. Baumgartner, WA: Infection in cardiac transplantation. Heart Transplant 3:75, 1983.

29. Hofflin, JM, Potasman, I, Baldwin, JC, et al: Infectious complications in heart transplant recipients receiving cyclosporine and corticosteroids. Ann Intern Med 106:209, 1987.

30. Rogers, AJ, Griffith, BP, Hardesty, RL, et al: Management of pulmonary infarction in cardiac transplantation. J Heart Transplant (in press).

31. Thompson, ME, Shapiro, AP, Johnsen, AM, et al: New onset hypertension following cardiac transplantation: A preliminary report and analysis. Transplant Proc 15:2573, 1983.

32. Myers, BD, Ross, J, Newton, L, et al: Cyclosporine associated chronic nephropathy. N Engl J Med 311:699, 1984.

33. Schwartz, GJ, and Gautheir, B: A simple estimate of glomerular filtration rate in adolescent boys. J Pediatr 106:522, 1985.

34. Tomlanovich, S, Golbetz, H, Perlroth, M, et al: Limitations of creatinine in quantifying the severity of cyclosporine-induced chronic nephropathy. Am J Kidney Dis 8:332, 1986.

35. Starzl, TE, Porter, KA, Nalesnik, MA, et al: Reversibility of lymphomas and lymphoproliferative lesions developing under cyclosporine-steroid therapy. Lancet 1:583, 1984.

36. Billingham, ME: Cardiac transplant atherosclerosis. Transplant Proc 19:19, 1987.

37. Uretsky, BF, Murali, S, Reddy, PS, et al: Development of coronary artery disease in cardiac transplant patients receiving immunosuppressive therapy with cyclosporine and prednisone. Circulation 76:827, 1987.

38. Hess, ML, Hastillo, A, Mohanakumar, T, et al: Accelerated atherosclerosis in cardiac transplantation: Role of cytotoxic B-cell antibodies and hyperlipidemia. Circulation 68 (Suppl II):II-94, 1983.

39. Lawrence, KS and Fricker, FJ. Pediatric heart transplantation: The quality of life. J Heart Transplant 6:329, 1987.

40. Bailey, LL, Neilsen-Cannarella, SL, Concepcion, W, et al: Baboon-to-human cardiac xenotransplantation in a neonate. JAMA 254:3321, 1985.

41. Bailey, LL, Neilsen-Cannarella, SL, Doroshow, RW, et al: Cardiac allotransplantation in newborns as therapy for hypoplastic left heart syndrome. N Engl J Med 315:949, 1986.

42. Bailey, LL: Personal communication, 1988.

43. Botkin, JR: Anencephalic infants as organ donors. Pediatrics 82:250, 1988.

44. Landwirth, J: Should anencephalic infants be used as organ donors? Pediatrics 82:257, 1988.

CHAPTER 16

Transplantation of Other Organs with the Heart

Henry T. Bahnson, M.D.
Robert D. Gordon, M.D.

As the art and science of transplantation have advanced over the last two decades, greater success has been obtained with an increasing number of organs—first the kidney, followed by the liver, heart, lungs, pancreas, and intestines. Initially, the ideal candidate for transplantation of any organ was a patient with disease limited to that specific organ. Success has bred confidence with the procedure, however, and, as a consequence, indications have expanded and contraindications diminished. Thus it was a natural extension to separately transplant multiple organs in a patient who was well otherwise and whose disease was largely limited to transplantable organs.

At the University Health Center of Pittsburgh, in addition to the heart-lung transplants referred to elsewhere in this volume, a heart has been transplanted in five patients along with another separately transplanted organ from the same donor.

COMBINED TRANSPLANTATION OF HEART AND LIVER

Combined transplantation of heart and liver has been done in three instances.[1] Two of the patients suffered from hypercholesterolemia and secondary severe coronary artery disease. The liver was transplanted with the expectation of correcting the hypercholesterolemia, and the heart was transplanted to correct the severe ischemic cardiomyopathy. A third patient had biliary cirrhosis and idiopathic cardiomyopathy.

Case Report

The first patient, S.J., is alive and well 5 years following the combined procedure. She was 6¾ years old at the time of transplantation and had been extensively studied at the University of Texas, Southwestern Medical School, in Dallas. Homozygous familial hypercholesterolemia was well established, the first evidence of which had been progressive development of xanthomas on the contact areas of her buttocks and extremities at 3 months of age. Her disease rapidly progressed in the 4 months prior to operation. At 6½ years of age she developed angina pectoris. An apical myocardial infarction was complicated by pulmonary edema, which required prolonged ventilatory support. Stenosis of the left main coronary artery was found and treated by coronary artery bypass to the anterior descending and first circumflex marginal arteries. Over the next 2 months angina recurred, and another acute myocardial infarction led to reoperation and bypass to a more distal circumflex marginal artery, the original graft to the circumflex marginal artery having been found occluded on repeat arteriography. At this operation, she could not be weaned from bypass until the mitral valve was replaced. Papillary muscles were infarcted. Recurrence of angina pectoris several weeks later led to the conclusion that the only hopeful option was replacement of both liver and heart, and she was transferred to Children's Hospital and the University Health Center of Pittsburgh where the operation was performed on February 13 and 14, 1984. Transplantation of the liver was deemed to be indicated to correct the deficiency or absence of low-density lipoprotein (LDL) receptors on the liver cells, which deficiency interferes with binding and mediating the uptake of LDL into the cells, thus leading to their accumulation in plasma and to acceleration of atherosclerosis.[2] Cardiac damage was beyond treatment except by transplantation.

The donor, age 4½ years, weighed 3 kg less (at 16.5 kg) than the patient, and was blood type O. The recipient was type A. There was a mismatch at HLA A, B, and DR loci. Techniques for combined procurement of multiple organs from the same donor have been extensively outlined in previous reports.[3] Preliminary dissection of the liver and kidneys is performed first, followed by dissection of the heart and great vessels. Cannulae are inserted into the donor's splenic vein, distal abdominal vena cava, and aorta. The liver is then precooled by infusion of cold Ringer's lactate solution via the splenic vein cannula. Almost simultaneously the distal ascending aorta is clamped and cold cardioplegic solution of electrolytes is infused through a cannula into the ascending aorta. Simultaneously, cold (4°C) EuroCollins solution is infused through the abdominal aortic cannula, and the inferior vena caval cannula is opened and allowed to drain into a container placed on the floor. After this *in situ* cooling, the heart is removed, followed by the liver and finally the kidneys. The organs are promptly immersed individually in iced Ringer's lactate solution and transported in crushed ice to the University Health Center, in this case arriving 90 minutes after the aorta had been clamped.

Recipient Procedure

Operation on the recipient was timed so that final dissection and removal of the recipient's heart and liver was completed as the donor organs arrived. In the absence of previous operation and adhesions, the donor hepatectomy was relatively easy. Adhesions about the heart, two previous vein bypasses from the ascending aorta, and two cannulation sites made preparation for the recipient heart more difficult. The right common iliac artery was selected for arterial return. It was severely atheromatous and sclerotic, but the ascending aorta was later seen to be greatly thickened also with soft atheroma. Venous cannulation was to the superior vena cava via the sinus venosus and a second cannula was inserted through the left common iliac vein to the inferior vena cava. Except for cannulation, implantation of the donor heart was performed in the usual manner at 28°C and with intermittent instillation of cold blood cardioplegic solution[4] (Figs. 16–1, 16–2, and 16–3). Flow was restored to the aorta 150 minutes after the donor aorta had been clamped. The patient was rewarmed as implantation was completed and cardiac action gradually returned.

Removal of the patient's liver and implantation of that of the donor was performed as usual (Figs. 16–4 through 16–6). Cardiopulmonary bypass was continued throughout with a cannula draining the portal vein to the pump oxygenator. Cardiopulmonary bypass offered this special advantage of drainage and decompression of the portal vein during completion of the two caval and hepatic arterial anastomoses. Arterial and portal flows were restored simultaneously to the liver approximately 3½ hours after devascularization of the liver in the donor. Cardiopulmonary bypass was used for 135 minutes for the two implantations.

The coagulopathy associated with heparin, bypass, and hepatic transplantation required several hours to correct. During this time, bile duct reconstruction was accomplished by an end-to-end anastomosis. At the completion of the 15-hour operation, minimal inotropic support was required, the liver was making large quantities of bile, and the patient's coagulation had returned to normal.

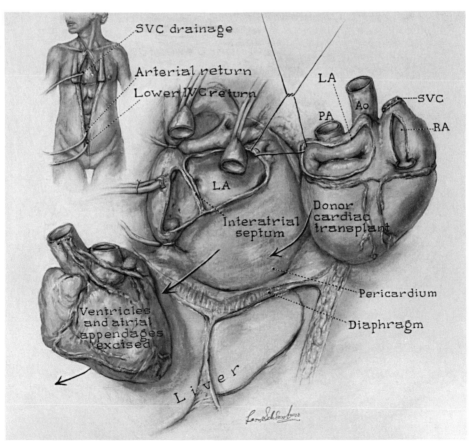

Figure 16–1. Beginning of cardiac implantation. The iliac vein and artery were cannulated, along with the superior vena cava, for cardiopulmonary bypass. (From Shaw et al.,[1] with permission.)

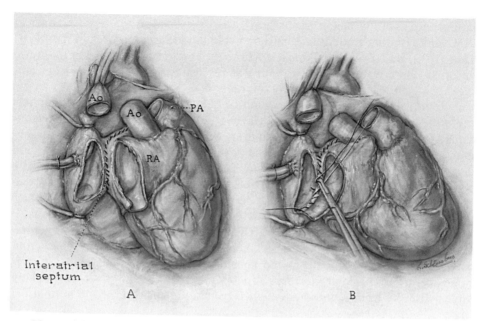

Figure 16–2. Completion of left (*A*) and then right (*B*) atrial anastomoses. Cardioplegic solution was infused on completion of each anastomosis. The heart was frequently bathed with iced saline. (From Shaw et al.,[1] with permission.)

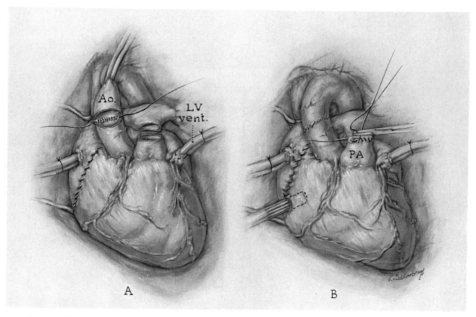

Figure 16–3. *A,* Completion of aortic anastomosis, following which arterial flow was restored and then the pulmonary arteries were anastomosed. *B,* Venting the right atrium facilitated the pulmonary anastomosis. (From Shaw et al.,[1] with permission.)

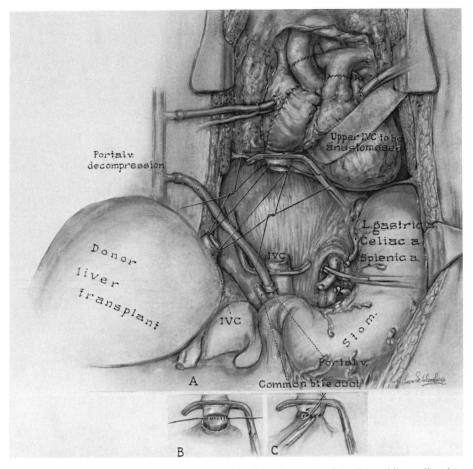

Figure 16–4. Inferior vena caval anastomosis and implantation of the liver while cardiopulmonary bypass continued and the portal vein was drained. (From Shaw et al.,[1] with permission.)

Subsequent Course

The patient was exquisitely dependent on catecholamines early after the operation, and the initial doses of 5 mcg/kg of dopamine and 7.5 mcg/kg of dobutamine were supplemented with a calcium chloride drip at 1.5 mg/min. The need for these drugs diminished rapidly, and they were discontinued 48 hours after surgery.

Cyclosporine and steroids were used for immunosuppression. Immunosuppression and clinical course are plotted in Figure 16–7. Intravenous cyclosporine was replaced by oral dosage (15 mg/kg daily) on the third day, when ileus had resolved. Intravenous methylprednisolone succinate was replaced by oral prednisone as soon as it was tolerated. The inital daily dose of 100 mg/day was tapered to 20 mg/day by the end of the second week. A bolus of 0.5 g methylprednisolone succinate was given on the second postoperative day because of a rise in serum transaminase, and a second bolus of 1 g hydrocortisone was given on the seventh postoperative day because of a rise in bilirubin on two successive days.

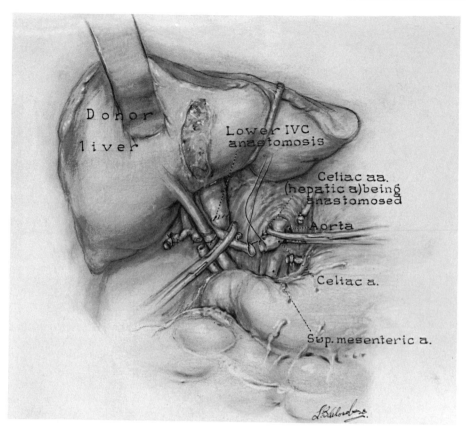

Figure 16–5. Anastomosis of celiac arteries while the portal vein was drained to the machine. Portal vein drainage was then stopped, and portal anastomosis was done. (From Shaw et al.,[1] with permission.)

Cardiac function appeared to be normal throughout the hospital course following the patient's initial brief stay in the intensive care unit. Endomyocardial biopsy, which is done weekly in other patients following cardiac transplantation, was used only once on the 18th postoperative day when it showed evidence of resolving rejection. Otherwise, hepatic function was used to monitor rejection. In the absence of clinical or laboratory evidence of rejection, aggressive treatment was not undertaken. The patient had one episode of mild hepatic rejection 5 months after operation, which was reversed by transiently increasing her immunosuppression. There was no evidence of cardiac rejection.

The patient's total cholesterol and low-density lipoprotein (LDL)-cholesterol levels fell dramatically after operation but remained elevated for her age and sex. Lipid levels fell to normal range with addition of mevinolin. She has continued growth at the 25th percentile in height and at the 50th percentile in weight, which is consistent with both parents being of short stature.[5]

Other Cases

A similar procedure was subsequently attempted in two other instances. One involved a 2-year-old child, K.C., weighing 7.2 kg, with end-stage cardiomyopa-

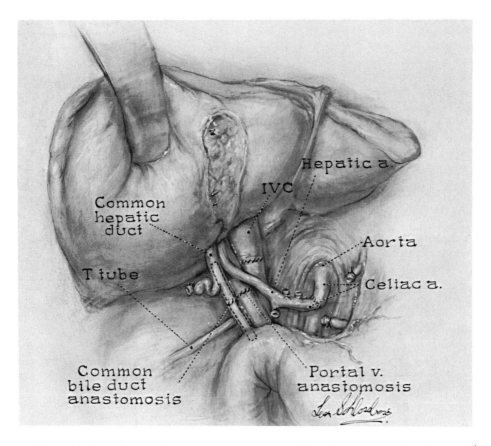

Figure 16–6. Completion of common duct anastomosis with T-tube drainage. (From Shaw et al.,[1] with permission.)

thy and biliary hypoplasia. The procedure was more difficult. Because of her small size, the inferior cava was cannulated instead of the iliac vein, and she was kept cold while the liver was implanted. The donor also weighed 7.2 kg but was younger, and the heart seemed small for the recipient. Her condition deteriorated and retransplantation was performed 24 hours later from a donor weighing 18 kg. Initial improvement was followed by deterioration and death.

The other procedure was on a 17-year-old girl, M.C., with familial hypercholesterolemia, which had been treated with portacaval shunt 10 years earlier. Eight years previously the aortic valve had been replaced, the adjacent aorta patched, and two coronary artery bypass grafts were sewn to the patch. The mitral valve was replaced. After a bout with endocarditis the prosthetic valve was replaced with a larger one 3 years later. Angina had recurred and the patient was severely limited in activity when she was referred to the University Health Center of Pittsburgh. She weighed 54.5 kg; the donor weighed 78.2 kg, but the donor heart was slightly smaller than the dilated heart of the recipient. After operation the chest was opened twice when there seemed to be compression of the heart, and there was transient improvement each time. The second time only the skin was closed. Serial electrocardiogram showed evidence of an inferior wall infarction. Because

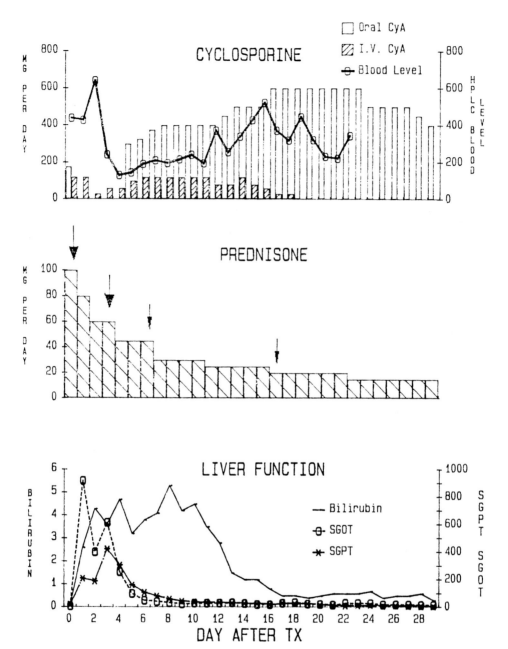

Figure 16–7. Clinical course following heart and liver transplantation. *Large arrows* indicate methylprednisolone succinate, 500 mg intravenous boluses, *small arrows,* 1000 mg hydrocortisone intravenous boluses. (From Shaw et al.,[1] with permission.)

the liver had swelled and seemed to be contributing to the compression, the left lobe of the liver was resected. Central lobular necrosis was found on histologic examination of the specimen. Thus, when another donor became available, a decision was made to retransplant, but after this was done the patient could not be removed from cardiopulmonary bypass. Lymphocytes from the first donor did not match recipient serum, the cross-match being done during implantation. However, histologic examination of the first donor heart, when it was removed at retransplantation, showed focal necrosis characteristic of ischemia without histologic evidence of rejection.

Although rejection cannot be excluded, appropriateness of size of the donor organs appeared to be important in these two failures. When heart and liver from different donors are individually transplanted, one would desire a donor heart slightly larger than the recipient's but a liver slightly smaller. When the procedures are combined, a compromise must be made, usually accepting a larger donor than recipient.

TRANSPLANTATION OF HEART AND KIDNEY

Heart and kidney transplantation from the same donor has been combined in two patients. The first, T.J., was a 44-year-old man with a history of idiopathic cardiomyopathy 1 year before orthotopic cardiac transplantation was performed in January 1983. His early course was complicated by three episodes of cardiac arrest and by subsequent mediastinitis that required drainage on several occasions. Immunosuppression was undertaken with cyclosporine and prednisone but repeated episodes of acute rejection were treated with increases in dosage, pulses of steroids, and rabbit antithymocytic globulin. Tonic-clonic seizures were treated with Dilantin 1 month after operation. When discharged from the hospital, 10 weeks after transplantation, serum creatinine and blood urea nitrogen levels were normal. He was rehospitalized several times during that year for recurrent mediastinal infection, evaluation of inguinal node hypertrophy (thought to be related to infection, possibly to the Dilantin, but not lymphoproliferative disease), and for acute rejection of the heart. Hypertension was treated initially with hydralazine, and subsequently with prazosin and clonidine. At 11 months his creatinine had risen to 3.2 mg/dl, and 6 weeks later about 1 year after operation, was 10.2 mg/dl. Clinical and catheterization evidence showed that cardiac function was progressively impaired, presumably due to chronic rejection. The patient was started on dialysis, and repeat cardiac transplantation with kidney transplantation was advised and accepted. Retransplantation of the heart was performed on April 14, 1984, 15 months after the initial transplantation, and the kidney was transplanted the following day, both organs coming from the same donor. Both procedures followed the usual practice. The excised heart showed focal myocyte dropout with fibrosis but no necrosis or evidence of active rejection. Immunosuppressive therapy again consisted of cyclosporine and prednisone but when renal function became impaired again with rising creatinine, and renal biopsy on July 3, 1984, showed changes more consistent with cyclosporine effect than with rejection, cyclosporine was replaced with Imuran. However, renal function progressively deteriorated over the next 6 months and dialysis was resumed. Cardiac function, assessed both clinically and by evaluation with catheterization, continued satisfactorily. Retransplantation of the kidney was planned but the patient died of respiratory distress with bilateral gram-negative pneumonia 6 months after the combined transplantation.

The second patient, N.B., had been on peritoneal dialysis for chronic glomerulonephritis for 1 year. Six months before operation, subsequent to a presumed viral illness, severe cardiomyopathy occurred. Cardiac ejection fraction on two occasions was measured at 9 percent and 10 percent.

Heart and kidney transplantation were performed in the usual manner for the individual organs, sequentially, 12 hours apart, on January 11, 1986. Cardiac function required significant support with cardiotonic drugs, including epinephrine, and the patient was getting this drug when renal transplantation was performed. The kidney never functioned satisfactorily and dialysis was resumed on the third postoperative day. His postoperative course was protracted and complicated with acute hemorrhagic pancreatitis and formation of pseudocyst. Three months after operation he developed refractory gram-negative pneumonia and bacteremia, further complicated by disseminated intravascular coagulation, and died.

DISCUSSION

From the literature and our own experience we know of 12 instances in which the heart has been transplanted along with another organ (exclusive of heart-lung transplantation)—five times with the liver,[6,7] and seven times with the kidney.[8-12] In all but one instance, that of Figuera and associates reporting a heart-liver combination,[7] both organs came from the same donor.

The most commonly performed double-organ transplant consists of transplantation of a liver and kidney. In such instances the more difficult and stressful operation, transplantation of the liver, is done first and the kidney from the same donor can be preserved 48 hours or longer and implanted once the patient's condition has stabilized. Nine of such cases were reported by Gonwa and associates,[13] and 13 have been performed at the University of Pittsburgh. Similarly with transplantation of the heart from the same donor, the kidney from the same donor can be preserved safely for 48 or more hours. Such staging is not possible with transplantation of heart and liver from the same donor, because of the shorter tolerable period of ischemia.

Starzl performed the first case of cardiac transplantation with another organ from the same donor in September 1968.[8] The patient lived for 3½ months, during which time episodes of apparent rejection of both organs occurred, independently of each other. Norman, Cooley, and 12 other authors reported the second case in 1978.[9] Their patient had developed the "stone heart syndrome" following open heart surgery, and this condition was followed by acute anuria. Heart and kidney were replaced on the fifth postoperative day, and although the heart worked well, the kidney never did, and the patient died 2 weeks later of multiple organ failure. Faggian and associates[10] reported a successful heart-kidney combination in a 41-year-old man with advanced glomerulosclerosis and coronary artery disease. The authors thought that observing renal function helped in the early diagnosis of cardiac rejection after operation. Livesey and colleagues[11] reported a successful case of a 17-year-old boy with renal failure. While on chronic ambulatory peritoneal dialysis he developed heart failure due to familial cardiomyopathy. Gonwa and associates[12] also were successful in a young person with diabetes, severe renal failure, and ischemic cardiomyopathy.

English and Calne successfully performed a combined heart-lung and liver transplant with organs from the same donor.[6] Figuera and associates[7] transplanted a heart in a 12-year-old boy with homozygous familial type IIa hypercholesterolemia, and a few weeks later they transplanted a liver from a different donor.

Several advantages are attributed to combined transplantation with organs from the same donor: antigenetically different grafts and the probable greater immunologic burden are avoided. Easier monitoring of rejection may be obtained, such as use of endomyocardial biopsy of the heart. However, it has been shown with transplantation of the heart and lungs that either organ may be rejected, by our present criteria, without rejection of the other. When the liver is the second organ, it may provide a protective effect inasmuch as previous work in animals has shown that transplantation of either the liver or spleen from the same donor provides an advantage of less severe and less frequent episodes of rejection.[14-16] There is evidence that multiple organs protect each other when transplanted in experimental animals, but the final answer is still awaited from experience in humans. When the liver and heart are transplanted, the same cardiopulmonary bypass can be used during the anhepatic state of implantation of the liver, thus relieving the portal and inferior vena caval obstruction. This was advantageous in our experience, but in the case of severe liver disease the problem of heparin would be added to the troublesome coagulopathy of liver disease.

Undoubtedly more multiple organ transplants will occur. Initially complex, as suggested by the long list of 14 authors of the first report of combined transplantation of heart and kidney, the precedure will become more easily accomplished and more widely done. Benefit has already been demonstrated, but the long-term results remain to be determined.

REFERENCES

1. Shaw, BW, Bahnson, HT, Hardesty, RL, et al: Combined transplantation of the heart and liver. Ann Surg 202:667, 1985.
2. Goldstein, JL and Brown, MS: Familial hypercholesterolemia. In Stanbury, JB, Wyngaarden, JB, Frederickson DS, et al: (eds): The Metabolic Basis of Inherited Disease, McGraw Hill, New York, 1983, pp 672–712.
3. Starzl, TE, Hakala, TR, Shaw, BW, et al: A flexible procedure for multiple cadaveric organ procurement. Surg Gynecol Obstet 158:223, 1984.
4. Griffith, BP: Heart and heart-lung transplantation. In Welch, KJ, Randolph, JG, Ravitch, MM, et al (eds): Pediatric Surgery. Year Book Publishers, Chicago, 1986, pp 386–391.
5. East, C, Grundy, SM, and Bilheimer, DW: Normal cholesterol levels with lovastatin (mevinolin) therapy in a child with homozygous familial hypercholesterolemia following liver transplantation. JAMA 256:2843, 1986.
6. Footnote to Livesay SA, et al (Reference 11).
7. Figuera, D, Ardaiz, J, Martin-Judez, V, et al: Combined transplantation of heart and liver from two different donors in a patient with familial Type IIa hypercholesterolemia. J Heart Transplant 5:327, 1986.
8. Starzl, TE: Personal communication, 1988.
9. Norman, JC, Cooley, DA, Kahan, BD, et al: Total support of the circulation of a patient with post-cardiotomy stone-heart syndrome by a partial artifical heart (ALVAD) for 5 days followed by heart and kidney transplantation. Lancet 1:1125, 1978.
10. Faggian, G, Bortolotti, V, Stellin, G, et al: Combined heart and kidney transplantation: A case report. J Heart Transplant 5:480, 1986.
11. Livesey, SA, Rolles, K, Calne, RY, et al: Successful simultaneous heart and kidney transplantation using the same donor. Clin Transplant 2:1, 1988.
12. Gonwa, T: Personal communication, 1988.
13. Gonwa, TA, Nery, JR, Husberg, BS, and Klintmalm, GB: Simultaneous liver and renal transplantation in man. Transplantation 46:690, 1988.

14. Gordon, RD, Fung, JJ, Markus, B, et al: The antibody crossmatch in liver transplantation. Surgery 100:705, 1986.
15. Roser, BJ, Kamada, N, Zimmerman, F, et al: Immunosuppressive effect of experimental liver allografts. In Calne, RY (ed): Liver Transplantation. Grune and Stratton, London, 1983, pp 35–54.
16. Starzl, TE, Tzakis, A, Makowka, L, et al: Combined liver and kidney transplantation: With particular reference to positive cytotoxic crossmatches. In Giodano, C and Friedman, EA (eds): Progress and Prevention of Uremia. Field and Wood, Philadelphia, 1989.

CHAPTER 17

Pulmonary Transplantation Status in 1989

Bartley P. Griffith, M.D.

Cardiopulmonary, single, and double lung transplantation have emerged from the past to the present decade as successful clinical procedures, and they are now recognized as reasonable alternatives to end-stage pulmonary and cardio-pulmonary diseases. [1-6] Much excitement exists among those interested in pulmonary transplantation today because, just as cardiac transplantation became a therapeutic modality early in this decade, it is believed that with additional experimental and clinical research, pulmonary transplantation in its various forms can assume a similar status. Before this is possible, investigators must select medical indications for the various types of pulmonary transplant procedures, expand the extremely limited number of donors by understanding pulmonary injury associated with brain death, develop operative schemes that will minimize the risk of dehiscence and stenosis of sutured airways, reduce the propensity for perioperative thoracic infection, and, importantly, study the allogeneic response, including early perivascular rejection and its more insidious form resulting in obliterative bronchiolitis. The purpose of this chapter is to review the current status of the various forms of pulmonary transplantation, combining the experience in Pittsburgh (which includes 70 heart-lung, 7 double-lung, and 2 single-lung procedures) and that of 12 other centers currently actively involved with the procedures (Table 17–1).

CLINICAL EXPERIENCE AND RESULTS

The collective experience reviewed includes 51 single-lung, 37 double-lung, and 457 heart-lung procedures (Table 17–2). The large percentage of operations performed in 1988 indicates the high level of interest in pulmonary transplantation. The experience in cardiopulmonary transplantation, which resumed in 1982 after a decade-long hiatus, has been heavily influenced of late by the almost incredible productivity of Yacoub and colleagues of Harefield Hospital, where 209 of these procedures have been performed, 67 in 1988 alone. Rates of survival

TABLE 17-1

CLINICAL EXPERIENCE—13 CENTERS

UNIVERSITY OF PITTSBURGH

BAYLOR	JOHNS HOPKINS
STANFORD	TORONTO GENERAL
HAREFIELD	UNIVERSITY OF TEXAS
PAPWORTH	UNIVERSITY OF ARIZONA
VANDERBILT	UNIVERSITY OF MISSISSIPPI
BARNES ST. LOUIS	UNIVERSITY OF MINNESOTA

following the various procedures have varied according to the centers' individual experiences but overall have been acceptable. The absolute 50 percent survival following heart-lung transplantation reflects a significantly longer average patient follow-up and more total patient days than either single or double lung transplantation.

The survival following heart and lung transplantation in Pittsburgh between 1982 and 1988 is 64 percent at 1 year and 42 percent at 5 years and is favorably compared with survival following cardiac transplantation (Fig. 17–1). Review of the deaths and morbidity provides a useful description of the clinical problems and suggests where additional study is required before the various forms of pulmonary transplantation can be considered along with cardiac transplantation as truly therapeutic.[3] Eighty-three percent of our deaths occurred in the first 3 perioperative months and were most commonly due to infection (13 patients), followed by inadequate *ex vivo* preservation of the heart-lung bloc (9 patients), perioperative exsanguination (7 patients), and miscellaneous causes (5 patients). Following double and single lung transplantation, healing of sutured airways is problematic because of a lack of bronchial arterial circulation (Table 17–3).[7] Although complete dehiscence of the sutured airway has generally been associated with death, stenosis of a scarred or ischemic anastomosis has been managed by resection by laser or reoperation and (most commonly in the Toronto series) by a Silastic stent. The potential for problems with the tracheal anastomosis is less following cardiopulmonary transplantation, perhaps because cardiopulmonary recipients are partially protected by collateral channels that are transplanted from

TABLE 17-2

CLINICAL EXPERIENCE
13 CENTERS

	TOTAL	ALIVE	1988
SINGLE LUNG	51	29 (57%)	28
DOUBLE LUNG	37	21 (57%)	22
HEART-LUNG	457	288 (50%)	136
DOMINO H/L	37	——	34

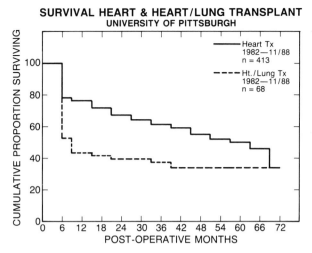

Figure 17–1. Survival following cardiopulmonary transplantation in Pittsburgh (67 cases).

the heart with the heart-lung bloc. These collaterals have been noted late on annual cardiac arteriography from the right coronary artery to surround the supracarinal-tracheal anastomosis,[8] but our autopsy studies have failed to demonstrate their presence acutely in a donor heart-lung bloc.[9] The use of encircling wraps of omentum about the tracheal and bronchial anastomoses is strongly recommended when double or single lung transplantation is performed, and is added prophylactically in our heart-lung series.[10]

DESCRIPTION AND CHOICE OF OPERATIVE PROCEDURES

Cardiopulmonary transplantation was successfully reintroduced by Reitz in 1982.[1] He suggested that the heart and lungs of the recipient be removed following sternotomy *en bloc* and that the anastomosis of the airways be performed 1 or 2 cartilaginous rings above the carina (Fig. 17–2). The cardiac attachments of the right atrium and aorta were made in a fashion similar to that established for cardiac transplantation. Cardiopulmonary transplantation avoids the necessity for pulmonary arterial and left atrial suture lines. With experience, it has been learned that removal of the recipient's heart and each lung separately facilitates exposure and subsequent hemostasis and lessens the risk of injury to phrenic

TABLE 17–3

AIRWAY PROBLEMS
TRACHEAL DEHISCENCE

	DEHISCENCE	TOTAL
SINGLE LUNG	2	2/51
DOUBLE LUNG	6	6/36
HEART-LUNG	10	10/451

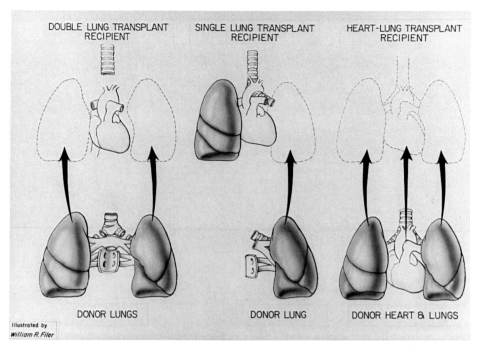

Figure 17-2. Various forms of surgical techniques of pulmonary transplantation.

nerves.[2,3] In cyanotic recipients, it can be especially difficult to maintain hemostasis in the mediastinum engorged with enlarged bronchial arteries and other collateral vessels. Postoperative hemorrhage or exsanguination has not only been common in this group of patients, but is the rule in patients previously operated upon by thoracotomy or median sternotomy. To encourage the healing of airways, the recipient's trachea is transected above the carina with minimal dissection. Constant awareness of the intrathoracic vagi and recurrent laryngeal and phrenic nerves is required. Injury to the latter has occurred bilaterally in two of our recipients and has ultimately proved lethal.

Single-lung transplantation was introduced by Hardy in 1963[11] and has recently been modified by Cooper,[4] who showed the benefit of wrapping the bronchial anastomosis with a tongue of omentum (see Fig. 17-2). While a diseased lung remains *in situ,* proponents of single-lung transplantation strongly suggest the procedure is less complicated and extensive than heart-lung transplantation, because it avoids cardiopulmonary bypass and heparinization and because the operation is limited to a single hemithorax. A left or right allograft may be sutured to the recipient's respective distal mainstem bronchus, mid pulmonary artery, and unilateral pulmonary veins. For simplicity, and to lessen the risk of thrombosis, the pulmonary venous connection is by anastomosis of a cuff of the donor's left atrium harvested to contain the unilateral pulmonary veins to an opening in the recipient's left atrium fashioned between transected pulmonary veins. The bronchial anastomosis is made in its midportion and is always wrapped with a tongue of omentum that has been delivered from the abdomen through the hemidiaphragm. Most surgeons prefer to interrupt the anastomosis of the mainstem and utilize a biodegradable braided suture to minimize the risk of scar formation.

The choice of either a left or right lung transplantation is based upon details of the individual recipient and/or donor.

Double-lung transplantation evolved with the belief that many recipients of cardiopulmonary allografts might not require excision of the heart, variably affected by predominating pulmonary parenchymal or pulmonary vascular diseases (see Fig. 17–2).[5] The proper questioning of the need to remove the heart of the recipient with moderate cor pulmonale was strengthened when it was shown that after surgical removal of chronic pulmonary emboli, patients suffering even advanced cor pulmonale improved dramatically as a consequence of a reduced pulmonary vascular resistance.[12] A possible obstacle confronting successful double-lung transplantation was concern over whether a supracarinal tracheal anastomosis would heal in the absence not only of bronchial arteries but also of those collaterals proposed to emanate from an intact heart-lung bloc. The double-lung procedure was introduced clinically by Patterson and associates in 1987.[6] Unlike the simpler, single-lung procedure, it requires median sternotomy and an extensive intrathoracic mediastinal dissection and the use of cardiopulmonary bypass. The double-lung bloc is removed from the donor after transection of the main pulmonary artery, supracarinal trachea, and posterior left atrial cuff, which includes the entering pulmonary veins. At transplantation, sequential anastomoses are made between the supracarinal tracheas, the donor's posterior and recipient's anterior left atrial cuffs, and main pulmonary arteries. As in single-lung transplantation, the omentum is used to encourage blood flow to the potentially ischemic anastomosis and provide containment of possible dehiscence. Because of their concern for the adequacy of tracheal healing with double-lung transplantation and for maximum utilization of donor organs, Yacoub and Baumgartner performed the "domino" procedure in which a standard cardiopulmonary transplantation is combined with donation of that recipient's heart, if suitable, to a candidate for cardiac transplantation. The domino procedure has been accepted by most and now has been performed 37 times in the centers listed in this chapter. While transplantation of the heart-lung bloc lessens the risk of problems with tracheal healing, it is not likely that the domino procedure will have an impact upon the shortage of donors for candidates of cardiopulmonary and double-lung transplantation, because, with the explosion of centers performing cardiac transplantation, few combined heart and lung donors are referred from outside local procurement agencies. In practice, this encourages the development of single and double lung transplantation in a few centers that might benefit from donors offered from those interested in cardiac transplantation alone.

With the success of the three clinically distinct operations, selection of the most appropriate procedure for any one recipient is currently unresolved. Initially, cardiopulmonary transplantation was introduced for primary or secondary diseases of the lung, including primary pulmonary hypertension and Eisenmenger's syndrome.[1] Soon, however, in the absence of proven alternatives, many centers, including Pittsburgh, expanded indications for this procedure to include all forms of pulmonary parenchymal disease with or without accompanying cor pulmonale.[3,13] With the emergence of single and double lung transplantation, indications for cardiopulmonary transplantation have generally returned to those candidates with pulmonary vascular disease and severe cor pulmonale or Eisenmenger's syndrome. Generally, double-lung transplantation now is seen as a procedure for those individuals without severe cor pulmonale who suffer from any form of pulmonary parenchymal and vascular disease. It appears to be especially indicated for patients with parenchymal diseases associated with pulmonary sepsis, such as cystic fibrosis and immotile cilia syndrome. Centers appear to be divided over the possible virtues of cardiopulmonary transplantation versus double-lung transplantation. Issues evolve around the possible greater availability of double-lung allografts versus the risks of poor healing at the tracheal anastomosis. In response to the latter, the double-lung procedure has recently been modified in some centers to include bilateral bronchial anastomoses. Not only may this lessen the risk of an ischemic suture line, but it also might reduce operative hemorrhage, since mediastinal dissection is avoided. Of course, these benefits must be weighed against the presence of bilateral bronchial anastomoses, each of which is at risk of stenosis, dehiscence, or both (see Table 17–3). The concern for acute perioperative right ventricular failure in the double-lung recipient with moderate cor pulmonale seems to be balanced by the greater availability of the double-lung donor and by the freedom from rejection and coronary artery disease in a transplanted heart.

The simplicity of single-lung transplantation has captured the attention of many new centers, and the procedure has been applied not only for its originally intended indication of fibrotic parenchymal disease but also for obstructive and pulmonary vascular diseases. Early experience with the expanded application of single-lung transplantation suggests that many of the traditionally held concepts regarding the likelihood of ventilation perfusion imbalance following single-lung transplantation for obstructive and vascular diseases might have been overemphasized. Aggressive application of single and double lung transplantation in association with repair of congenital heart defects as a treatment for Eisenmenger's syndrome already has been attempted with some success, but more procedures and time must pass for a more complete evaluation of their appropriateness (A. Patterson, personal communication).

It appears that the only absolutes regarding the selection of procedures include the advisability of cardiopulmonary transplantation in the face of severe cor pulmonale and the avoidance of single-lung transplantation for pulmonary diseases complicated by chronic pulmonary sepsis. Much of the excitement in the field of pulmonary transplantation involves the issues of proper selection of procedures, and it is likely a few years will pass before more specific procedure-related criteria will be formed.

INFECTION

The experience in Pittsburgh with cardiopulmonary transplantation has taught that the recipients of pulmonary allografts are predisposed to a greater risk of perioperative pneumonia and mediastinitis than are cardiac recipients.[14] Pulmonary allografts may transmit infection acquired by the cascade of events subsequent to brain injury, including aspiration of gastric contents, prolonged mechanical ventilation, and neurogenic pulmonary injury and edema. In spite of strict criteria for selection of donors, including a normal chest radiograph and a clear sputum, 67 percent of our cardiopulmonary donors have had positive bacterial cultures of their airways at the time of transplantation.[15] A significant association of infection has been noted when those cultures showed mixed oral flora, suggesting aspiration, and when moderate to heavy *Candida* has been found. Of interest, infection has not been correlated to the length of time that a donor has been maintained on mechanical ventilatory assistance, to the cause of brain death, or to the *ex-vivo* ischemic time of the donor heart-lung bloc. In addition to donor-acquired infection, cardiopulmonary and double-lung transplant recipients require operations with extensive dissection and associated hemorrhage and mediastinal contamination from anastomoses of open airways. Other factors increasing the risk of early infection include the loss of innervation and subsequent elimination of a cough reflex from the donor airways, abnormal mucociliary clearance, severance of lymphatic connections, and confusion in host defense brought on by the allogeneic response and required multiple immunosuppressants.

It is likely that most of the defects in immune defense are overcome after the first few operative weeks, since the risk of late infection is significantly less. The most common pathogens found early after operation have been bacterial, followed by viral and fungal agents (Fig. 17–3).[14] Perioperative prophylaxis of infection in Pittsburgh currently includes Clindamycin, 900 mg every 8 hours, and ceftazidime, 1 g every 8 hours, each for 3 days. Amphotericin B, 0.3 mg/kg per day for 14 days, has been added to reduce the likelihood of mediastinal and anastomotic fungal infections. Immune globulin, 200 mg/kg, is given postoperatively every 2 weeks for 3 months in those recipients who demonstrate seronegativity to cytomegalic viral antigen. Because we have noted significant clinical and subclinical infections with *Pneumocystis carinii,* we maintain all patients on chronic prophylaxis with sulfa, generally a double-strength Septra tablet once daily for 1 week of every month. Epstein-Barr virus-related lymphoma has occurred in six surviving patients; and although a pulmonary recipient may be uniquely predis-

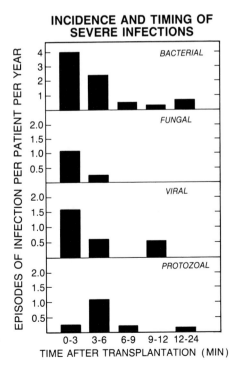

Figure 17–3. Incidence of infection after cardipulmonary transplantation in Pittsburgh.

posed because of the large amount of tissue transplanted, we believe the combination of cytolytic therapy with antithymocyte globulin and cyclosporine, plus seronegativity to the Epstein-Barr virus, places recipients at high risk.[16] Currently, we avoid cytolytic immune prophylaxis in the seronegative recipient. A few of our late-surviving recipients with obliterative bronchiolitis have associated bronchiectasis with purulent bronchitis. These patients require intense physiotherapy and often cyclic antibiotics directed against predominating *Pseudomonas* organisms. As will be elaborated upon in the subsequent section, we believe that obliterative bronchiolitis is related to an immune-mediated injury that results in epithelial damage and in loss of structural muscular support of the medium and small airways.[17]

IMMUNOSUPPRESSION AND REJECTION

More than anything else, the powerful immunosuppressant cyclosporine (CsA) has been responsible for the resurgent success of pulmonary transplantation. Early after operation, in an attempt to improve healing of the airways, steroids are avoided and CsA is combined with azathioprine (AZA). Many centers, including Pittsburgh, use an induction or prophylactic cytolytic therapy with antithymocyte globulin or the monoclonal antibody OKT3. After 3 weeks, prednisone is added (0.15 mg/kg every day), and the dose of CsA is adjusted to blood levels and AZA to a white blood cell count greater than 3500. Initially, AZA was deleted from the chronic regimen, but the success of triple-drug immunosuppression in cardiac transplantation, and the recognition that obliterative bronchiolitis might be limited with additional immunosuppression, has caused most to adopt AZA in the chronic immunosuppression regimen.[18] An attempt is made to balance the maintenance therapy so that the toxicities of individual components might be minimized.

Acute perioperative rejection of the lung has been diagnosed in approximately one third of our cardiopulmonary recipients and has not been recognized in our series after 4 weeks. It is interesting that it has been diagnosed often in the absence of significant abnormalities detected on the endomyocardial biopsy.[19] Recipients with acute rejection develop radiographic opacification of the lung parenchyma over a period of 24 to 36 hours. During the mild phases of this process, cough, shortness of breath, and low-grade fever are minimal; but as the infiltrate progresses, patients become markedly short of breath, with accompanying reductions in arterial oxygen saturation. Histologically, acute rejection is marked by perivascular inflammation in which leukocytes predominate (Fig. 17–4). The interstitium and air spaces are variably infiltrated and edematous. Inflammation of the small and larger airways typical of the more insidious obliterative bronchiolitis is variably present in the acute perioperative process. In the absence of evidence of infection, including a negative bronchoalveolar lavage, it is reasonable to treat the radiographic change expectantly with intravenous methylprednisolone. Rapid clearing of the infiltrate has been the rule, but when the diagnosis is in doubt, trans-bronchial biopsy has provided adequate tissue and is preferable to the morbidity of an open biopsy of the lung.

Within 3 months of successful cardiopulmonary or double-lung transplantation, our recipients have been able to function normally and are usually unrestricted from physical tasks. A moderate restrictive abnormality and a mild impairment in diffusing capacity have been detected by spirometric examination

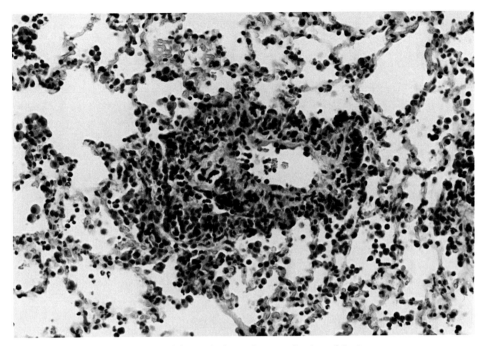

Figure 17-4. Histopathology of acute rejection of the lung.

within the first 3 months, perhaps due to operative factors. Only a mild restrictive defect seems to persist unless the recipient has developed obliterative bronchiolitis. Tests of airway function are difficult to interpret after single-lung transplantation, because the values are complicated by the combination of the transplanted organ and the remaining diseased lung. Little information currently exists regarding the usefulness of spirometric examination in these patients. In 11 of our 36 surviving recipients, we have noticed a progressive decline in forced expiratory volumes.[17] In these patients, biopsy of the lung has demonstrated obliterative bronchiolitis. We believe that this destructive process begins with allogeneically activated leukocytes, which cause a bronchiolar epithelial injury and subsequent necrosis. Sloughing of the epithelial cells into the lumen of the airways follows, and fibroblasts organize with the intraluminal debris into polypoid masses of granulation tissue. This granulation tissue may be reabsorbed or, unfortunately, organized into plaques of dense collagen that obliterate the lumen of the bronchioles (Fig. 17-5).[20] We have diagnosed obliterative bronchiolitis with an associated clinical syndrome of purulent bronchiectasis and believe injury to the small bronchi may predispose them to dilatation due to loss of muscular support. An immune basis for this chronic process is likely because it has been predicted by the presence of donor-specific alloreactivity of lung lymphocytes and has been, at least temporarily, responsive to augmented immunosuppression.[17,18,21,22] A slight relationship between the occurence of bronchiolitis and human leukocyte antigen incompatibility has been suggested,[23] but these observations have not been confirmed in our larger population. The incidence in Pittsburgh has been related to antecedent early perivascular rejection and viral-plus-protozoa infections that might up-regulate the allogeneic response. It is of interest that obliterative bronchiolitis as yet has not been diagnosed in the Toronto group's series of

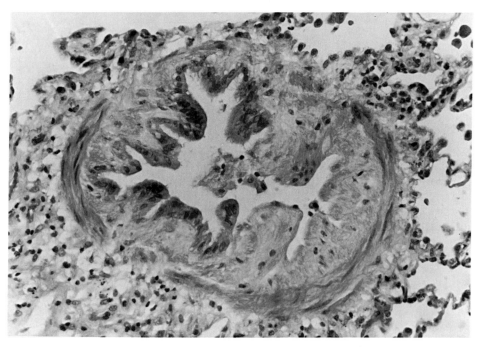

Figure 17–5. Histopathology of obliterative bronchiolitis.

single- and double-lung transplant recipients. We, however, have been treating a double-lung recipient for the obliterative process, and it has been associated with the death of another patient after single-lung transplantation (C. McGregor, personal communication, 1989). The lower incidence following single and possibly double lung transplantation might relate to the fact that less donor lymphatic tissue is transplanted with single and even double lung transplantation. But more likely, it is due to fewer patients at risk and fewer patient days accumulated with these newer procedures. Because of the complexities in interpretation of spirometric tests following single-lung transplantation, a mild obliteraitve bronchiolitis might easily be missed in this group of patients.

No patient with obstructive airway disease has ever experienced a complete recovery, and most follow a relentless downhill course. It may well be, however, that treatment will be more effective earlier, at the peak of the alloreactive response, when donor-specific activation in the airway is first present. We currently recommend the combined use of transbronchial biopsy and tests of donor-specific alloreactivity of lung lymphocytes as the mainstay in following patients after the various forms of pulmonary transplantation. Although considerable damage may occur in the absence of abnormal spirometry, we continue to recommend frequent measurement of forced expiratory volumes at home on a portable device, much as blood pressure is observed after cardiac transplantation.

REFERENCES

1. Reitz, BA, Burton, WA, Jamieson, SW, et al: Heart and lung transplantation. J Thorac Cardiovasc Surg 80:360, 1981.

2. Jamieson, S, Baldwin, J, Stinson, E, et al: Clinical heart-lung transplantation. Transplantation 37:81, 1984.

3. Griffith, BP, Hardesty, RL, Trento, A, et al: Heart-lung transplantation-lessons learned and future hopes. Ann Thorac Surg 43:6, 1987.

4. Cooper, JD, Pearson, FG, Patterson, GA, et al: Technique of successful lung transplantation in humans. J Thorac Cardiovasc Surg 94:173, 1988.

5. Patterson, GA, Cooper, JD, Dark, JH, Jones, MT (Toronto Lung Transplant Group): Experimental and clinical double-lung transplantation. J Thorac Cardiovasc Surg 95:70, 1988.

6. Patterson, GA, Cooper, JD, Goldman, B, et al: Technique of successful clinical double-lung transplantation. Ann Thorac Surg 45:628, 1988.

7. Cooper JD: Lung transplantation. Ann Thorac Surg 47:28, 1989.

8. Sadeghi, AM, Gunthaner, DF, Wexler, L, et al: Healing and revascularization of the tracheal anastomosis following heart-lung transplantation. Surg Forum 33:236, 1982.

9. Ladowski, JS, Hardesty, RL, and Griffith, BP: The pulmonary artery blood supply to the supracarinal trachea. Heart Transplant 4(1):40, 1984.

10. Dubois, P, Choiniere, L, and Cooper, JD: Bronchial omentopexy in canine lung allotransplantation. Ann Thorac Surg 38:211, 1984.

11. Hardy, JD, Webb, WR, Dalton, ML, et al: Lung homotransplantation in man. JAMA 186:1065, 1963.

12. Daily, PO, Dembitsky, WP, Peterson, KL, et al: Modifications of techniques and early results of pulmonary thromboendarterectomy for chronic pulmonary embolism. J Thorac Cardiovasc Surg 93:221, 1987.

13. Griffith, BP: Cardiopulmonary transplantation: Growing pains. Int J Cardiol 17:119, 1987.

14. Dummer, JS, White, LT, Ho, M, et al: Morbidity of cytomegalovirus infection in recipients of heart or heart-lung transplants who received cyclosporine. J Infect Dis 152:1182, 1985.

15. Zenati, M, Dowling, RD, Dummer, JS, et al: Influence of donor lung on the development of early infections in heart-lung transplant recipients. J Heart Transpl 8:95, 1989.

16. Ho, M, Miller, G, Atchison, RW, et al: Epstein-Barr virus infections and post-transplantation lymphoma and lymphoproliferative lesions. J Infect Dis 152:876, 1985.

17. Griffith, BP, Paradis, IL, Zeevi, A, et al: Immunologically mediated disease of the airways after pulmonary transplantation. Ann Surg 208:371, 1988.

18. Glanville, AR, Baldwin, JC, Burke, CM, et al: Obliterative bronchiolitis after heart-lung transplantation: Apparent arrest by augmented immunosuppression. Ann Intern Med 107:300, 1987.

19. Griffith, BP, Hardesty, RL, Trento A, et al: Asynchronous rejection of heart and lungs following cardiopulmonary transplantation. Ann Surg 40:488, 1985.

20. Yousem, DA, Conor, BM, Billingham, ME, et al: Pathologic pulmonary alterations in long-term human heart-lung transplantation. Hum Pathol 16:911, 1985.

21. Zeevi, A, Fung, JJ, Paradis, IL, et al: Lymphocytes of bronchoalveolar lavages from heart-lung transplant recipients. Heart Transplant 4:417, 1985.

22. Allen, MD, Burke, CM, McGregor, CGA, et al: Steroid-responsive bronchiolitis after human heart-lung transplantation. J Thorac Cardiovasc Surg 92:449, 1986.

23. Romaniuk, A, Propp, J, Petersen, AH, et al: Increased expression of class II major histocompatibility complex antigens in untreated and cyclosporine-treated rat lung allografts. Heart Transplant 5:455, 1986.

Index

A page number in *italics* indicates a figure. A "t" following a page number indicates a table.